Health Literacy Development among People with Chronic Diseases: Advancing the State of the Art and Learning from International Practices

Health Literacy Development among People with Chronic Diseases: Advancing the State of the Art and Learning from International Practices

Editors

Marie-Luise Dierks
Jonas Lander
Melanie Hawkins

MDPI • Basel • Beijing • Wuhan • Barcelona • Belgrade • Manchester • Tokyo • Cluj • Tianjin

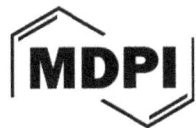

Editors
Marie-Luise Dierks
Institute for Epidemiology,
Social Medicine and Health
Systems Research
Hannover Medical School
Hannover
Germany

Jonas Lander
Institute for Epidemiology,
Social Medicine and Health
Systems Research
Hannover Medical School
Hannover
Germany

Melanie Hawkins
Centre for Global Health and
Equity
Swinburne University of
Technology
Melbourne
Australia

Editorial Office
MDPI
St. Alban-Anlage 66
4052 Basel, Switzerland

This is a reprint of articles from the Special Issue published online in the open access journal *International Journal of Environmental Research and Public Health* (ISSN 1660-4601) (available at: www.mdpi.com/journal/ijerph/special_issues/health_literacy_chronic_diseases).

For citation purposes, cite each article independently as indicated on the article page online and as indicated below:

LastName, A.A.; LastName, B.B.; LastName, C.C. Article Title. *Journal Name* **Year**, *Volume Number*, Page Range.

ISBN 978-3-0365-4921-7 (Hbk)
ISBN 978-3-0365-4922-4 (PDF)

Cover image courtesy of Marianne Bos on Unsplash

© 2022 by the authors. Articles in this book are Open Access and distributed under the Creative Commons Attribution (CC BY) license, which allows users to download, copy and build upon published articles, as long as the author and publisher are properly credited, which ensures maximum dissemination and a wider impact of our publications.

The book as a whole is distributed by MDPI under the terms and conditions of the Creative Commons license CC BY-NC-ND.

Contents

About the Editors . . . . **vii**

Jonas Lander, Marie-Luise Dierks and Melanie Hawkins
Health Literacy Development among People with Chronic Diseases: Advancing the State of the Art and Learning from International Practices
Reprinted from: *Int. J. Environ. Res. Public Health* **2022**, *19*, 7315, doi:10.3390/ijerph19127315 . . . **1**

Wagida A. Anwar, Nayera S. Mostafa, Sally Adel Hakim, Dalia G. Sos, Christina Cheng and Richard H. Osborne
Health Literacy Co-Design in a Low Resource Setting: Harnessing Local Wisdom to Inform Interventions across Fishing Villages in Egypt to Improve Health and Equity
Reprinted from: *Int. J. Environ. Res. Public Health* **2021**, *18*, 4518, doi:10.3390/ijerph18094518 . . . **7**

Elena Castarlenas, Elisabet Sánchez-Rodríguez, Rubén Roy, Catarina Tomé-Pires, Ester Solé and Mark P. Jensen et al.
Electronic Health Literacy in Individuals with Chronic Pain and Its Association with Psychological Function
Reprinted from: *Int. J. Environ. Res. Public Health* **2021**, *18*, 12528, doi:10.3390/ijerph182312528 . **21**

Anna Isselhard, Laura Lorenz, Wolfgang Mayer-Berger, Marcus Redaélli and Stephanie Stock
How Can Cardiac Rehabilitation Promote Health Literacy? Results from a Qualitative Study in Cardiac Inpatients
Reprinted from: *Int. J. Environ. Res. Public Health* **2022**, *19*, 1300, doi:10.3390/ijerph19031300 . . . **33**

Svea Gille, Lennert Griese and Doris Schaeffer
Preferences and Experiences of People with Chronic Illness in Using Different Sources of Health Information: Results of a Mixed-Methods Study
Reprinted from: *Int. J. Environ. Res. Public Health* **2021**, *18*, 13185, doi:10.3390/ijerph182413185 . **43**

Shyam Sundar Budhathoki, Melanie Hawkins, Gerald Elsworth, Michael T. Fahey, Jeevan Thapa and Sandeepa Karki et al.
Use of the English Health Literacy Questionnaire (HLQ) with Health Science University Students in Nepal: A Validity Testing Study
Reprinted from: *Int. J. Environ. Res. Public Health* **2022**, *19*, 3241, doi:10.3390/ijerph19063241 . . . **59**

Mona Voigt-Barbarowicz, Günter Dietz, Nicole Renken, Ruben Schmöger and Anna Levke Brütt
Patients' Health Literacy in Rehabilitation: Comparison between the Estimation of Patients and Health Care Professionals
Reprinted from: *Int. J. Environ. Res. Public Health* **2022**, *19*, 3522, doi:10.3390/ijerph19063522 . . . **73**

Julia von Sommoggy, Eva-Maria Grepmeier and Janina Curbach
Health Literacy-Sensitive Counselling on Early Childhood Allergy Prevention: Results of a Qualitative Study on German Midwives' Perspectives
Reprinted from: *Int. J. Environ. Res. Public Health* **2022**, *19*, 4182, doi:10.3390/ijerph19074182 . . . **87**

Johanna Sophie Lubasch, Mona Voigt-Barbarowicz, Nicole Ernstmann, Christoph Kowalski, Anna Levke Brütt and Lena Ansmann
Organizational Health Literacy in a Hospital—Insights on the Patients' Perspective
Reprinted from: *Int. J. Environ. Res. Public Health* **2021**, *18*, 12646, doi:10.3390/ijerph182312646 . **103**

Maiken Meldgaard, Rikke Damkjær Maimburg, Maiken Fabricius Damm, Anna Aaby, Anna Peeters and Helle Terkildsen Maindal
The Health Literacy in Pregnancy (HeLP) Program Study Protocol: Development of an Antenatal Care Intervention Using the Ophelia Process
Reprinted from: *Int. J. Environ. Res. Public Health* **2022**, *19*, 4449, doi:10.3390/ijerph19084449 . . . **117**

Constanze Hübner, Mariya Lorke, Annika Buchholz, Stefanie Frech, Laura Harzheim and Sabine Schulz et al.
Health Literacy in the Context of Implant Care—Perspectives of (Prospective) Implant Wearers on Individual and Organisational Factors
Reprinted from: *Int. J. Environ. Res. Public Health* **2022**, *19*, 6975, doi:10.3390/ijerph19126975 . . . **131**

About the Editors

Marie-Luise Dierks

Marie-Luise Dierks is a Professor in public health at Hannover Medical School, where she founded the "Hannover Medical School Patient University" to support the knowledge and skills of individuals about medicine, health behaviour and disease prevention. Her main research interests include, but are not limited to, self-management for chronic diseases, health literacy, patient empowerment and user needs.

Jonas Lander

Jonas Lander is a postdoctoral researcher at Hannover Medical School, where he does research on health literacy and patient and public involvement. In his PhD, he assessed current practices of selecting participants for involvement in health research and how these practices are reported in scientific publications. Currently, he seeks to better understand how parents of infant children search and apply disease prevention recommendations, to inform tailored and evidence-based approaches of providing health information.

Melanie Hawkins

Melanie Hawkins is a postdoctoral researcher at Swinburne University of Technology. Her research focuses on health program evaluation, qualitative research methods, and methodology to the development and testing of patient self-report questionnaires. As part of the postdoc role, she manages the Crohn's & Colitis Australia Ophelia project to improve health information and services for people with inflammatory bowel disease. Dr. Hawkins also contributes to unit work for the World Health Organization.

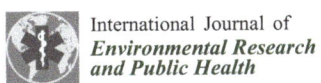

Editorial

Health Literacy Development among People with Chronic Diseases: Advancing the State of the Art and Learning from International Practices

Jonas Lander [1,*], Marie-Luise Dierks [1] and Melanie Hawkins [2]

1. Institute for Epidemiology, Social Medicine and Health Systems Research, Hannover Medical School, 30625 Hannover, Germany; dierks.marie-luise@mh-hannover.de
2. Centre for Global Health and Equity, Faculty of Health, Arts and Design, Department of Health and Biostatistics, Swinburne University of Technology, Melbourne, VIC 3122, Australia; melaniehawkins@swin.edu.au
* Correspondence: lander.jonas@mh-hannover.de

Citation: Lander, J.; Dierks, M.-L.; Hawkins, M. Health Literacy Development among People with Chronic Diseases: Advancing the State of the Art and Learning from International Practices. *Int. J. Environ. Res. Public Health* **2022**, *19*, 7315. https://doi.org/10.3390/ijerph19127315

Received: 13 June 2022
Accepted: 14 June 2022
Published: 14 June 2022

Publisher's Note: MDPI stays neutral with regard to jurisdictional claims in published maps and institutional affiliations.

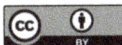

Copyright: © 2022 by the authors. Licensee MDPI, Basel, Switzerland. This article is an open access article distributed under the terms and conditions of the Creative Commons Attribution (CC BY) license (https://creativecommons.org/licenses/by/4.0/).

1. Introduction

Chronic diseases account for a considerable part of the strain on health care systems [1]. They are also burdensome for each affected individual and their families. In recent years, the concept of health literacy has been substantially elaborated on, particularly regarding the development and implementation of interventions at different levels, efforts to improve its measurement, and the role of communities and organizations. While a range of advancements are uncontested, specific challenges still revolve around: Thoroughly implementing modern practices of health literacy that do not focus on individual deficits but societal support of health literacy strengths and response to health literacy challenges [2]; developing, testing, and evaluating strategies for organizational health literacy responsiveness [3]; understanding the impact of eHealth literacy on health outcomes [4]; improving the co-design, local ownership, and integration of health literacy actions and interventions in communities experiencing vulnerability and disadvantage [5–7]; further refining measurement instruments, e.g., with less focus on self-assessments [8]; and addressing current health literacy support strategies by healthcare professionals [9].

This Special Issue was open to submissions about research addressing these aspects and more about advancing health literacy, and had a specific focus on developing health literacy among people with chronic diseases. Health literacy development is about advancements in health practices, organizations, and policies that create enabling environments in which people have the necessary knowledge and feel confident and comfortable accessing, understanding, and using health information and services. Enabling environments are especially necessary for people who are managing health conditions (often more than one condition) over long periods of time, more so for people experiencing vulnerability and disadvantage. This Special Issue includes 10 articles from five countries, which we discuss here according to the distinct perspectives from which health literacy might be approached or developed: individual, professional, and organizational.

2. Articles in the Special Issue

2.1. Health Literacy Development as an Individuals' Effort and/or as a Combined Effort between Target Populations and Professionals

In "Health Literacy Co-Design in a Low Resource Setting: Harnessing Local Wisdom to Inform Interventions across Fishing Villages in Egypt to Improve Health and Equity", Anwar et al. [5] describe how researchers and a local fishing community used the Ophelia (Optimising Health Literacy and Access) process [10] to co-design ideas for health literacy interventions in a low-resource setting. The article highlights that health literacy development is likely to be more effective and feasible if a community identifies its own diverse health literacy strengths, needs, and preferences and has local ownership of the actions that are subsequently integrated into intervention planning. Unfortunately, this type of genuine co-design of health literacy interventions seems to be an exception rather than a standard. The authors also point out the need for focusing on groups and communities experiencing disadvantage who may be more difficult to reach but who benefit most from appropriate, meaningful, and useful approaches for strengthening health literacy.

The cross-sectional survey study "Electronic Health Literacy in Individuals with Chronic Pain and its Association with Psychological Function" by Castarlenas et al. [11] examines the association between electronic health literacy (eHealth literacy) and health-related behaviours in people with chronic pain, not least because people with chronic illnesses make more frequent use of and rely on health information and services more than individuals without such conditions. According to the authors, the "good news" for clinical implications is that eHealth literacy can be learned, which is important for (electronic) health literacy development given the challenges that people have in finding good quality health information in the seemingly endless online information landscape. With respect to the special role, i.e., the importance of navigational health literacy and hence, strategies to improve navigation skills among individuals, needs not to be forgotten, given the number of recent studies pointing at challenges for individuals when trying to find targeted and information landscape, particularly in online environments.

"How Can Cardiac Rehabilitation Promote Health Literacy? Results from a Qualitative Study in Cardiac Inpatients" by Isselhard et al. [12] contributes to the exploration and discussion of relevant, already existing, and "hidden", i.e., overlooked domains of the current concept and understanding of health literacy. The empirical investigation exemplifies the importance of integrating patient perspectives into health literacy conceptualizations. This is, on the one hand, to "approve" or consent to experts and healthcare professionals' accounts and understandings about health literacy, and on the other hand, to include patients' perspectives of health literacy, which is essential to revealing potentially important (new) components of the concept that would be otherwise invisible. The example of cardiac rehabilitation highlights that different target groups may place different emphasis on single components of health literacy, which supports, for instance, Anwar et al.'s argument against one-size-fits-all approaches.

In the mixed-methods study "Preferences and Experiences of People with Chronic Illness in Using Different Sources of Health Information" by Gille et al. [13], the authors investigate information-seeking behaviour and information preferences in a generic sample of chronically ill persons. The findings are valuable for the discussion about health literacy development in so far as, despite the wide availability of digital health information, chronically ill people still consider doctors and other healthcare professionals to be the most useful and trusted source of information. While calls for the role and responsibility of healthcare professionals as, for example, "health literacy mediators" [14] seem obvious, healthcare professionals' first and foremost (or traditional?) responsibility lies in providing diagnosis and treatment and, where relevant, prevention. The challenge for health literacy development may therefore lie in identifying what could be called "windows of opportunities" within established healthcare structures to promote feasible and resource-friendly health literacy interventions.

2.2. Health Literacy Development through Healthcare Professions

Budhatoki et al. [15] provide an argument for valid health literacy measurements as the foundation for any evidence-based approach to identifying health literacy needs, and based on that, developing suitable interventions in their validity testing study "Use of the English Health Literacy Questionnaire (HLQ) with Health Science University Students in Nepal". As the case of Nepali health science students illustrates, identifying the health literacy of (future) healthcare professionals is so important because only when individuals working in healthcare institutions are aware of their own health literacy resources can they better understand how to meaningfully support the health literacy of the people they serve. In terms of health literacy development, the authors also forward an argument for including health literacy training early in academic and medical education.

Combining a cross-sectional and longitudinal study design, Voigt-Barbarowicz and colleagues [16] asked in-clinic rehabilitation patients to estimate their health literacy (at the start and at the end of their rehabilitation stay) and compared the results with a health literacy estimation of the same patients by their respective treatment providers, i.e., physicians, physiotherapists, nurses, and social workers. Regarding health literacy development, one important finding of "Patients' Health Literacy in Rehabilitation: Comparison between the Estimation of Patients and Health Care Professionals" is that—in this study—initial improvements in patient's health literacy are difficult to maintain months after treatment termination, causing the authors to call for a more sustained way of fostering individual health literacy, for instance, in the phase after care. The other, maybe even more important, finding relates to the fact that healthcare professionals in this study overestimate their patients' health literacy—the comparison indicates only poor to fair agreements in accordance with previous research findings [17–19]. This has important implications for approaches to develop and strengthen health literacy in individuals because healthcare provider-related efforts to do so may only be targeted, reasonable, and meaningful once health literacy is accurately estimated by respective professionals.

In "Health Literacy-Sensitive Counselling on Early Childhood Allergy Prevention: Results of a Qualitative Study on German Midwives' Perspectives", von Sommoggy et al. [20] showcase concrete examples of how healthcare professionals—here, midwives—convey health literacy-related knowledge and competencies towards their clients. One encouraging point made by this study—based on the perspectives of interviewed midwives—is that there are actual "windows of opportunity", such as the phase of pregnancy, that seem particularly well suited to develop and strengthen health literacy in respective target populations. For example, understanding and applying effective early allergy prevention measures as a parent, using evidence-based health information. However, von Sommoggy and colleagues find that midwives do not explicitly counsel in a health literacy-sensitive way. That is, they do not emphasize health literacy as a standalone topic but usually only implicitly convey knowledge and competencies, e.g., regarding awareness about available allergy prevention guidelines. As such, the study provides another argument for focusing healthcare professionals' attention on health literacy, and according to the authors, this ideally happens already during the formal qualification and training phase.

2.3. Health Literacy Development through Healthcare Organizations

The importance of developing health literacy research and practice from the patients' perspective is revealed in "Organizational Health Literacy in a Hospital—Insights on the Patients' Perspective" by Lubasch et al. [21]. The authors investigate potential associations between individual patient characteristics, their perceptions, and health-literacy-sensitive communication by hospital staff and the respective organizational structures underlying such communication. One of the central findings, namely the strong association between a hospital's organization and health-literacy-sensitive communication towards patients, not only supports the argument for understanding health literacy as a relations construct between individuals and organizations—emphasizing institutional and organizational responsibility to create health-literate environments. Moreover, and in line with the arguments provided by, e.g., Anwar et al. [5] and Isselhard et al. [12], it may also be seen as a good and feasible opportunity for healthcare organizations struggling to create health-literacy-sensitive structures: target group perspectives on what constitutes a health literate organization may be used as starting point for any organizational, structural, or cultural change.

As organizational health literacy seems to lie in the hands of healthcare institutions and the professionals working within these institutions, Meldgaard et al. [22] outlined how (lay) target group perspectives may be integrated into processes that aim to foster individual HL through organizational efforts. Their study protocol reports on the intended use of the

Ophelia process (see above) to develop an antenatal care intervention, which, in turn, is intended to foster pregnant women's health literacy. Since pregnant women are in a specific phase of life, this needs to be accounted for when adapting health information services to their needs and preferences. Importantly, the authors do not only point to the various potential benefits of applying the Ophelia process towards health literacy development efforts. Moreover, they refer to the conditions and prerequisites required to make health literacy co-design approaches work, not least in terms of its' participants' confidence and capabilities to engage effectively in in-depth cooperation with researchers and vice versa.

Lastly, as shown by Huebner et al. [23], health literacy development will be increasingly related to ethical aspects, such as the dependence on technology to make "good" health decisions or the extent of actual responsibility of health professions and healthcare systems to support individuals in becoming health literate. To understand how health literacy and ethics are interrelated, the authors assess implant wearers' perspectives on responsibilities and challenges when accessing and applying information and advice about the integration of (implant) technology in everyday life, as well as how individual skills, as well as a healthcare system's responsiveness, impacts the dependence on a technological device. Though this research equally relates to individual health literacy, an important argument is made here regarding the organizational perspective: Healthcare organizations may not only allow information and technology to be medically comprehensible but acknowledge health literacy development as an inherently ethical task that requires consideration of an individuals' "lifeworld" and the values attached to living with a technological device on a daily basis.

3. Conclusions

The purpose of this Special Issue was to better understand how to develop health literacy for a population with specific, often increased, health literacy requirements, such as people living with chronic diseases. Given this, it seems warranted to invite perspectives on a broad range of health literacy research objectives, contents, and formats. By "learning from international practices", we hope to attract interest in and awareness of co-design methodologies, such as the use of the Ophelia process in different contexts, and of understanding dimensions of health literacy as perceived by people with lived experiences. Health literacy development is the ways in which health literacy promoting environments are created to enable people to access, understand, appraise, remember, and use information about health and health care, rather than putting the onus on individuals—especially those living in circumstances that perpetuate vulnerabilities—to always need to know how and be able to undertake the complex task of managing chronic disease. Ideally, the research findings in this Special Issue will provide a valuable addition to research or a change of perspective for those working in the field of health literacy. The articles reveal a clear argument for healthcare professionals, services, and researchers to dedicate resources and research priorities to actions that develop health literacy. Instead of expecting individuals to be responsible for navigating through an ever-growing and increasingly complex health information landscape, people living with chronic conditions will benefit from health literacy research that informs actions and policies that improve access to and use of health information and services.

Author Contributions: Writing—original draft preparation, J.L., M.H. and M.-L.D. Writing—review and editing, J.L., M.H. and M.-L.D. All authors have read and agreed to the published version of the manuscript.

Funding: This research received no external funding.

Conflicts of Interest: The authors declare no conflict of interest.

References

1. World Health Organization. *Global Status Report on Noncommunicable Diseases 2014*; World Health Organization: Geneva, Switzerland, 2014; ISBN 978-92-4-156485-4.
2. Okan, O.; Bauer, U.; Levin-Zamir, D.; Pinheiro, P.; Sørensen, K. (Eds.) *International Handbook of Health Literacy: Research, Practice and Policy across the Life-Span*, 1st ed.; Policy Press: Bristol, UK, 2019; ISBN 978-1-4473-4453-7.
3. Aaby, A.; Simonsen, C.B.; Ryom, K.; Maindal, H.T. Improving Organizational Health Literacy Responsiveness in Cardiac Rehabilitation Using a Co-Design Methodology: Results from the Heart Skills Study. *Int. J. Environ. Res. Public Health* **2020**, *17*, 1015. [CrossRef]
4. Cheng, C.; Beauchamp, A.; Elsworth, G.R.; Osborne, R.H. Applying the Electronic Health Literacy Lens: Systematic Review of Electronic Health Interventions Targeted at Socially Disadvantaged Groups. *J. Med. Internet Res.* **2020**, *22*, e18476. [CrossRef]
5. Anwar, W.A.; Mostafa, N.S.; Hakim, S.A.; Sos, D.G.; Cheng, C.; Osborne, R.H. Health Literacy Co-Design in a Low Resource Setting: Harnessing Local Wisdom to Inform Interventions across Fishing Villages in Egypt to Improve Health and Equity. *Int. J. Environ. Res. Public Health* **2021**, *18*, 4518. [CrossRef]
6. Dias, S.; Gama, A.; Maia, A.C.; Marques, M.J.; Campos Fernandes, A.; Goes, A.R.; Loureiro, I.; Osborne, R.H. Migrant Communities at the Center in Co-design of Health Literacy-Based Innovative Solutions for Non-communicable Diseases Prevention and Risk Reduction: Application of the OPtimising HEalth LIteracy and Access (Ophelia) Process. *Front. Public Health* **2021**, *9*, 639405. [CrossRef]
7. Boateng, M.A.; Agyei-Baffour, E.; Angel, S.; Asare, O.; Prempeh, B.; Enemark, U. Co-creation and prototyping of an intervention focusing on health literacy in management of malaria at community-level in Ghana. *Res. Involv. Engagem.* **2021**, *7*, 55. [CrossRef]
8. Elbrink, S.H.; Elmer, S.L.; Osborne, R.H. Are communities of practice a way to support health literacy: A study protocol for a realist review. *BMJ Open* **2021**, *11*, e048352. [CrossRef]
9. Leslie, C.J.; Hawkins, M.; Smith, D.L. Using the Health Literacy Questionnaire (HLQ) with Providers in the Early Intervention Setting: A Qualitative Validity Testing Study. *Int. J. Environ. Res. Public Health* **2020**, *17*, 2603. [CrossRef]
10. Batterham, R.W.; Buchbinder, R.; Beauchamp, A.; Dodson, S.; Elsworth, G.R.; Osborne, R.H. The OPtimising HEalth LIterAcy (Ophelia) process: Study protocol for using health literacy profiling and community engagement to create and implement health reform. *BMC Public Health* **2014**, *14*, 694. [CrossRef]
11. Castarlenas, E.; Sánchez-Rodríguez, E.; Roy, R.; Tomé-Pires, C.; Solé, E.; Jensen, M.P.; Miró, J. Electronic Health Literacy in Individuals with Chronic Pain and Its Association with Psychological Function. *Int. J. Environ. Res. Public Health* **2021**, *18*, 2528. [CrossRef]
12. Isselhard, A.; Lorenz, L.; Mayer-Berger, W.; Redaélli, M.; Stock, S. How Can Cardiac Rehabilitation Promote Health Literacy? Results from a Qualitative Study in Cardiac Inpatients. *Int. J. Environ. Res. Public Health* **2022**, *19*, 1300. [CrossRef]
13. Gille, S.; Griese, L.; Schaeffer, D. Preferences and Experiences of People with Chronic Illness in Using Different Sources of Health Information: Results of a Mixed-Methods Study. *Int. J. Environ. Res. Public Health* **2021**, *18*, 3185. [CrossRef] [PubMed]
14. Spencer, M.; Kemp, N.; Cruickshank, V.; Otten, C.; Nash, R. An International Review to Characterize the Role, Responsibilities, and Optimal Setting for Health Literacy Mediators. *Glob. Pediatr. Health* **2021**, *8*, 2333794X211025401. [CrossRef] [PubMed]
15. Budhathoki, S.S.; Hawkins, M.; Elsworth, G.; Fahey, M.T.; Thapa, J.; Karki, S.; Basnet, L.B.; Pokharel, P.K.; Osborne, R.H. Use of the English Health Literacy Questionnaire (HLQ) with Health Science University Students in Nepal: A Validity Testing Study. *Int. J. Environ. Res. Public Health* **2022**, *19*, 3241. [CrossRef]
16. Voigt-Barbarowicz, M.; Dietz, G.; Renken, N.; Schmöger, R.; Brütt, A.L. Patients' Health Literacy in Rehabilitation: Comparison between the Estimation of Patients and Health Care Professionals. *Int. J. Environ. Res. Public Health* **2022**, *19*, 3522. [CrossRef] [PubMed]
17. Dickens, C.; Lambert, B.L.; Cromwell, T.; Piano, M.R. Nurse overestimation of patients' health literacy. *J. Health Commun.* **2013**, *18* (Suppl. S1), 62–69. [CrossRef] [PubMed]
18. Storms, H.; Aertgeerts, B.; Vandenabeele, F.; Claes, N. General practitioners' predictions of their own patients' health literacy: A cross-sectional study in Belgium. *BMJ Open* **2019**, *9*, e029357. [CrossRef]
19. Zawilinski, L.L.; Kirkpatrick, H.; Pawlaczyk, B.; Yarlagadda, H. Actual and perceived patient health literacy: How accurate are residents' predictions? *Int. J. Psychiatry Med.* **2019**, *54*, 290–295. [CrossRef]
20. Von Sommoggy, J.; Grepmeier, E.-M.; Curbach, J. Health Literacy-Sensitive Counselling on Early Childhood Allergy Prevention: Results of a Qualitative Study on German Midwives' Perspectives. *Int. J. Environ. Res. Public Health* **2022**, *19*, 4182. [CrossRef]
21. Lubasch, J.S.; Voigt-Barbarowicz, M.; Ernstmann, N.; Kowalski, C.; Brütt, A.L.; Ansmann, L. Organizational Health Literacy in a Hospital-Insights on the Patients' Perspective. *Int. J. Environ. Res. Public Health* **2021**, *18*, 2646. [CrossRef]
22. Meldgaard, M.; Maimburg, R.D.; Damm, M.F.; Aaby, A.; Peeters, A.; Maindal, H.T. The Health Literacy in Pregnancy (HeLP) Program Study Protocol: Development of an Antenatal Care Intervention Using the Ophelia Process. *Int. J. Environ. Res. Public Health* **2022**, *19*, 4449. [CrossRef]
23. Huebner, C.; Lorke, M.; Buchhol, A.; Frech, S.; Harzheim, L.; Schulz, S.; Juenger, S.; Woopen, C. Health Literacy in the context of implant care—Perspectives of (prospective) implant wearers on individual and organisational factors. *Int. J. Environ. Res. Public Health* **2022**, *19*, 6975. [CrossRef]

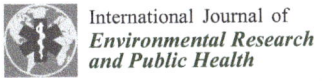

Article

Health Literacy Co-Design in a Low Resource Setting: Harnessing Local Wisdom to Inform Interventions across Fishing Villages in Egypt to Improve Health and Equity

Wagida A. Anwar [1], Nayera S. Mostafa [1,*], Sally Adel Hakim [1], Dalia G. Sos [1], Christina Cheng [2] and Richard H. Osborne [2]

1 Department of Community, Environmental and Occupational Medicine, Faculty of Medicine, Ain Shams University, Cairo 11566, Egypt; wagidaanwar@med.asu.edu.eg (W.A.A.); drsallyhakim7@gmail.com (S.A.H.); daliagabesos@gmail.com (D.G.S.)
2 Centre for Global Health and Equity, Swinburne University of Technology, Melbourne, VIC 3122, Australia; cccheng@swin.edu.au (C.C.); rosborne@swin.edu.au (R.H.O.)
* Correspondence: nayera_samy@med.asu.edu.eg

Abstract: Fishermen in low resource settings have limited access to health services and may have a range of health literacy-related difficulties that may lead to poor health outcomes. To provide solutions and interventions based on their needs, co-design is considered best practice in such settings. This study aimed to implement a co-design process as a step towards developing health literacy interventions to improve health and equity in the Borollos Lake region of northern Egypt, a low resource setting with a high prevalence of chronic diseases. This study was guided by the Ophelia (Optimising Health Literacy and Access) process, a widely used and flexible co-design process that seeks to create local and fit-for-purpose health literacy solutions through genuine engagement and participation of community members and relevant stakeholders. Following a health literacy survey using the Health Literacy Questionnaire (HLQ), cluster analysis was conducted to identify the diverse health literacy profiles among the fishing communities. Seven health literacy profiles were identified. Vignettes, representing these profiles, were presented and discussed in ideas generation/co-design workshops with fishermen and health workers to develop intervention ideas. Seventeen fishermen, 22 wives of fishermen, and 20 nurses participated in four workshops. Fifteen key strategies across five themes, including 'Enhancing education among fishing communities', 'Provide good quality health services', 'Financial support for health', 'Social support for health', and 'Promote better health-related quality of life among fishermen', were generated. The ideas did not only target the individuals but also required actions from the government, non-government organizations, and fishermen syndicates. By harnessing local wisdom, the Ophelia process has created meaningful engagement with the local communities, leading to a wide range of practical and feasible solutions that match the special needs and environment of a low resource setting.

Keywords: health literacy; fishermen; co-design; Borollos lake; health literacy questionnaire (HLQ); health inequality; Ophelia (optimising health literacy and access) process

Citation: Anwar, W.A.; Mostafa, N.S.; Hakim, S.A.; Sos, D.G.; Cheng, C.; Osborne, R.H. Health Literacy Co-Design in a Low Resource Setting: Harnessing Local Wisdom to Inform Interventions across Fishing Villages in Egypt to Improve Health and Equity. *Int. J. Environ. Res. Public Health* **2021**, *18*, 4518. https://doi.org/10.3390/ijerph18094518

Academic Editors: Marie-Luise Dierks, Jonas Lander, Melanie Hawkins and Joanna Mazur

Received: 9 March 2021
Accepted: 21 April 2021
Published: 24 April 2021

Publisher's Note: MDPI stays neutral with regard to jurisdictional claims in published maps and institutional affiliations.

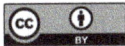

Copyright: © 2021 by the authors. Licensee MDPI, Basel, Switzerland. This article is an open access article distributed under the terms and conditions of the Creative Commons Attribution (CC BY) license (https://creativecommons.org/licenses/by/4.0/).

1. Introduction

Fishing is considered one of the most dangerous occupations in the world due to the constant exposure to unpredictable weather, regular use of heavy machinery in unstable environments and long working hours [1,2]. Smoking and poor diet are also among the common behaviour health risks in fishermen [3,4]. The Borollos Lake in northern Egypt, located in Kafr el-Sheikh Governorate east of Rosetta, bordered by the Mediterranean Sea, has many islands separated by great distances inhabited by fishermen communities. These communities are typically poor, with low education (including high rates of illiteracy), and have limited access to health services because of the remote location. Fishermen are at high risk of musculoskeletal disorders, hearing problems, sunburn, physical trauma as well as psychological stress arising from job instability [2,5,6]. Our recent health literacy survey using the Health Literacy Questionnaire (HLQ), a commonly used questionnaire used to support health literacy intervention development, found that people in this region have remarkably low health literacy on most dimensions of health literacy. The findings clearly show that fishermen and their families are experiencing health literacy challenges that will likely lead to poor health outcomes [5] and efforts are needed to improve health and equity outcomes for the fishing communities living in low resource settings.

Literacy varies globally, from a country to another and even in the same country [7]. Health literacy is a multidimensional mechanism that determines people's knowledge, confidence, and comfort (which accumulate through daily activities, social interactions and across generations) to access, understand, appraise, remember, and use information about health and health care [8]. It is closely linked to health equity and can be used to understand who is missing out on current services, why individuals and groups are being left behind, and how health policy, programs and interventions can be developed and/or improved to accelerate impacts on health and equity [9]. The HLQ, developed using a grounded approach and demonstrated to have robust psychometric properties, measures nine domains of health literacy:

1. Feeling understood and supported by healthcare providers.
2. Having sufficient information to manage my health.
3. Actively managing my health.
4. Social support for health.
5. Appraisal of health information.
6. Ability to actively engage with healthcare providers.
7. Navigating the healthcare system.
8. Ability to find good health information.
9. Understand health information well enough to know what to do [10].

By assessing the nine dimensions of health literacy, the HLQ provides insights into an individual's experiences when engaging with health information, health practitioners and health services [10], and it provides a comprehensive picture about how individual, social and cultural contexts influence an individual's health literacy [11]. Through the Ophelia (Optimising Health Literacy and Access) process, the HLQ informs the development and implementation of interventions by healthcare organizations to meet the health literacy needs of their communities.

The Ophelia process is a widely used method developed with community engagement and co-design as the core principles to improve access, equity and outcomes by addressing health literacy needs [12]. The development of interventions to serve community needs must take into consideration the contexts and needs of those living in the community. To achieve this purpose, a co-design approach harnessing local wisdom and collective creativity [13] is considered best practice, especially when working with vulnerable populations [14]. Local wisdom is highly regarded as it refers to the knowledge and values gained through experiences and activities by a group of people. It may pass on from one generation to the next generation. The Ophelia process has been applied mainly in European and Western settings with considerable success, including within the World Health Organization (WHO) National Health Literacy Development Program and in a digital health context [15–21].

Given the unique features of the fishing communities in the Borollos Lake region of northern Egypt, the importing of externally developed public health interventions, either from the published literature or from other sources, may not match what might be needed and useful for fishermen and their families. Consequently, we applied the Ophelia process to provide in-depth assessment of community needs and deep community engagement in the context of fishing village life for the development of potentially useful interventions.

The aim of this study was to implement the co-design process where university staff engaged with fishermen and healthcare provider representatives through the Ophelia process to develop health literacy interventions that meet the needs of fishing communities, with the ultimate aim to improve health and equity outcomes.

2. Materials and Methods

This study was set in the remote Borollos Lake region in Kafr El Shiekh, Egypt and the methods were guided by the Ophelia process. This process was developed based on intervention mapping, quality improvement collaboratives and realist synthesis to improve individual and organizational health literacy responsiveness [12]. The process includes three phases: (1) identifying local needs; (2) co-design of interventions; and (3) implementation, evaluation and ongoing improvement [12,21]. This study represents phase 1 of the Ophelia process, which involves three steps: (1) health literacy survey; (2) cluster analysis and develop vignettes; and (3) ideas generation/co-design workshops. See Figure 1 of the study process.

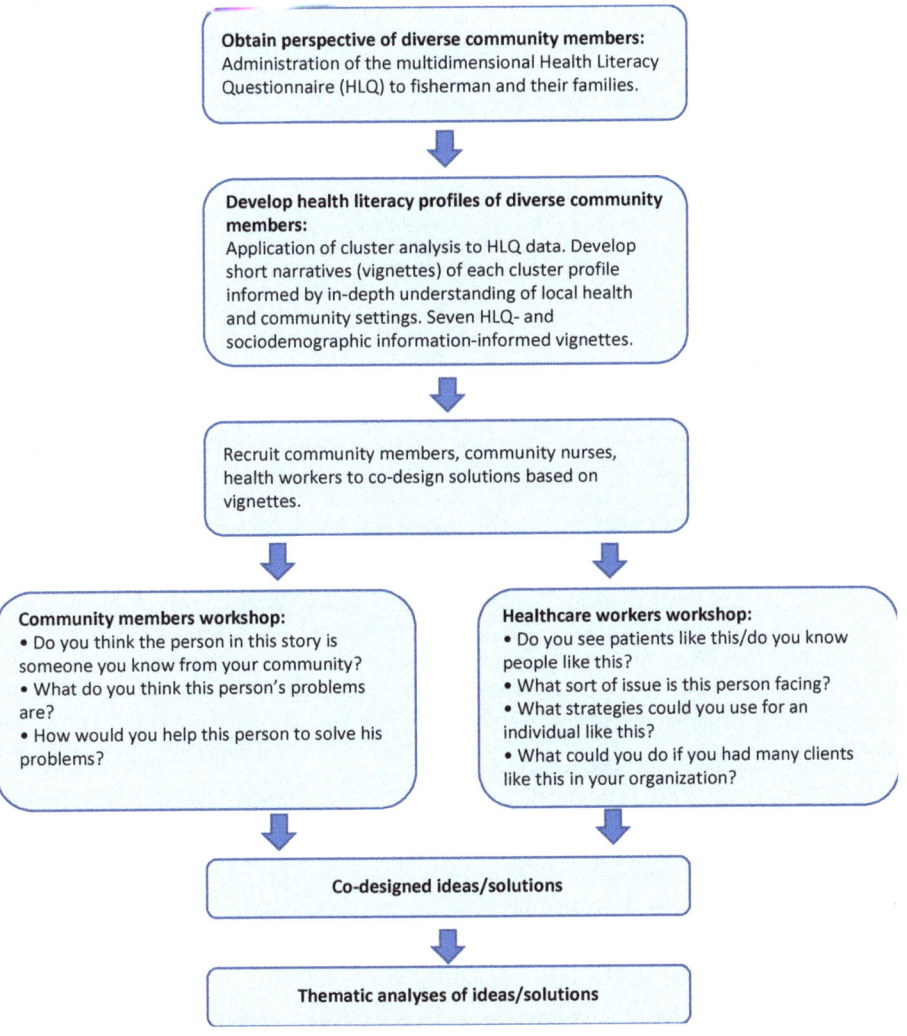

Figure 1. Study process.

The first step of health literacy survey was conducted from January–May 2018 and the results are described elsewhere [5]. Study data is available in the Supplementary Material. In summary, data were collected from five villages where the majority of their inhabitants were fishermen. The socio-demographic data collected included age, sex, living alone or with others, internet usage, family income, occupation (fisherman or other), educational attainment (illiterate, primary level, or above primary level) [5]. A total of 436 participants, including fishermen and their families, completed the survey by face-to-face interview. The age range was 18–89 with 65.2% aged under 50 years and 50% were males. Over a third of the sample (37.1%) were illiterate and 42.4% were active fishermen. The results showed that they had relatively low to very low scores for most of the health literacy dimensions but had some strengths in terms of social support and communication with health professionals [5]. See Table 1.

Table 1. Health Literacy Questionnaire (HLQ) scores of people from fishing communities in Borollos Lake region, Northern Egypt.

HLQ Scale	Mean (SD) [95% CI]
	Range: 1 (lowest)–4 (highest) *
1. Feeling understood and supported by healthcare providers	2.51 (0.83) [2.43–2.58]
2. Having sufficient information to manage my health	2.23 (0.76) [2.16–2.30]
3. Actively managing my health	2.37 (0.75) [2.30–2.44]
4. Social support for health	2.95 (0.69) [2.89–3.03]
5. Appraisal of health information	2.37 (0.79) [2.29–2.44]
	Range: 1 (lowest)–5 (highest) ^
6. Ability to actively engage with healthcare providers	3.50 (0.96) [3.41–3.59]
7. Navigating the healthcare system	3.11 (1.03) [3.01–3.21]
8. Ability to find good health information	2.78 (1.10) [2.67–2.88]
9. Understand health information well enough to know what to do	3.26 (0.88) [3.18–3.35]

SD = standard deviation; CI = confidence interval. * 1 = strongly disagree, 2 = disagree, 3 = agree, 4 = strongly agree. ^ 1 = cannot do or usually difficult, 2 = very difficult, 3 = quite difficult, 4 = easy, 5 = very easy.

2.1. Cluster Analysis and Vignette Development

The cross-sectional survey provided a glimpse of the health literacy of fishermen and their families. Given the diverse demographic characteristics which may lead to different health literacy strengths or weaknesses among subgroups within the sample, the Ophelia process recommends using cluster analysis, based on the nine scale scores of the HLQ, to identify groups with similar patterns for equity planning [12,19,21]. To generate groups of participants with similar HLQ strengths and weaknesses (i.e., profiles), hierarchical cluster analysis using Ward's method for linkage was used. Ward's method is also known as Ward's minimum variance method and aims to join elements into clusters while minimizing the variance within clusters [22]. Therefore, the optimal number of clusters was also guided by the aims to minimize the variance within each domain of each cluster (SD <0.6) and ensure the clusters represent different patterns of health literacy strengths and needs. Besides, the demographics and clinical data of subgroups also needed to be considered when determining the optimal number of clusters [12]. The cluster analysis was conducted using SPSS Version 21.

The clusters and related demographic characteristics were then combined to create personal stories/vignettes to represent how a typical person of each cluster accesses and uses health information and services. In addition to the empirical data, in-depth knowledge and experience of working with the local communities from the researchers and public health practitioners were drawn on to develop the vignettes. The vignettes would further be validated at the ideas generation/co-design workshops (see Section 2.2 for details).

2.2. Ideas Generation/Co-Design Workshops

The Ophelia ideas generation/co-design workshop is a brainstorm session when the vignettes are presented, and participants are asked to consider ideas/solutions that can be used to help the vignettes. Workshops are usually run separately for community members and for healthcare professionals [12,19,21].

The workshops started with a brief overview of the Ophelia process. It was then clarified that the vignettes to be presented were not real persons but did represent the challenges people in their own community faced in accessing and using health information and services. Participants were encouraged to come up with solutions to help these vignettes based on their personal experiences as a way to harness local wisdom. The following questions were asked to guide the discussion following presentation of each vignette:

Questions for community members:
1. Do you think the person in this story is someone you know from your community?
2. What do you think this person's problems are?
3. How would you help this person to solve his problems?

Questions for healthcare worker:
1. Do you see clients like this/ do you know people like this?
2. What sort of issues is this person facing?
3. What strategies could you use for an individual like this?
4. What could you do if you had many clients like this in your organization?

These questions are standard questions in the Ophelia process. The first question is used to allow workshop participants to see the characters in the story as someone real and help them identify with the characters. It also serves as a grounded and frontline form of validation of the vignettes. The second question encourages participants to see how health literacy can affect the life of people and the challenges people are facing. Based on these problems, participants can then suggest solutions to help the character on an individual or clinician level. The fourth question is asked to encourage healthcare workers to think of solutions at the organizational or community level so that a holistic approach can be taken to help people with health literacy needs. See Figure 1 for the workshop process to generate co-design solutions.

The first workshop was facilitated by experienced facilitators (RHO, WAA) and attended by the project team. The other workshops were facilitated by the trained project team from the Faculty of Medicine, Ain Shams University. All workshops were audio-recorded with participants' consent. Two note-takers were also present to record the insights and ideas generated for each vignette. During the discussion, main ideas were written on a flip chart that was used at the end of the workshop to sum up the ideas generated.

2.2.1. Participant Recruitment

Recruitment was conducted by phone to invite community members, including fishermen and wives of fishermen, living in the region, as well as Radaat Refeyat (female nurses of primary health centers serving the fishing communities).

Community members were encouraged to participate through the help of community leaders. In addition, some free medical services to participants or their families preceding the workshops were provided as incentives to participate. They were informed that their suggestions and solutions would help policy makers to improve their living conditions over the coming years. Transportation was provided should participants agree to attend. As a small community and the participants were usually well acquainted with each other, such as neighbours, family and friends, they were generally willing to share their ideas during the workshops. For the one workshop joined by government officials, community members recruited to this workshop were senior fisherman leaders and were familiar with the officials and were comfortable to share their ideas and suggestions. Regarding the Radaat Refeyat, all the teams working in the selected community were invited to participate at the healthcare professionals workshop.

2.2.2. Data Analysis

The solutions generated from the workshops were first coded across three theoretical themes by DGS:

1. Governmental level
2. Non-government organizations (NGOs) and fishermen syndicates level
3. Individual level

Further thematic analysis based on the content was undertaken by the research team and reviewed by the principal investigator (WAA), and the international collaborator (RHO). Thematic analysis is a reflective process. To ensure that the conclusions drawn accurately reflected the content of the workshops, two authors (SAH and DGS) separately coded all the workshop data using an iterative constant comparative method [23]. The process involved three stages which included initial coding, focused coding to reduce overlap and redundancy of coding, and theoretical coding using the themes identified above [24]. Two cross-checks to compare emerging themes was performed to assess for the accuracy of inferences at each stage. Where a difference was found, the authors were asked to demonstrate from the raw data how their interpretation was determined until agreement was reached. A pragmatic approach was adopted when drawing final inferences from this study, with a focus on the development of useful knowledge directly related to health literacy for the fishermen communities. Final inferences were verified by NSM and WAA. To ensure consistency with the co-design process, the data were then referred back to those who attended the workshops to provide respondent validation.

3. Results

The cluster analysis was undertaken for a subset of the health literacy survey, with 178 survey participants. Seven clusters were identified with different health literacy profiles. Cluster A had the highest scores across all nine scales compared to the other clusters. The other clusters all had some higher scores in certain scales but lower scores in other scales, indicating varying strengths and weaknesses in different health literacy domains. See Table 2. The average age of Cluster A was 40.6 and 65% of the people in this cluster were male. About 55% of them were fishermen, with 95% lived in a family and 18% were illiterate. The illiterates represented 20%, 63%, 59%, 57%, 62%, and 80% of Clusters B–G respectively (see Table 3 for other demographic details). Seven vignettes were developed for the seven clusters and were translated into simple Arabic for presentation at the workshops. Refer to Table 4 for an example of a vignette from Cluster G.

Four workshops were held during 2019 and in early 2020. Almost all invited participants attended the sessions. People who did not participate had personal reasons rather than being unwilling to participate. A total of 25 participants joined the first two workshops. Participants included 17 fishermen, five representatives of fishermen syndicate, two representatives of the Health Directorate, Ministry of Health from the same governorate and one representative of the Cooperative Union of Egyptian Water Resources. The mean age of the 17 fishermen was 50 and all of them did not complete secondary school. Each of them had at least 25 years of experience in the fishing industry. Two of the fishermen had cardiovascular disease. Workshop 3 included 20 Radaat Refeyat (mean age: 40) and workshop 4 was attended by 22 wives of fishermen (mean age: 45). Ten of the 22 wives of fishermen reported having two or more chronic conditions.

With the first question about whether participants recognized this kind of person in their community, participants universally and strongly agreed that the vignettes were common in their community. This provided grounded validation that the vignettes presented were appropriately developed to represent the experience of local community members when accessing and using health information and services.

Across the workshops, a total of 80 intervention ideas to improve the care and services for the vignettes were generated. The number of ideas ranged from 10 to 25 per workshop. Five themes with 15 general strategies emerged from the analysis and were then grouped across the three theoretical themes of governmental level, NGO and syndicates level, and individual level (See Table 5).

Table 2. Health literacy seven cluster solution.

Cluster			A	B	C	D	E	F	G
Cluster N			20	30	52	22	21	8	25
% of sample in cluster			11.2	16.9	29.2	12.4	11.8	4.5	14.0
Mean age			40.6	41.5	43.8	45.2	39.0	39.1	49.3
1. Feeling understood and supported by healthcare providers	Mean Score	Range: 1 (lowest)–4 (highest)	3.75	2.02	2.85	2.85	2.15	1.31	1.18
2. Having sufficient information to manage my health			3.42	2.66	2.54	1.74	2.15	1.06	1.07
3. Actively managing my health			3.27	3.10	2.91	2.31	2.28	3.55	1.90
4. Social support for health			3.73	3.46	3.16	3.15	2.20	3.75	2.87
5. Appraisal of health information			3.63	3.12	2.75	1.86	2.26	1.10	1.08
6. Ability to actively engage with healthcare providers		Range: 1 (lowest)–5 (highest)	4.68	4.35	4.04	3.51	2.70	2.90	2.66
7. Navigating the healthcare system			4.32	3.97	3.38	2.89	2.48	1.92	1.54
8. Ability to find good health information			4.34	4.04	2.97	1.93	2.39	1.57	1.16
9. Understand health information well enough to know what to do			4.36	4.35	3.23	2.79	2.53	3.20	2.60
1. Feeling understood and supported by healthcare providers	Standard Deviation		0.30	0.85	0.66	0.64	0.76	0.35	0.41
2. Having sufficient information to manage my health			0.42	0.79	0.49	0.50	0.59	0.18	0.18
3. Actively managing my health			0.48	0.86	0.40	0.47	0.64	0.42	0.69
4. Social support for health			0.29	0.44	0.48	0.38	0.54	0.41	0.47
5. Appraisal of health information			0.33	0.71	0.52	0.50	0.56	0.19	0.24
6. Ability to actively engage with healthcare providers			0.26	0.53	0.50	0.61	0.73	0.81	0.66
7. Navigating the healthcare system			0.47	0.67	0.53	0.56	0.66	0.68	0.66
8. Ability to find good health information			0.43	0.69	0.65	0.51	0.53	0.31	0.29
9. Understand health information well enough to know what to do			0.49	0.59	0.62	0.53	0.69	0.83	0.61

Note: The scores are highlighted using the traffic light system of colour coding as recommended in the Ophelia process. Cells coloured in green represented higher scores, the range of yellow represents medium scores and red indicates lower scores.

Table 3. Demographic characteristics of clusters.

Cluster Group	Mean Age	% Male	% Fisherman	% Housewife	% Other	% Lives in a Family	% Illiterate	% Low Income	% Average Income	% High Income
A	40.6	65	55	20	25	95	18	26	58	16
B	41.53	53	27	40	33	100	20	40	37	23
C	43.79	46	42	38	19	96	63	82	16	2
D	45.18	55	50	18	32	100	59	82	9	9
E	39	62	52	33	14	86	57	76	19	5
F	39.12	62	62	38	0	100	62	0	25	75
G	49.32	92	88	8	4	96	80	24	60	16

Table 4. Example of a vignette (Cluster G).

% of Sample in Cluster G		14	Hassan is a Male fisherman aged 49. Illiterate, did 1–2 years of schooling. Moderate health, has some inflammatory disease. He is a smoker and quite overweight. Not an internet user, moderate income. Very low health literacy, struggles with most aspects. Has some social support for health, and his other relative strengths are in being able to talk with health providers and understand health information, but these are still low. Would have great difficulty finding information—he doesn't feel he has enough information but as his health is not at all a priority to him, he may not see this as a problem.
1. Feeling understood and supported by healthcare providers	Score range: 1 (lowest)–4 (highest)	1.18	
2. Have sufficient information to manage my health		1.07	
3. Actively managing my health		1.9	
4. Social support for health		2.87	
5. Appraisal of health information		1.08	
6. Actively engage with healthcare providers	Score range: 1 (lowest)–5 (highest)	2.66	
7. Ability to navigate the healthcare system		1.54	
8. Ability to find good health information		1.16	
9. Understand health information well enough to know what to do		2.6	

Note: The scores are highlighted using the traffic light system of colour coding as recommended in the Ophelia process. Cells coloured in green represented higher scores, the range of yellow represents medium scores and red indicates lower scores.

Table 5. Workshop thematic analysis.

Theoretical Theme	Emergent Theme	Issue	Solutions	Fishermen Workshop	Wives of Fishermen Workshop	Raedat Refyeat Workshop
Governmental level	*Theme 1: Enhancing education among fishing communities*	Literacy classes are usually in the morning and at fixed time	Establish literacy classes on weekends of the fishermen and afternoon classes Educational sessions in primary health centers visited by wives of fishermen Provide health educational tips during home visits done by Raedat Refyeat Health Educational programs on television that target pressing issues (e.g., family planning, personal hygiene)	✓	✓ ✓	✓
	Theme 2: Provide good quality health care services	Lack of specialized staff in certain specialties	Increase number of trained specialized health care workers	✓		✓
		Fishermen are not satisfied with service provided	Training programs for doctors and physicians to ensure effective communication Monitoring staff performance and conducting frequent audit visits of health care services	✓		
	Theme 3: Financial support for health	Fishermen (private carrier) do not have salaries and no pension	Fixed pension should be provided or social security after fishermen retire	✓		
		Fishermen are unable to pay for the health services	Health insurance cover should encompass the fishing communities.	✓		
NGOs and Fishermen syndicates	*Theme 1: Enhancing education among fishing communities*	Lack of basic education	Assigning an educational course at their yearly vacation and provide certificate of pass	✓		✓
	Theme 2: Provide good quality health care services	Most fishing communities suffer from chronic diseases that needs frequent follow up	Increase numbers of medical convoys from NGOs and co-ordination between different NGOs to provide regular services Provision of screening services and provision of medication supply especially for chronic cases	✓	✓	
	Theme 3: Financial support for health	All fishermen wives do not work although they are capable	Financial support for starting small projects that can be managed at home		✓	✓
	Theme 4: Social support for health	No clubs or spaces to practice any kind of sport or walking	NGOs should collaborate with locals to build youth centers and clubs for the elderly Health promotion sessions on how to keep fit and should include diet as well as simple physical exercises.			✓
Individual level	*Theme 5: Promoting better health-related Quality of life among fishermen*	Lack of exercise	Fishermen should include walking for half an hour twice weekly to stay healthy			✓
		Fishermen do not follow healthy dietary pattern	Wives of fishermen should be encouraged to avoid junk food and cook healthy food daily, such as green vegetables and fresh salad			✓

Levels are in bold. Themes are in bold and italics.

Theme 1: Enhancing education among fishing communities.

This theme included ideas at both governmental level and NGOs and fishermen syndicates level. Participants from both community members and healthcare workers workshops agreed that the four main requirements for enhancing education among fishing communities were:

(1) Establishing national programs for literacy and adult education that suit their working career. "providing a suitable educational program for adults that suit them will even enable them to acquire a driving license and enable him to stand on solid floor"—Workshop 2
(2) Initiating a basic educational course through fishermen syndicate at a reasonable and affordable price. "Fishermen syndicate knows our basic needs and the level of education that we should start from"—Workshop 1
(3) Health education sessions in the primary health centers and through home visits that can be conducted by Raedat Refyeat. "We usually conduct home visits and know all the fishermen housewives through the vaccination campaigns which could be good opportunity to deliver health education tips for them"—Workshop 3
(4) Establishing awareness campaign using the mass media (television) to provide health education regarding different health topics such as family planning, healthy diet and how to quit risky behaviors such as smoking. "TV is on the whole day, if it can be an educational source instead of entertainment for some time, it will help us a lot"—Workshop 4

Theme 2: Provide good quality health care services.

Participants reported facing difficulties in accessing health services at the right time or simply unable to reach acceptable quality care. The following strategies, including at the governmental level and NGOs and fishermen syndicates levels, were suggested:

(5) Increase number of well-trained physicians and specialists in government hospitals. "Usually fresh graduated doctors are found, and we face difficulty reaching senior expert in the field"—Workshop 1
(6) Healthcare providers to undergo effective communication skills training. "Sometimes we don't feel that the doctor understands our suffering and in many times I don't understand the doctor's instructions and hence don't take or follow his prescriptions"—Workshop 4
(7) Enhance service quality to ensure customer satisfaction through continuous monitoring and auditing of service providers. "Having a frequent audit visit will ensure better service to achieve our satisfaction"—Workshop 1
(8) Frequent medical convoys from non-governmental organizations that provide both diagnostic and treatment services. "NGOs can reach us easily and communicate with us effectively and even provide all the required medications for us immediately after diagnosis"—Workshop 2 and 4

Theme 3: Financial support for health.

Participants in the workshop identified that financial support as the main enabler to access health service and ensure better health related quality of life. Three overall strategies involving both government, NGOs and fishermen syndicates were suggested:

(9) Pension for fishermen from governmental and non-governmental sources. "Although we face many accidents during our fishing career, yet we don't have any pension later. We don't have a fixed income, hence ensuring food on the table is number1 priority"—Workshops 1 and 2
(10) Financial support for starting small projects that can be managed at home. "We can work from home through small projects as making clothes, but we need a sum of money to start. If we can have this, we will help our husbands"—Workshop 4 "Most of fishermen wives are talented and have many skills but they need support to start their dreams"—Workshop 3

(11) Health insurance cover for the fishermen and their families. "There is no health insurance at all, so we seek doctors in late stages and never at an early stage"—Workshop 1 and 2

Theme 4: Social support for health.

Wives of fishermen mentioned that social support will encourage them to acquire healthy behaviors, which could be undertaken by NGOs and fishermen syndicates. The following strategies were suggested:

(12) Availability of clubs for sports and exercise to improve health and enable weight reduction. "We don't have a place to walk or even for our children to practice any sport, we are sitting all the time in our homes and get fat"—Workshop 4

(13) Group physical therapy and education sessions for people going through the same health experience to allow for sharing of information, resources, and strategies from others' lived experience. "When we talk together and hear others similar situation and their success, we feel that there is a hope and we can change our habits"—Workshop 4

Theme 5: Promoting better health-related quality of life among fishermen.

This theme was mainly targeted at the individuals. Radaat Refeyat suggested that individuals could promote better quality of life through the following two strategies:

(14) Female household members can serve nutritious diet and keep their family healthier. "If every mother prevented junk food and served salad daily—especially that television now provides many healthy food channels that can support a lot—all members of her family will acquire healthy diet behaviors"—Workshop 4

(15) Walking twice daily for half an hour as regular exercise. "We live in villages, everything is near, and the air is clean that encourages walking"—Workshop 4

4. Discussion

This study undertook the Ophelia process, a co-design approach, to identify potential interventions to improve health and equity outcomes for the fishing communities in the Borollos Lake region of Northern Egypt. The results of 15 key strategies across five themes indicate that the Ophelia process can be effectively applied in a low resource setting [25]. By following the Ophelia process, it is expected that this research can be reproduced in other similar community settings.

The health literacy survey found that most people scored at the 'disagree' or 'difficult'/'very difficult' end of the scales even for people with higher income or education, particularly for scales about having enough information, being able to find good information, being able to appraise information and actively managing their health while they tend to score higher in social support and communicating with health professionals, reflecting a culture of communal practice [5]. Hence, health literacy development in community settings such as the unique rural fishing communities of this study requires an understanding of the ways in which families, friends, and peers interact and how these social networks influence how people think and act in relation to their health [26].

Although many of the participants had limited education, this study engaged them in the design and development of locally relevant programs for their own community. Instead of providing participants with statistical data, they heard stories of people whom they recognized. This was useful because they could relate to the same problems, challenges, and limited resources, as well as understand the negative impacts on their health. In spite of limited education, the results showed that participants did have deep understanding of their own contexts and can generate realistic low-cost local solutions. Through meaningful community participation irrespective of people's education level or social status, this study has captured the essence of communal culture common in rural communities.

This study used the HLQ to understand the health literacy strengths and weaknesses of people living in low resources setting. Instead of focusing only on health-related literacy or numerical skills as in other health literacy studies, or simplistic health literacy data expressed as inadequate vs adequate, this study revealed nuanced challenges people have when accessing and using health information and services. This study also found that people could have diverse health literacy needs and a one-size-fits-all approach is inappropriate to address these needs.

By using the Ophelia process to engage with and provide a voice for the communities through the ideas generation/co-design workshops, the unique limitations and resources available in the communities can be identified to support the health literacy needs of people living in these communities. For example, the two fishermen workshops indicated that organized literacy programs must suit their working hours. Both fishermen and Radaat Refeyat had identified television as the appropriate channel for delivering health education, unlike the many digital interventions proposed in high-income countries these days. Walking should be promoted as a regular exercise, suggested by the wives of fishermen, because they pointed to the clean and fresh air in the villages. The wives of fishermen also noted that children did not have access to any facilities to exercise and therefore sporting facilities were required. By harnessing local knowledge and wisdom, uptake of interventions generated from the co-design process will likely be higher as they suit the special needs or environment of the communities.

Two of the strategies commonly raised at different workshops were 'Increasing the numbers of medical convoys from NGOs and co-ordination between different NGOs to provide regular services' (proposed at the fishermen and Radaat Refeyat workshops) and 'Financial support for starting small projects that can be managed at home' (proposed at the wives of fishermen and Radaat Refeyat workshops). On the other hand, the other strategies were uniquely suggested by different groups, representing the different perspectives of fishermen, wives of fishermen and Radaat Refeyat in meeting the health literacy needs of the fishing communities. The findings indicate that both community members and healthcare professionals are important players in the co-design process.

The overall HLQ mean score indicated weaknesses around health information (Scales 2, 5, 8, and 9) while the demographics further showed that 37.1% of the sample were illiterate [5]. These weaknesses were also identified among the majority of the sample (71.9%) from Clusters C–G. In response to the vignettes representing these data, the strategies such as health education sessions and awareness campaigns were suggested. These ideas echoed the recommendation of an earlier research brief to organize training programs to improve the skills, knowledge and behaviour among the Kafr El Sheikh population [27].

The difficulties in navigating the healthcare system (Scale 7), strongly expressed in Clusters C–G, led to the idea of frequent medical convoys from NGOs to provide regular healthcare services. The need for convoys is in fact urgent because convoys can complement the diagnostic and medication services of hospitals, primary healthcare centers and clinics. As such, this strategy is an opportunity to provide equal access to health services in the region.

While strengths in social support are found in the overall sample, reflecting the communal culture of the fishing communities, the cluster analysis identified two clusters (Clusters E and G) that did not seem to have adequate social support. These two clusters represented a quarter (25.8%) of the sample. By using the Ophelia process to ensure health equity and that disadvantaged groups were not overlooked, the needs of the people in these two clusters were reflected in the vignettes. The strategy of 'Group sessions to allow for sharing of information, resources, and strategies from others' lived experience' will likely meet the need for social support among people of Clusters E and G.

The financial needs voiced by the fishermen and wives of fishermen represented real-life issues that need to be tackled in order to achieve better health outcomes. Fishing is an unpredictable occupation and the tough environment leads fishermen to make their work a priority to secure income instead of making their health a priority [1,5]. Therefore, poverty is a problem that needs to be addressed. Without financial security, such as a pension, health insurance cover, or support for small projects proposed at the workshops, fishermen will continue to prioritize work instead of their health.

The range of strategies identified in the Ophelia workshops showed that meeting health literacy needs should not only be the responsibility of the individuals. The results have identified action areas for government, NGOs, fishermen syndicates, and families and communities as collaborators in the effort of health literacy development. As many individuals at this fishing community are either illiterate or have limited education, individuals may need to receive education and take action with family to enhance health. However, ideas involving governments and NGOs were also generated based on local wisdom in this study. While education is closely related to improving health literacy of communities and several reports originated from developing countries highlighted the positive impact of education on health and pointed out that a lack of literacy contributes significantly to disease burden, others suggested that a higher level of education or literacy does not necessarily ensure a high level of health literacy [28]. As such, ideas from this study, such as involving governments and NGOs to improve health services, deliver quality care, establish enabling environments, and provide financial support, are needed to achieve better health and equity outcomes for the community.

Egypt has gone through several steps to promote health equity, which includes providing care that does not vary in quality because of personal characteristics such as gender, ethnicity, geographic location, and socioeconomic status. This is being achieved through constructing new hospitals that are well equipped, allocating more budget resources to health, supporting primary health care, conducting convoys that provide medical examination and treatment, and maintaining several presidential initiatives, such as raising awareness against hepatitis C, early diagnosis of breast cancer, and non-communicable diseases.

This study added another step towards improvement of health equity in Egypt. The intervention ideas generated through community participation lay the foundation for the next phase of the Ophelia process to select and implement interventions. Based on the findings from this study, several intervention ideas were initiated, mainly focused on the establishment of health education in different health fields with special consideration to diet and nutrition as well as healthy lifestyles and self-care. A report was also submitted to government authorities that included the community's ideas and suggestions.

Limitations

A limitation of this study was that some groups of community leaders in governmental organizations and NGOs did not participate in the ideas generation/co-design workshops. Recruitment of community members workshop participants also did not undergo formal sampling processes. This may have affected the representativeness of community members. Another limitation was that only researchers and healthcare workers were involved in the development of vignettes but not community members. However, the universal agreement that the vignettes were well-recognized during the workshops indicated the vignettes did capture the lived experience of people in their community. A further limitation to the co-design strategy was that workshop participants or community members had yet to be involved in the subsequent process of intervention ideas implementation. Future co-design studies should consider engaging community members in the design, development, and even refinement of health literacy interventions.

5. Conclusions

Fishing communities in low resource settings are at risk of lower health literacy and hence poor health. This study applied the Ophelia process to understand health literacy needs and used local wisdom to generate intervention ideas to address these needs. A total of 15 strategies across five themes that suit local needs were developed. Health literacy actions were identified for government, NGOs, fishing syndicates, fishermen and their families, providing a holistic approach to promote health literacy development for the community. By harnessing local knowledge and wisdom, practical and doable solutions that matched the special needs and environment of the community were generated. These ideas are ready to be selected, tested, and implemented to improve health and equity outcomes for the fishing community.

Supplementary Materials: The following are available online at https://www.mdpi.com/article/10.3390/ijerph18094518/s1, Table S1: Data.

Author Contributions: Conceptualization, N.S.M.; data curation, D.G.S.; formal analysis, D.G.S.; funding acquisition, N.S.M.; investigation, W.A.A.; methodology, N.S.M., S.A.H., D.G.S., and R.H.O.; project administration, W.A.A. and N.S.M.; resources, W.A.A.; supervision, N.S.M.; writing—original draft, W.A.A., N.S.M., S.A.H., and D.G.S.; writing—review and editing, W.A.A., N.S.M., S.A.H., D.G.S., C.C., and R.H.O. All authors have read and agreed to the published version of the manuscript.

Funding: Science and Technology Development Fund (STDF) by the Egyptian Ministry of Higher Education and Research: None.

Institutional Review Board Statement: The study was conducted according to the guidelines of the Declaration of Helsinki, and approved by Faculty of Medicine, Ain Shams University Research Ethics (FMASU R 2/2017).

Informed Consent Statement: Informed consent was obtained from all subjects involved in the study.

Data Availability Statement: The data presented in this study are available in Supplementary Material.

Acknowledgments: The project is funded by an initiative of Science and Technology Development Fund (STDF) by the Egyptian Ministry of Higher Education and Research, which aims to improve the health status of Egyptian communities especially the less developed ones. The scientific approach is a partnership between Ain Shams University, Egypt and Deakin University, Australia. Richard Osborne was funded in part through a National Health and Medical Research Council (NHMRC) of Australia Principal Research Fellowship #APP1155125.

Conflicts of Interest: The authors declare no conflict of interest.

References

1. Woodhead, A.J.; Abernethy, K.E.; Szaboova, L.; Turner, R.A. Health in fishing communities: A global perspective. *Fish Fish.* **2018**, *19*, 839–852. [CrossRef]
2. Eckert, C.; Baker, T.; Cherry, D. Chronic Health Risks in Commercial Fishermen: A Cross-Sectional Analysis from a Small Rural Fishing Village in Alaska. *J. Agromed.* **2018**, *23*, 176–185. [CrossRef] [PubMed]
3. Lawrie, T.; Matheson, C.; Ritchie, L.; Murphy, E.; Bond, C. The health and lifestyle of Scottish fishermen: A need for health promotion. *Health Educ. Res.* **2004**, *19*, 373–379. [CrossRef]
4. Matheson, C.; Morrison, S.; Murphy, E.; Lawrie, T.; Ritchie, L.; Bond, C. The health of fishermen in the catching sector of the fishing industry: A gap analysis. *Occup. Med.* **2001**, *51*, 305–311. [CrossRef]
5. Anwar, W.A.; Mostafa, N.S.; Hakim, S.A.; Sos, D.G.; Abozaid, D.A.; Osborne, R.H. Health literacy strengths and limitations among rural fishing communities in Egypt using the Health Literacy Questionnaire (HLQ). *PLoS ONE* **2020**, *15*, e0235550. [CrossRef]
6. El-Saadawy, M.; Soliman, N.E.; El-Tayeb, I.M.; Hammouda, M.A. Some occupational health hazards among fishermen in Alexandria city. *Gaziantep Med. J.* **2014**, *20*, 71–78. [CrossRef]
7. The World Bank. Literacy Rate. 2021. Available online: https://data.worldbank.org/indicator/SE.ADT.LITR.ZS (accessed on 31 March 2021).
8. World Health Organization. *Health Literacy Development for the Prevention and Control of Noncommunicable Diseases*; World Health Organization: Geneva, Switzerland, 2021; forthcoming.
9. Osborne, R.H.; Batterham, R.; Melwani, S.; Elmer, S. Health literacy and education to empower the individual to make informed choices and promote healthy lifestyles. In *WHO Independent High-Level Commission on Noncommunicable Diseases. Final Report—WHO Independent High-Level Commission on Noncommunicable Diseases Working Group 1*; Final Report 2019; Available online: https://www.who.int/ncds/governance/high-level-commission/HLC2-WG1-report.pdf (accessed on 2 June 2020).
10. Osborne, R.; Batterham, R.W.; Elsworth, G.R.; Hawkins, M.; Buchbinder, R. The grounded psychometric development and initial validation of the Health Literacy Questionnaire (HLQ). *BMC Public Health* **2013**, *13*, 658. [CrossRef]
11. Batterham, R.W.; Hawkins, M.; Collins, P.A.; Buchbinder, R.; Osborne, R.H. Health literacy: Applying current concepts to improve health services and reduce health inequalities. *Public Health* **2016**, *132*, 3–12. [CrossRef] [PubMed]
12. Batterham, R.W.; Buchbinder, R.; Beauchamp, A.; Dodson, S.; Elsworth, G.R.; Osborne, R.H. The OPtimising HEalth LIterAcy (Ophelia) process: Study protocol for using health literacy profiling and community engagement to create and implement health reform. *BMC Public Health* **2014**, *14*, 694. [CrossRef] [PubMed]
13. Sanders, E.B.N.; Stappers, P.J. Co-creation and the new landscapes of design. *CoDesign* **2008**, *4*, 5–18. [CrossRef]

14. Goodyear-Smith, F.; Jackson, C.; Greenhalgh, T. Co-design and implementation research: Challenges and solutions for ethics committees. *BMC Med. Ethics* **2015**, *16*, 1–5. [CrossRef]
15. Bakker, M.M.; Putrik, P.; Aaby, A.; Debussche, X.; Morrissey, J.; Råheim Borge, C.; Nascimento do Ó, D.; Kolarčik, P.; Batterham, R.; Osborne, R.H.; et al. Acting together–WHO National Health Literacy Demonstration Projects (NHLDPs) address health literacy needs in the European Region. *Public Health Panor.* **2019**, *5*, 123–329.
16. Beauchamp, A.; Mohebbi, M.; Cooper, A.; Pridmore, V.; Livingston, P.; Scanlon, M.; Davis, M.; O'Hara, J.; Osborne, R. The impact of translated reminder letters and phone calls on mammography screening booking rates: Two randomised controlled trials. *PLoS ONE* **2020**, *15*, e0226610. [CrossRef] [PubMed]
17. Bakker, M.M.; Putrik, P.; Rademakers, J.; van de Laar, M.; Vonkeman, H.; Kok, M.R.; Voorneveld-Nieuwenhuis, H.; Ramiro, S.; de Wit, M.; Buchbinder, R.; et al. Addressing health literacy needs in rheumatology—Which patient health literacy profiles need the attention of health professionals? *Arthritis Care Res.* **2020**, *73*, 100–109. [CrossRef]
18. Aaby, A.; Simonsen, C.B.; Ryom, K.; Maindal, H.T. Improving Organizational Health Literacy Responsiveness in Cardiac Rehabilitation Using a Co-Design Methodology: Results from the Heart Skills Study. *Int. J. Environ. Res. Public Health* **2020**, *17*, 1015. [CrossRef]
19. Cheng, C.; Elsworth, G.R.; Osborne, R.H. Co-designing eHealth and Equity Solutions: Application of the Ophelia (Optimizing Health Literacy and Access) Process. *Front. Public Health* **2020**, *8*, 792. [CrossRef]
20. Spillane, A.; Belton, S.; McDermott, C.; Issartel, J.; Osborne, R.H.; Elmer, S.; Murrin, C. Development and validity testing of the Adolescent Health Literacy Questionnaire (AHLQ): Protocol for a mixed methods study within the Irish school setting. *BMJ Open* **2020**, *10*, e039920. [CrossRef] [PubMed]
21. Beauchamp, A.; Batterham, R.W.; Dodson, S.; Astbury, B.; Elsworth, G.R.; McPhee, C.; Jacobson, J.; Buchbinder, R.; Osborne, R.H. Systematic development and implementation of interventions to OPtimise Health Literacy and Access (Ophelia). *BMC Public Health* **2017**, *17*, 1–18. [CrossRef]
22. Everitt, B. *Cluster Analysis*, 5th ed.; Wiley: Chichester, UK, 2011.
23. Glaser, B.G. The constant comparative method of qualitative analysis. *Soc. Probl.* **1965**, *12*, 436–445. [CrossRef]
24. Charmaz, K. *Constructing Grounded Theory*; Sage: Sonoma, CA, USA, 2014.
25. World Health Organization SEARO. *Health Literacy Toolkit for Low and Middle-Income Countries: A Series of Information Sheets to Empower Communities and Strengthen Health Systems*; World Health Organization SEARO: New Delhi, India, 2015.
26. Harris, J.; Springett, J.; Booth, A.; Campbell, F.; Thompson, J.; Goyder, E.; Van Cleemput, P.; Wilkins, E.; Yang, Y. Can community-based peer support promote health literacy and reduce inequalities? A realist review. *Public Health Res.* **2015**, *3*. [CrossRef]
27. Khamis, M.I. *Poverty and Developmental Practices in Rural Areas: An Exploratory Study in Sohag and Kafr El Sheikh, in Research Brief No. 11*; American University in Cairo Social Research Center: Cairo, Egypt, 2001.
28. Schrauben, S.J.; Wiebe, D.J. Health literacy assessment in developing countries: A case study in Zambia. *Health Promot. Int.* **2015**, *32*, 475–481. [CrossRef] [PubMed]

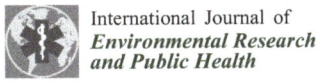

Article

Electronic Health Literacy in Individuals with Chronic Pain and Its Association with Psychological Function

Elena Castarlenas [1,2], Elisabet Sánchez-Rodríguez [1,2], Rubén Roy [1,2], Catarina Tomé-Pires [1,2], Ester Solé [1,2], Mark P. Jensen [3] and Jordi Miró [1,2,*]

[1] Universitat Rovira i Virgili, Department of Psychology, Research Center for Behavior Assessment (CRAMC), Chair in Pediatric Pain Universitat Rovira i Virgili-Fudación Grünenthal, Unit for the Study and Treatment of Pain—ALGOS, 43007 Tarragona, Catalonia, Spain; elena.castarlenas@urv.cat (E.C.); elisabet.sanchez@urv.cat (E.S.-R.); ruben.roy@urv.cat (R.R.); jamnista@gmail.com (C.T.-P.); ester.sole@urv.cat (E.S.)
[2] Institut d'Investigació Sanitària Pere Virgili, 43007 Tarragona, Catalonia, Spain
[3] Department of Rehabilitation Medicine, University of Washington, Seattle, WA 98104, USA; mjensen@uw.edu
* Correspondence: jordi.miro@urv.cat

Abstract: Electronic health literacy skills and competences are important for empowering people to have an active role in making appropriate health care decisions. The aims of this cross-sectional study were to (1) examine the frequency of use of the Internet for seeking online information about chronic pain, (2) determine the level of eHealth literacy skills in the study sample, (3) identify the factors most closely associated with higher levels of eHealth literacy, and (4) examine self-efficacy as a potential mediator of the association between eHealth literacy and measures of pain and function in a sample of adults with chronic pain. One-hundred and sixty-one adults with chronic pain completed measures assessing internet use, eHealth literacy, pain interference, anxiety, depression, and pain-related self-efficacy. Results indicated that 70% of the participants are active users of the Internet for seeking information related to their health. The level of eHealth literacy skills was not statistically significantly associated with participants' age or pain interference but was significantly negatively associated with both anxiety and depression. In addition, the findings showed that self-efficacy fully explained the relationship between eHealth literacy and depression and partially explained the relationship between eHealth literacy and anxiety. Self-efficacy should be considered as a treatment target in eHealth literacy interventions, due to its role in explaining the potential benefits of eHealth literacy.

Keywords: eHealth literacy; chronic pain; self-efficacy; psychological function

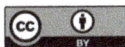

1. Introduction

Chronic pain is a common health condition worldwide, associated with financial, physical, and emotional burdens [1–4]. It is also one of the most common reasons for individuals seeking health care [5]. Given the evidence that the severity and impact of chronic pain is associated with biological, psychological, and social variables, it is often managed with multidisciplinary and multicomponent programs that address all of these factors [6–8]. Among the effective components of most, if not all, pain treatment programs is pain education [9,10]. Pain education is designed to increase patients' knowledge about pain, which is thought to lead to increases in adaptive coping responses and reductions in pain and its negative impact [11].

Specific knowledge domains addressed by pain education include information about the possible causes of pain, treatment options, effective self-management strategies, and prognosis [12]. Patients can obtain this information from a variety of sources, including the Internet [13]. For example, de Boer and colleagues [14] found that 39% of a sample of 200 patients attending a university pain center used the Internet to obtain information about their pain condition. However, although the Internet has become a common source of information about pain, the quality and usefulness of the information available on the Internet can be questioned [15,16].

Electronic health literacy (eHealth literacy) is a relatively new construct that extends the study of the traditional health literacy to encompass health literacy as it relates to the Internet. Specifically, eHealth literacy has been defined by Norman and Skinner as "... the ability to seek, find, understand, and appraise health information from electronic sources and apply the knowledge gained to addressing or solving a health problem" [17] (p. 2). Thus, eHealth literacy goes beyond the individual's ability to simply obtain relevant information about health from the Internet. It also includes the ability to apply that information to one's health care [18].

Although a considerable amount of research has examined traditional health literacy in individuals with chronic pain [19–23], and research on eHealth literacy has been conducted with individuals with other health conditions such as cancer, diabetics, epilepsy, cardiovascular diseases, recent fractures, or dental disease [24–27], none of those studies included pain-related variables as an outcome variables. As a whole, this research has found that being younger and having a higher level of education is associated with higher eHealth literacy skills [24–28]. Findings related to sex are less consistent; some studies have reported that eHealth literacy skills are similar between females and males [25], while others have found significant sex differences, with female predilection [24].

Research has also shown that having higher levels of eHealth literacy skills is associated with better health outcomes, as indicated by greater medication adherence, higher levels of quality of life and psychosocial well-being, and the adoption of adaptive health behaviors [29–32]. Self-efficacy, which is an individual's judgment of his or her ability to engage in or perform a specific activity, is a key component in the conceptual framework study of eHealth literacy, and has been hypothesized to mediate the associations between eHealth literacy skills and health outcomes [33]. To our knowledge, however, only one study has examined self-efficacy as a potential mediator of the effects of eHealth literacy in chronic pain samples. Specifically, Rabenbauer and Mevenkamp [34] found that self-efficacy mediated the association between eHealth literacy skills and healthy habits (e.g., organized physical exercise) in a sample of 207 adults with chronic back pain who used eHealth interventions for the management of chronic pain. However, these initial findings have yet to be replicated.

Given these considerations, the current study had four primary aims. First, we sought to examine the frequency of use of the Internet for seeking online information about chronic pain. Second, we wanted to better understand the association between eHealth literacy skills related to pain (i.e., seeking and understanding information about pain, and applying this information to own pain problems) and measures of pain and function in a sample of adults with chronic pain. Third, we sought to identify the factors most closely associated with higher levels of eHealth literacy in the study sample. Finally, we sought to test pain-related self-efficacy as a possible mediator of the associations between eHealth literacy and measures of function. On the basis of the research published to date, we hypothesized that seeking health information online would be common in a substantial subset of participants (i.e., that 33% or more would report that they sought health information online about their problem [14]). We also hypothesized that the levels of eHealth literacy would be negatively associated with participants' age and their levels of anxiety, depression, and pain interference. Finally, we hypothesized that self-efficacy would mediate the associations between eHealth literacy and anxiety, depression, and pain interference.

2. Materials and Methods

2.1. Participants

Study participants were recruited from the general population through sending an invitation via associations of patients or groups of patients with chronic pain in social networks. For individuals to be considered as potential participants, they had to (1) be aged

18 years old or older, (2) report having a pain problem of at least three months' duration, (3) be able to understand Spanish, and (4) have access to an electronic device connected to the Internet to be able to respond to the online survey.

Sample size estimation was calculated using G*Power [35]. The results revealed that at least 89 participants should be needed to address the study objectives with the planned analyses (effect size $f^2 = 0.15$; $\alpha = 0.05$ at 2-tailed; power = 0.95; two predictors).

2.2. Procedure

A cross-sectional study was conducted to address the objectives of the study. We created an online survey using the LimeSurvey program (https://www.limesurvey.org/es/, accessed on 24 November 2021) that included all the variables and instruments of interest for this study. The survey was made available during the months of November 2019 through January 2020. A short description of the study, which included a link for contacting research staff if a potential participant was interested in participating, was shared via social networks mainly through the profiles of associations of patients. We also encouraged individuals to share the study information through their own social networks to reach a wider audience. Once individuals clicked on the survey link, they could read additional details about the objectives and procedures of the study. The description of the study provided information about the study's aims. Specifically, participants were told that the study aimed to examine what people do, feel, or think when they have pain. They were also informed that participation in this study was anonymous and voluntary. After providing their consent to participate, they were able to respond to the survey questions. Participants did not receive any compensation for completing the survey. As no follow-up was planned, we decided to collect responses anonymously. On average, participants spent 17 min to respond to the survey. Participants were requested to respond to each question in the survey. Responses from 18 individuals were excluded from the planned analyses due to their failing to respond to all questions (the completion rate in this study was 90%).

All study procedures were approved by the Internal Review Board of the Universitat Rovira i Virgili.

2.3. Measures

Demographic and descriptive variables: Participants were asked to provide information regarding their gender, age, and maximum education level.

Pain information: We asked participants whether they had been experiencing pain for 3 or more months to ensure that their pain condition met the temporal criteria to be considered as chronic [36]. Participants were also asked to indicate the location of their most frequent pain problem, if they did or did not have a specific pain diagnosis, and if they were or were not on medical leave due to their pain problem(s).

Use of the Internet for seeking health information: Participants were asked to provide the frequency of their use of the Internet to seek information about their chronic pain condition, using a 5-point scale (1 = "never," 2 = "almost never," 3 = "sometimes," 4 = "almost always," and 5 = "always").

Health Literacy in an Electronic Context: We used a modified version of the 8-item eHealth Literacy Scale (eHEALS) [37] to assess the participants' perception of their knowledge, comfort, and resources at finding, evaluating, and applying electronic health information related to their chronic pain problem(s). Specifically, we modified the original instructions slightly by asking participants to respond to the items on the scale with respect to their chronic pain health problem (sample items: "I know how to use the Internet to answer my health questions about chronic pain," "I have the skills I need to evaluate the health resources about chronic pain that I find on the Internet"). Respondents indicated their level of agreement with each item using a 5-point Likert scale, ranging from 1 ("strongly disagree") to 5 ("strongly agree"). Responses were summed to create a total score that can range from 8 to 40, with higher scores representing higher self-perceived eHealth literacy related to chronic pain. Previous studies have identified a score of 26 or higher on this scale as indicative of high eHealth literacy skills [38,39]. eHEALS scores have been shown to be reliable and valid in a wide range of populations and contexts [40–42], and the Spanish version was translated and shown to be valid by Paramio and colleagues [43]. The Cronbach's alpha coefficient of the scale in the current sample was 0.94, indicating an excellent internal consistency.

Anxiety and depression symptom severity: The Hospital Anxiety and Depression Scale (HADS) originally developed by Zigmond and Snaith [44] was used to assess anxiety and depression symptoms severity. The questionnaire includes seven questions for assessing anxiety (HADS Anxiety) and seven for assessing depression (HADS Depression) symptom severity. Respondents were asked to indicate the frequency or severity (depending on the item) of each anxiety or depression symptom listed on a 4-point Likert scale (e.g., 0 = "not at all" or "only occasionally"; 3 = "very often" or "very much indeed"). The items of each subscale were summed to obtain a total score, which can range from 0 to 21; higher scores represent higher levels of depression or anxiety symptom severity. The Spanish version used in this study has been shown to provide valid and reliable scores [45]. In the current study, the internal consistency coefficients (Cronbach's alpha) for the anxiety and the depression subscales were 0.88 and 0.87, respectively, indicating a good internal consistency for both.

Pain self-efficacy: We used the 10-item Pain Self-Efficacy Questionnaire (PSEQ) [46] to measure the confidence in performing activities despite pain. With the PSEQ, responders are asked to rate their level of confidence for performing at present each activity described on a 7-point Likert scale, where 0 = "not at all confident" and 6 = "completely confident". The total PSEQ score is calculated by summing the responses; thus, the total score can range from 0 to 60, with higher scores indicating higher levels of pain self-efficacy. Scores on the PSEQ have shown good validity and reliability properties when used with samples of adults with chronic pain, including our population [47]. The Cronbach's alpha in the current sample indicated excellent internal consistency (α = 0.94).

Pain interference with daily activities: The Pain Interference Scale of the Brief Pain Inventory (BPI) [48] was used to assess the pain impact on functioning. The BPI has 7 items describing daily activities, and respondents are asked to indicate the extent that pain interfered with the activity in the past 24 h on a 0 ("does not interfere") to 10 ("completely interferes") scale. The total score is obtained by computing the mean for the seven items, resulting in an interference score that could range from 0 to 10. The BPI is a widely used tool with multiples studies supporting its reliability and validity [49–52], including studies with Spanish-speaking individuals [53–55]. The Cronbach's alpha of the pain interference scale in the current sample was 0.92, indicating excellent internal consistency.

2.4. Data Analysis

We first computed the means and standard deviations (continuous variables), as well as number and percentages (categorical variables) of the demographic and study variables to describe the sample and address the first two study aims (that is, to examine the frequency of use of the Internet for seeking online information about chronic pain and the level of eHealth literacy skills in the sample). We computed a Pearson correlation coefficient between participants' age and scores on the eHEALS to test the hypotheses that these variables would be positively associated. We then computed Pearson correlation coefficients between the eHealth literacy score and the measures of pain interference, depression, and anxiety symptoms to test the third hypothesis, with the plan to only proceed with a formal mediational analysis if these associations were statistically significant (i.e., in order to ensure that there was an association to explain). Finally, we performed mediation analyses to test the hypothesized mediating role of pain-related self-efficacy between eHealth literacy (independent variable) and criterion variables using the PROCESS macro version 3.4 for SPSS developed by Hayes (available at https://www.processmacro.org, accessed on 24 November 2021). For bootstrap, 5000 samples were computed. All statistical analyses were performed using the Statistical Package for Social Sciences (SPSS) for Windows Version 23.

3. Results

3.1. Sample Description

Participants consisted of a sample of 161 adults with chronic pain problems who were recruited from the general population. The overwhelming majority of participants were women ($N = 154$, 96%), ranging in age from 24 to 68 years, with a mean age of 44.63 years (SD = 9.55). The most common pain sites were the lower back ($N = 57$, 35%), the shoulder, and the upper limbs ($N = 48$, 30%). Table 1 provides additional information about the participants.

Table 1. Descriptive characteristics of the study participants.

Descriptive Characteristic		
Participants (N)		161
Mean age in years (range; SD)		44.63 (24–68; 9.55)
Gender, N (%)	Female	154 (96)
	Male	7 (4)
Education level, N (%)	Did not complete primary education	63 (39)
	Completed primary education	20 (12)
	Completed secondary education	52 (32)
	Completed bachelor's degree	17 (11)
	Post-bachelor education	4 (3)
On medical leave due to pain? N (%)	No	113 (70)
	Yes	48 (30)
Have a specific pain diagnoses? N (%)	No	17 (11)
	Yes	144 (89)
Location of the most frequent chronic pain, N (%)	Head, face, and mouth	11 (7)
	Cervical region	17 (11)
	Upper shoulder and upper limbs	48 (30)
	Thoracic region	4 (3)
	Abdominal region	3 (2)
	Lower back, lumbar spine, sacrum, and coccyx	57 (35)
	Lower limbs	2 (1)
	Pelvic region	2 (1)
	Anal, perineal, and genital region	17 (11)

3.2. Internet Use for Seeking Health Information and eHealth Literacy Skills

One-hundred and thirteen (70%) participants in our study reported that they used the Internet "almost always" or "always" for seeking information related to their chronic pain problem (specifically: never = 1 (1%), almost never = 3 (2%), sometimes = 44 (27%), almost always = 38 (24%), and always = 75 (46%) of the total participants). The mean score on the eHEALS scale for the whole sample was 29.53 (SD = 6.54; range = 9–40) and 42 (26%) of the participants had scores below 26, indicating low levels of eHealth literacy skills [38,39].

3.3. Association between eHealth Literacy Skills, Participants' Age, and Health-Related Outcomes

No statistically significant association was found between participants' age and the total score of the eHEALS scale ($r = 0.02$, $p = 0.845$). In addition, the measure of eHealth literacy was not statistically significantly associated with pain interference ($r = -0.13$, $p = 0.113$). However, it was significantly associated with both anxiety and depression (r's = -0.23 and -0.24, respectively, p's < 0.001). We therefore proceeded to evaluate the extent to which general self-efficacy mediated the association between eHealth literacy and anxiety and depression symptoms.

3.4. Self-Efficacy as a Mediator of the Relationship between eHealth Literacy and Health-Related Outcomes

Figure 1 depicts the results of the mediational analyses as hypothesized when depression is considered the criterion variable. Path a, that is, the effect of eHealth literacy (independent variable) on pain-related self-efficacy (mediator variable), was statistically significant (path a: β = 0.54, t = 3.09, $p < 0.01$). The data indicated a direct and negative association between pain-related self-efficacy and depressive symptoms (path b: β = −0.19, t = −9.16, $p < 0.001$). Moreover, the relationship between eHealth literacy and depression is fully explained by self-efficacy (path c: β = −0.17, t = −3.01, $p < 0.01$). Bootstrapping using confidence intervals not including zero confirmed that the mediating role of pain self-efficacy was statistically significant (β = 0.01, 95% confidence interval = −0.1722 to −0.0366, 5000 bootstrap resamples).

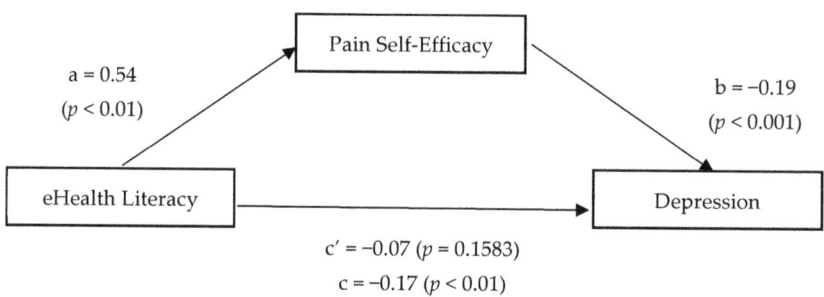

Figure 1. Relationship between eHealth literacy and depression mediated by pain-related self-efficacy.

A summary of the results of the mediational analyses when examining the role of pain-related self-efficacy as a mediator on the relation between eHealth literacy and anxiety symptoms is shown in Figure 2. The direct and significant effect of the independent variable on the mediator has been previously reported. We also found a negative and significant effect of pain-related self-efficacy on anxiety (path b: β = −0.09, t = −3.86, $p < 0.001$). Unlike the previous models, the effect of eHealth literacy on the criterion variable (i.e., anxiety) was found to be statistically significant (path c′: β = −0.10, t = −1.99, $p < 0.05$). In this case, the findings support partial mediation for pain-related self-efficacy on the relationship between the level of eHealth literacy and anxiety, that is, the indirect effect (path c: β = −0.15, t = −2.88, $p < 0.01$) explains part of the relationship between eHealth literacy and anxiety. Bootstrapping method with confidence intervals not including zero value confirms that the mediating role of pain self-efficacy was statistically significant (β = −0.05, 95% confidence interval = −0.0899 to −0.0126, 5000 bootstrap resamples).

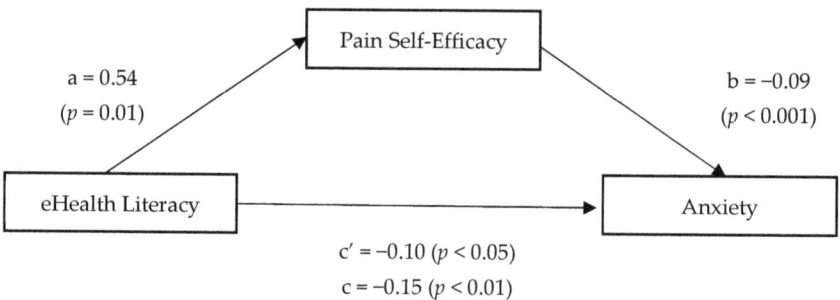

Figure 2. Relationship between eHealth literacy and anxiety mediated by pain-related self-efficacy.

4. Discussion

This study contributes knowledge about the eHealth literacy in individuals with chronic pain, as well as on the association between chronic pain-related eHealth literacy and function in these individuals. Consistent with the study hypothesis, a large number of participants in this sample (70%) were active in seeking information related to their chronic pain condition on the Internet. This percentage is considerably higher than that found by other authors [14] and it might be due to the characteristics of the sample. Participants in this study were recruited via social networks mainly through the profiles of associations of patients. Therefore, it seems likely that these participants were familiar with online resources, and that they were used to seek information on the Internet, health-related or otherwise. Moreover, more than 10 years has passed between de Boer and colleagues' study and ours; in the last few years, internet use for obtaining information about health conditions has increased exponentially [56].

Most of the participants in this study (74%) obtained a score of 26 or higher on the eHEALS scale, indicating high levels of eHealth literacy skills on the basis of the cutoff used in previous studies [38,39]. In our study, the mean score of eHEALS was 29.5 (out of 40), which is similar to those reported by Richtening and colleagues [38] in a sample of 453 adults at risk for cardiovascular diseases, who found a mean score on the eHEALS of 27.2 and that 66% of their participants had a high level of eHealth literacy ($\geq$26 out of 40).

The results did not support the hypothesis that participants' age would be negatively associated with higher eHealth literacy skills. Although the majority of previous studies have found that being younger is associated with a higher level of eHealth literacy [24–28], other researchers have obtained results similar to ours. For example, Milne and colleagues [57] did not find a statistically significant association between eHealth literacy and age in a sample of 83 primary lung cancer survivors.

On the other hand, the hypothesis that eHealth literacy would be associated with health outcomes was partially supported. eHealth literacy was significantly and negatively associated with anxiety and depression but was not significantly associated with pain interference. Finally, the data partially supported the hypothesis that self-efficacy mediated the association between eHealth literacy and patient function (here, depression and anxiety, although not pain interference). As noted in the Introduction section, self-efficacy has been identified as a mediator of the association between eHealth literacy and health status both in clinical and community samples (e.g., [34,58]). Moreover, self-efficacy beliefs have been found to be a mediator in the association between measures of "traditional" health literacy skills and health-related outcomes (e.g., [59–62]). For example, Jones and colleagues [61] found that self-efficacy mediated the association between oral health literacy and self-rated oral health in a sample of 278 indigenous adults from South Australia.

The results of this study have important research and clinical implications. First, this study contributes to a better understanding of the relationship between eHealth literacy and psychological health status in a sample of adults with chronic pain, a target population in which these associations have not yet been thoroughly explored. In addition, the direct associations found between measures of electronic literacy and psychological function highlight the potential importance of having adequate electronic literacy skills. This finding is consistent with the results of others that show that higher electronic literacy skills are more likely to be associated with better health-related outcomes [63].

With respect to the clinical implications of the study findings, eHealth literacy encompasses a set of abilities that can be learned. The current studies suggest that eHealth literacy interventions should emphasize increases in self-efficacy as a component of intervention, in order to maximize the potential benefits of the intervention on psychological function. Research to evaluate the efficacy of treatments that could enhance eHealth literacy, as well as to enhance self-efficacy for using the Internet in adaptive ways to better manage pain, is warranted. Although some eHealth literacy interventions have demonstrated benefits for patients and community samples, more efforts are required to develop these interventions in ways that are informed by eHealth literacy conceptual models [33]. This is of special relevance when considering that high levels of eHealth literacy skills have been found to be associated with variables that predict better treatment outcomes, such as treatment adherence, motivation, adaptive health behaviors, and the degree of trust in health care providers [64,65]. It is also possible that treatments which target non-eHealth literacy skills as primary outcomes—such as those that target depression or anxiety—might have an indirect impact on eHealth skills, which could then help to maintain treatment gains. Research examining this possibility is also warranted.

A number of limitations of this study should be considered when interpreting the results. First, the sample was composed by adults with chronic pain problems recruited from patients' associations with an active role in social networks who were responding to an online survey. Thus, the extent to which they generalize to other adults with chronic pain who would not be interested or willing to participate in a study such as this one, or to adults with chronic pain seen in clinics and health care centers (i.e., patients), is not known. Future studies should be conducted with other samples of individuals with chronic pain to help determine the generalizability of the findings. Second, and also related to the characteristics of the sample, almost all the participants in our study were females. As a result, we were not able to examine gender-related differences in the variables studied. Research is needed to study eHealth literacy in more balanced samples and looking at other variables that could help explain the quality of the experience in using the Internet for health-related purposes among individuals with chronic pain. For example, it would have been interesting to include some additional measures examining the attitudes and experience in the use of electronic sources for seeking health-related information, beyond the frequency in which they do that. Further research needs also to examine the role of the eHealth literacy skills as moderators between sociodemographic variables (e.g., socioeconomic or education level) and health care habits and outcomes.

5. Conclusions

This study provides new information about eHealth literacy and its association with psychosocial variables in individuals with chronic pain. The data showed that seeking information about health is a common practice. However, contrary to what was hypothesized, participants' age was not significantly associated with eHealth literacy. In addition, the findings of this study showed the potential role of this literacy on emotional symptoms and the role of self-efficacy as a mediator between eHealth literacy and function in adults with chronic pain. Future efforts should be focused on the development and assessment of effective educational programs which enhance electronic health literacy in individuals with chronic health conditions as well as for the population from the community. Further studies examining the association between eHealth literacy and function and its mediators are also warranted.

Author Contributions: Conceptualization, E.C., E.S.-R., R.R., C.T.-P., E.S., M.P.J. and J.M.; methodology, E.C., M.P.J. and J.M.; formal analysis, E.C.; investigation, E.C., E.S.-R., R.R., C.T.-P., E.S., M.P.J. and J.M.; data curation, E.C.; writing—original draft preparation, E.C., E.S.-R., R.R., C.T.-P., E.S., M.P.J. and J.M.; writing—review and editing, E.C., E.S.-R., R.R., C.T.-P., E.S., M.P.J. and J.M.; funding acquisition, J.M. All authors have read and agreed to the published version of the manuscript.

Funding: This work was partly supported by grants from the Spanish Ministry of Economy, Industry and Competitiveness (RTI2018-09870-B-I00; RED2018-102546-T), the European Regional Development Fund (ERDF), the Government of Catalonia (AGAUR; 2017SGR-1321), and Universitat Rovira i Virgili (PFR program). J.M.'s work is also supported by ICREA-Acadèmia and Fundación Grünenthal (Spain).

Institutional Review Board Statement: The study was conducted according to the guidelines of the Declaration of Helsinki and approved by the Internal Review Board of the Universitat Rovira i Virgili (CEIM: 136/2018).

Informed Consent Statement: Informed consent was obtained from all subjects involved in the study.

Data Availability Statement: The dataset used and analyzed in this study is available from the corresponding author upon request.

Conflicts of Interest: The authors declare no conflict of interest. The funders had no role in the design of the study; in the collection, analyses, or interpretation of data; in the writing of the manu.

References

1. Vos, T.; Abajobir, A.A.; Abbafati, C.; Abbas, K.M.; Abate, K.H.; Abd-Allah, F.; Abdulle, A.M.; Abebo, T.A.; Abera, S.F.; Aboyans, V.; et al. Global, regional, and national incidence, prevalence, and years lived with disability for 328 diseases and injuries for 195 countries, 1990-2016: A systematic analysis for the Global Burden of Disease Study 2016. *Lancet* **2017**, *390*, 1211–1259. [CrossRef]
2. Phillips, C.J. The Cost and Burden of Chronic Pain. *Rev. Pain* **2009**, *3*, 2–5. [CrossRef]
3. Henschke, N.; Kamper, S.J.; Maher, C.G. The epidemiology and economic consequences of pain. In *Mayo Clinic Proceedings*; Elsevier Ltd.: Amsterdam, The Netherlands, 2015; Volume 90, pp. 139–147.
4. Breivik, H.; Eisenberg, E.; O'Brien, T. The individual and societal burden of chronic pain in Europe: The case for strategic prioritisation and action to improve knowledge and availability of appropriate care. *BMC Public Health* **2013**, *13*, 1229. [CrossRef] [PubMed]
5. Finley, C.R.; Chan, D.S.; Garrison, S.; Korownyk, C.; Kolber, M.R.; Campbell, S.; Eurich, D.T.; Lindblad, A.J.; Vandermeer, B.; Allan, G.M. What are the most common conditions in primary care? Systematic review. *Can. Fam. Physician* **2018**, *64*, 832–840. [PubMed]
6. Scascighini, L.; Toma, V.; Dober-Spielmann, S.; Sprott, H. Multidisciplinary treatment for chronic pain: A systematic review of interventions and outcomes. *Rheumatology* **2008**, *47*, 670–678. [CrossRef] [PubMed]
7. Serrat, M.; Almirall, M.; Musté, M.; Sanabria-Mazo, J.P.; Feliu-Soler, A.; Méndez-Ulrich, J.L.; Luciano, J.V.; Sanz, A. Effectiveness of a Multicomponent Treatment for Fibromyalgia Based on Pain Neuroscience Education, Exercise Therapy, Psychological Support, and Nature Exposure (NAT-FM): A Pragmatic Randomized Controlled Trial. *J. Clin. Med.* **2020**, *9*, 3348. [CrossRef]
8. Aragonès, E.; López-Cortacans, G.; Caballero, A.; Piñol, J.L.; Sánchez-Rodríguez, E.; Rambla, C.; Tomé-Pires, C.; Miró, J. Evaluation of a multicomponent programme for the management of musculoskeletal pain and depression in primary care: A cluster-randomised clinical trial (the DROP study). *BMC Psychiatry* **2016**, *16*, 69. [CrossRef] [PubMed]
9. Burns, J.W.; Van Dyke, B.P.; Newman, A.K.; Morais, C.A.; Thorn, B.E. Cognitive behavioral therapy (CBT) and pain education for people with chronic pain: Tests of treatment mechanisms. *J. Consult. Clin. Psychol.* **2020**, *88*, 1008–1018. [CrossRef] [PubMed]
10. Gokhale, A.; Yap, T.; Heaphy, N.; McCullough, M.J. Group pain education is as effective as individual education in patients with chronic temporomandibular disorders. *J. Oral Pathol. Med.* **2020**, *49*, 470–475. [CrossRef] [PubMed]
11. Marris, D.; Theophanous, K.; Cabezon, P.; Dunlap, Z.; Donaldson, M. The impact of combining pain education strategies with physical therapy interventions for patients with chronic pain: A systematic review and meta-analysis of randomized controlled trials. *Physiother. Theory Pract.* **2019**, *37*, 461–472. [CrossRef]
12. Cooper, K.; Smith, B.H.; Hancock, E. Patients' perceptions of self-management of chronic low back pain: Evidence for enhancing patient education and support. *Physiotherapy* **2009**, *95*, 43–50. [CrossRef]
13. Ziebland, S.; Lavie-Ajayi, M.; Lucius-Hoene, G. The role of the internet for people with chronic pain: Examples from the DIPEx international project. *Br. J. Pain* **2014**, *9*, 62–64. [CrossRef] [PubMed]
14. de Boer, M.J.; Versteegen, G.J.; van Wijhe, M. Patients' use of the Internet for pain-related medical information. *Patient Educ. Couns.* **2007**, *68*, 86–97. [CrossRef]
15. Bailey, S.J.; Lachapelle, D.L.; Lefort, S.M.; Gordon, A.; Hadjistavropoulos, T. Evaluation of chronic pain-related information available to consumers on the internet. *Pain Med.* **2013**, *14*, 855–864. [CrossRef] [PubMed]
16. Corcoran, T.B.; Haigh, F.; Seabrook, A.; Schug, S.A. The quality of internet-sourced information for patients with chronic pain is poor. *Clin. J. Pain* **2009**, *25*, 617–623. [CrossRef] [PubMed]
17. Norman, C.D.; Skinner, H.A. eHealth literacy: Essential skills for consumer health in a networked world. *J. Med. Internet Res.* **2006**, *8*, e9. [CrossRef] [PubMed]
18. Paige, S.R.; Stellefson, M.; Krieger, J.L.; Anderson-Lewis, C.; Cheong, J.W.; Stopka, C. Proposing a transactional model of eHealth literacy: Concept analysis. *J. Med. Internet Res.* **2018**, *20*, e10175. [CrossRef] [PubMed]
19. Lacey, R.J.; Campbell, P.; Lewis, M.; Protheroe, J. The Impact of Inadequate Health Literacy in a Population with Musculoskeletal Pain. *HLRP Health Lit. Res. Pract.* **2018**, *2*, e215–e220. [CrossRef] [PubMed]
20. Rogers, A.H.; Bakhshaie, J.; Orr, M.F.; Ditre, J.W.; Zvolensky, M.J. Health Literacy, Opioid Misuse, and Pain Experience among Adults with Chronic Pain. *Pain Med.* **2020**, *21*, 670–676. [CrossRef] [PubMed]
21. Mackey, L.M.; Blake, C.; Casey, M.B.; Power, C.K.; Victory, R.; Hearty, C.; Fullen, B.M. The impact of health literacy on health outcomes in individuals with chronic pain: A cross-sectional study. *Physiotherapy* **2019**, *105*, 346–353. [CrossRef] [PubMed]
22. Mackey, L.M.; Blake, C.; Squiers, L.; Casey, M.B.; Power, C.; Victory, R.; Hearty, C.; Fullen, B.M. An investigation of healthcare utilization and its association with levels of health literacy in individuals with chronic pain. *Musculoskelet. Care* **2019**, *17*, 174–182. [CrossRef] [PubMed]

23. Turner, B.J.; Liang, Y.; Rodriguez, N.; Bobadilla, R.; Simmonds, M.J.; Yin, Z. Randomized Trial of a Low-Literacy Chronic Pain Self-Management Program: Analysis of Secondary Pain and Psychological Outcome Measures. *J. Pain* **2018**, *19*, 1471–1479. [CrossRef]
24. Valizadeh-Haghi, S.; Rahmatizadeh, S. eHealth literacy and general interest in using online Health information: A survey among patients with dental diseases. *Online J. Public Health Inform.* **2018**, *10*, e219. [CrossRef] [PubMed]
25. Cherid, C.; Baghdadli, A.; Wall, M.; Mayo, N.E.; Berry, G.; Harvey, E.J.; Albers, A.; Bergeron, S.G.; Morin, S.N. Current level of technology use, health and eHealth literacy in older Canadians with a recent fracture—a survey in orthopedic clinics. *Osteoporos. Int.* **2020**, *31*, 1333–1340. [CrossRef] [PubMed]
26. Shiferaw, K.B.; Tilahun, B.C.; Endehabtu, B.F.; Gullslett, M.K.; Mengiste, S.A. E-health literacy and associated factors among chronic patients in a low-income country: A cross-sectional survey. *BMC Med. Inform. Decis. Mak.* **2020**, *20*, 1–9. [CrossRef] [PubMed]
27. Hoogland, A.I.; Mansfield, J.; Lafranchise, E.A.; Bulls, H.W.; Johnstone, P.A.; Jim, H.S.L. eHealth literacy in older adults with cancer. *J. Geriatr. Oncol.* **2020**, *11*, 1020–1022. [CrossRef] [PubMed]
28. Hsu, W.C. The effect of age on electronic health literacy: Mixed-method study. *J. Med. Internet Res.* **2019**, *21*, e11480. [CrossRef] [PubMed]
29. Lin, C.Y.; Ganji, M.; Griffiths, M.D.; Bravell, M.E.; Broström, A.; Pakpour, A.H. Mediated effects of insomnia, psychological distress and medication adherence in the association of eHealth literacy and cardiac events among Iranian older patients with heart failure: A longitudinal study. *Eur. J. Cardiovasc. Nurs.* **2020**, *19*, 155–164. [CrossRef] [PubMed]
30. Filabadi, Z.; Estebsari, F.; Milani, A.; Feizi, S.; Nasiri, M. Relationship between electronic health literacy, quality of life, and self-efficacy in Tehran, Iran: A community-based study. *J. Educ. Health Promot.* **2020**, *9*, 175. [CrossRef]
31. Yang, S.C.; Luo, Y.F.; Chiang, C.H. The associations among individual factors, ehealth literacy, and health-promoting lifestyles among college students. *J. Med. Internet Res.* **2017**, *19*, e15. [CrossRef]
32. Mitsutake, S.; Shibata, A.; Ishii, K.; Oka, K. Associations of eHealth literacy with health behavior among adult internet users. *J. Med. Internet Res.* **2016**, *18*, e192. [CrossRef] [PubMed]
33. Pourrazavi, S.; Kouzekanani, K.; Bazargan-Hejazi, S.; Shaghaghi, A.; Hashemiparast, M.; Fathifar, Z.; Allahverdipour, H. Theory-based E-health literacy interventions in older adults: A systematic review. *Arch. Public Heal.* **2020**, *78*, 72. [CrossRef] [PubMed]
34. Rabenbauer, L.M.; Mevenkamp, N. Factors in the Effectiveness of e-Health Interventions for Chronic Back Pain: How Self-Efficacy Mediates e-Health Literacy and Healthy Habits. *Telemed. Health* **2020**, *27*, 184–192. [CrossRef] [PubMed]
35. Erdfelder, E.; Faul, F.; Buchner, A.; Lang, A.G. Statistical power analyses using G*Power 3.1: Tests for correlation and regression analyses. *Behav. Res. Methods* **2009**, *41*, 1149–1160. [CrossRef]
36. Raja, S.N.; Carr, D.B.; Cohen, M.; Finnerup, N.B.; Flor, H.; Gibson, S.; Keefe, F.J.; Mogil, J.S.; Ringkamp, M.; Sluka, K.A.; et al. The revised International Association for the Study of Pain definition of pain: Concepts, challenges, and compromises. *Pain* **2020**, *161*, 1976–1982. [CrossRef]
37. Norman, C.D.; Skinner, H.A. eHEALS: The eHealth literacy scale. *J. Med. Internet Res.* **2006**, *8*, e27. [CrossRef]
38. Richtering, S.S.; Hyun, K.; Neubeck, L.; Coorey, G.; Chalmers, J.; Usherwood, T.; Peiris, D.; Chow, C.K.; Redfern, J. eHealth Literacy: Predictors in a Population With Moderate-to-High Cardiovascular Risk. *JMIR Hum. Factors* **2017**, *4*, e4. [CrossRef] [PubMed]
39. Shiferaw, K.B.; Mehari, E.A. Internet use and ehealth literacy among health-care professionals in a resource limited setting: A cross-sectional survey. *Adv. Med. Educ. Pract.* **2019**, *10*, 563–570. [CrossRef]
40. Brørs, G.; Wentzel-Larsen, T.; Dalen, H.; Hansen, T.B.; Norman, C.D.; Wahl, A.; Norekvål, T.M. Psychometric properties of the norwegian version of the electronic health literacy scale (eheals) among patients after percutaneous coronary intervention: Cross-sectional validation study. *J. Med. Internet Res.* **2020**, *22*, e1731. [CrossRef] [PubMed]
41. Paige, S.R.; Krieger, J.L.; Stellefson, M.; Alber, J.M. eHealth literacy in chronic disease patients: An item response theory analysis of the eHealth literacy scale (eHEALS). *Patient Educ. Couns.* **2017**, *100*, 320–326. [CrossRef] [PubMed]
42. Lin, C.Y.; Broström, A.; Griffiths, M.D.; Pakpour, A.H. Psychometric Evaluation of the Persian eHealth Literacy Scale (eHEALS) Among Elder Iranians With Heart Failure. *Eval. Health Prof.* **2020**, *43*, 222–229. [CrossRef] [PubMed]
43. Paramio, G.; Almagro, B.J.; Hernando, Á.; Aguaded, J.I. Validación de la escala eHealth Literacy (eHEALS) en población universitaria española. *Rev. Esp. Salud Publica* **2015**, *89*, 329–338. [CrossRef] [PubMed]
44. Zigmond, A.S.; Snaith, R.P. The Hospital Anxiety and Depression Scale. *Acta Psychiatr. Scand.* **1983**, *67*, 361–370. [CrossRef] [PubMed]
45. Terol-Cantero, M.; Cabrera-Perona, V.; Martín-Aragón, M. Revisión de estudios de la Escala de Ansiedad y Depresión Hospitalaria (HAD) en muestras españolas. *Ann. Psicol.* **2015**, *31*, 494–503. [CrossRef]
46. Nicholas, M.K. The pain self-efficacy questionnaire: Taking pain into account. *Eur. J. Pain* **2007**, *11*, 153–163. [CrossRef] [PubMed]
47. Castarlenas, E.; Solé, E.; Galán, S.; Racine, M.; Jensen, M.P.; Miró, J. Construct Validity and Internal Consistency of the Catalan Version of the Pain Self-Efficacy Questionnaire in Young People With Chronic Pain. *Eval. Health Prof.* **2020**, *43*, 213–221. [CrossRef]
48. Cleeland, C.S.; Ryan, K.M. Pain assessment: Global use of the Brief Pain Inventory. *Ann. Acad. Med.* **1994**, *23*, 129–138.
49. Ger, L.P.; Ho, S.T.; Sun, W.Z.; Wang, M.S.; Cleeland, C.S. Validation of the brief pain inventory in a Taiwanese population. *J. Pain Symptom Manag.* **1999**, *18*, 316–322. [CrossRef]

50. Majedi, H.; Dehghani, S.S.; Soleyman-Jahi, S.; Emami Meibodi, S.A.; Mireskandari, S.M.; Hajiaghababaei, M.; Tafakhori, A.; Mendoza, T.R.; Cleeland, C.S. Validation of the Persian Version of the Brief Pain Inventory (BPI-P) in Chronic Pain Patients. *J. Pain Symptom Manag.* **2017**, *54*, 132–138.e2. [CrossRef] [PubMed]
51. Ferreira, K.A.; Teixeira, M.J.; Mendonza, T.R.; Cleeland, C.S. Validation of brief pain inventory to Brazilian patients with pain. *Support. Care Cancer* **2011**, *19*, 505–511. [CrossRef] [PubMed]
52. Miró, J.; Gertz, K.J.; Carter, G.T.; Jensen, M.P. Pain location and functioning in persons with spinal cord injury. *PM R* **2014**, *6*, 690–697. [CrossRef]
53. Badia, X.; Muriel, C.; Gracia, A.; Núñez-Olarte, J.M.; Perulero, N.; Gálvez, R.; Carulla, J.; Cleeland, C.S. Validación española del cuestionario Brief Pain Inventory en pacientes con dolor de causa neoplásica. *Med. Clin.* **2003**, *120*, 52–59. [CrossRef]
54. Ares, J.D.A.; Prado, L.M.C.; Verdecho, M.A.C.; Villanueva, L.P.; Hoyos, M.D.V.; Herdman, M.; Lugilde, S.T.; Rivera, I.V. Validation of the Short Form of the Brief Pain Inventory (BPI-SF) in Spanish Patients with Non-Cancer-Related Pain. *Pain Pract.* **2015**, *15*, 643–653. [CrossRef]
55. Expósito-Vizcaíno, S.; Sánchez-Rodríguez, E.; Miró, J. The role of physical, cognitive and social factors in pain interference with activities of daily living among individuals with chronic cancer pain. *Eur. J. Cancer Care* **2020**, *29*, e13203. [CrossRef] [PubMed]
56. Rouvinen, H.; Jokiniemi, K.; Sormunen, M.; Turunen, H. Internet use and health in higher education students: A scoping review. *Health Promot. Int.* **2021**. [CrossRef]
57. Milne, R.A.; Puts, M.T.E.; Papadakos, J.; Le, L.W.; Milne, V.C.; Hope, A.J.; Catton, P.; Giuliani, M.E. Predictors of High eHealth Literacy in Primary Lung Cancer Survivors. *J. Cancer Educ.* **2015**, *30*, 685–692. [CrossRef]
58. Choi, M. Association of ehealth use, literacy, informational social support, and health-promoting behaviors: Mediation of health self-efficacy. *Int. J. Environ. Res. Public Health* **2020**, *17*, 7890. [CrossRef] [PubMed]
59. Chen, A.M.H.; Yehle, K.S.; Plake, K.S.; Rathman, L.D.; Heinle, J.W.; Frase, R.T.; Anderson, J.G.; Bentley, J. The role of health literacy, depression, disease knowledge, and self-efficacy in self-care among adults with heart failure: An updated model. *Hear. Lung* **2020**, *49*, 702–708. [CrossRef] [PubMed]
60. Geboers, B.; De Winter, A.F.; Luten, K.A.; Jansen, C.J.M.; Reijneveld, S.A. The association of health literacy with physical activity and nutritional behavior in older adults, and its social cognitive mediators. *J. Health Commun.* **2014**, *19*, 61–76. [CrossRef] [PubMed]
61. Jones, K.; Brennan, D.S.; Parker, E.J.; Mills, H.; Jamieson, L. Does self-efficacy mediate the effect of oral health literacy on self-rated oral health in an Indigenous population? *J. Public Health Dent.* **2016**, *76*, 350–355. [CrossRef] [PubMed]
62. Kim, S.H.; Yu, X. The mediating effect of self-efficacy on the relationship between health literacy and health status in Korean older adults: A short report. *Aging Ment. Health* **2010**, *14*, 870–873. [CrossRef] [PubMed]
63. Xesfingi, S.; Vozikis, A. eHealth Literacy: In the Quest of the Contributing Factors. *Interact. J. Med. Res.* **2016**, *5*, e16. [CrossRef] [PubMed]
64. Lu, X.; Zhang, R. Association Between eHealth Literacy in Online Health Communities and Patient Adherence: Cross-sectional Questionnaire Study. *J. Med. Internet Res.* **2021**, *23*, e14908. [CrossRef] [PubMed]
65. Neter, E.; Brainin, E. eHealth literacy: Extending the digital divide to the realm of health information. *J. Med. Internet Res.* **2012**, *14*, e19. [CrossRef] [PubMed]

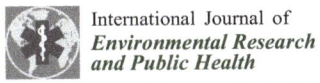

Article

How Can Cardiac Rehabilitation Promote Health Literacy? Results from a Qualitative Study in Cardiac Inpatients

Anna Isselhard [1,*], Laura Lorenz [1], Wolfgang Mayer-Berger [2], Marcus Redaélli [1] and Stephanie Stock [1]

1. Institute of Health Economics and Clinical Epidemiology, University Hospital of Cologne, 50935 Cologne, Germany; laura.lorenz@uk-koeln.de (L.L.); marcus.redaelli@uk-koeln.de (M.R.); stephanie.stock@uk-koeln.de (S.S.)
2. Centre for Cardiovascular Rehabilitation, 42799 Leichlingen, Germany; wolfgang.mayer-berger@klinik-roderbirken.de
* Correspondence: anna.isselhard@uk-koeln.de

Abstract: After acute care of a cardiac event, cardiac rehabilitation helps future disease management. Patients with low health literacy have been shown to have fewer knowledge gains from rehabilitation and higher all-cause mortality after acute cardiac events. Cardiac rehabilitation may be the best channel to target population with low health literacy, yet research on this topic is limited. Consequently, the main aim of the current study was to identify patient perceptions about the health literacy domains that are needed for successful rehabilitation of patients attending German cardiac rehabilitation clinics after an acute cardiac event. Five focus group interviews with 25 inpatients (80% male, 20% female) were conducted at a cardiac rehabilitation clinic in Germany. Patients were eligible to participate if they had sufficient understanding of the German language and had no other debilitating diseases. Patients identified five domains of health literacy for rehabilitation success: knowledge about their health condition; being able to find and evaluate health-related information, being able to make plans and sticking to them, assumption of responsibility over one's health and the ability to ask for and receive support. The results give an important insight into what patients perceive as important components of their cardiac rehabilitation, which can provide the basis for developing the health literacy of patients and how cardiac rehabilitation clinics respond to the recovery needs of their patients.

Keywords: health literacy; cardiac rehabilitation; heart attack; empowerment

Citation: Isselhard, A.; Lorenz, L.; Mayer-Berger, W.; Redaélli, M.; Stock, S. How Can Cardiac Rehabilitation Promote Health Literacy? Results from a Qualitative Study in Cardiac Inpatients. *Int. J. Environ. Res. Public Health* **2022**, *19*, 1300. https://doi.org/10.3390/ijerph19031300

Academic Editors: Marie-Luise Dierks, Jonas Lander, Melanie Hawkins and Paul B. Tchounwou

Received: 30 October 2021
Accepted: 20 January 2022
Published: 24 January 2022

Publisher's Note: MDPI stays neutral with regard to jurisdictional claims in published maps and institutional affiliations.

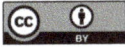

Copyright: © 2022 by the authors. Licensee MDPI, Basel, Switzerland. This article is an open access article distributed under the terms and conditions of the Creative Commons Attribution (CC BY) license (https://creativecommons.org/licenses/by/4.0/).

1. Introduction

Cardiovascular diseases such as coronary heart disease remain the number one cause of death globally, with close to 18 million deaths every year [1] and health-care costs of roughly 111€ billion just within the European Union [2]. The development of cardiovascular diseases can be linked to non-modifiable risk factors, such as family history, age, gender, or ethnicity [3]. Modifiable risk factors, such as unhealthy behavioral habits like cigarette smoking, a diet high in fat and sugar, and a lack of physical exercise have also been found to be strongly linked to its genesis [3]. There are also a variety of psychosocial risk factors that have been linked to cardiovascular disease, such as chronic stress, low levels of education and low income, or health literacy challenges [4–6].

In its infancy, health literacy has been defined as the skill to read and comprehend written medical information, a concept now known as functional health literacy [7]. Research nowadays has adopted a broader scope of the term: it is generally agreed upon that health literacy encompasses all abilities to understand, evaluate and apply health information in order to navigate the healthcare system and to make conscious decisions and subsequently to stay both physically and mentally healthy and subsequently maintain or increase quality of life [7,8]. This includes not only being able to locate health information, reading comprehension and numeracy, but also being able to communicate and understanding physicians' instructions and applying them. Accordingly, a person with health literacy challenges is often not able to access healthcare, read or understand basic information about health and illness, to communicate symptoms to their physician, to comprehend what they are being told to do, and to adhere to those instructions.

It has been shown that low levels of health literacy reliably predict detrimental health outcomes, such as lower uptake of preventive care [9], lower treatment adherence when in care [10], higher emergency room costs [11], and higher frequency of hospitalization [12,13]. In patients with cardiovascular diseases specifically, it has been shown that low health literacy is associated with lower disease-related knowledge [14,15], less well controlled blood pressure, less self-management behaviors, such as weight-monitoring, exercise behaviors, and salt consumption, as well as lower quality of life [15]. Two studies have shown that among patients with heart failure, those with low health literacy had a significantly higher all-cause mortality rates over the course of one year after hospitalization compared to those with adequate health literacy [16,17].

It is apparent that cardiovascular patients with low health literacy seem to have specific needs that are often not addressed in usual care. One channel to target this population is through cardiac rehabilitation. While originally created to recover patients from an acute cardiac event through exercise in the early 20th century, cardiac rehabilitation nowadays can be defined as a combination of medical and psychosocial interventions to assist patients with chronic or post-acute heart diseases [18,19].

In Germany, rehabilitation is usually initiated directly or shortly after acute care of a cardiac event, such as a heart attack or bypass surgery. It may be initiated by the hospital that provides acute care to the patient or through the patients' primary care provider or cardiologist. Since 1974, rehabilitation is guaranteed to patients by German law [18].

The program during rehabilitation typically consists of a three-week exercise and diet regimen, combined with psychological services and education under the supervision of a professional team of physicians, nurses, psychologists, physiotherapists, and dieticians. Special attention is paid to the imparting of complex medical content about the genesis of cardiovascular issues and prevention of further cardiac events in order to trigger behavioral changes. The majority of rehabilitation services take place in an inpatient form; however, outpatient services have recently been added to complement the existing structures [19]. The distribution among genders in German cardiac rehabilitation is heavily skewed, with men constituting approximately 75–80% of all patients consistently from 1990 to 2016 [18–20]. To support patients well, cardiac rehabilitation services need to be able to respond to the health literacy needs of their patients, which means understanding those needs from the patient perspective.

In Germany, the "National Action Plan Health Literacy" (NAP for HL) was initiated as a scientific guideline to strengthen health literacy on an individual and systemic level [21]. Given the weighty impact of health literacy on the genesis of chronic disease and the management thereof, it is advisable to consider tailoring health care services, such as cardiac rehabilitation, to the health literacy level of the patient. There is evidence that patients with low health literacy levels have lower disease related knowledge, but also fewer knowledge gains in rehabilitation when compared to patients with adequate or high health literacy levels [22]. In other words, patients who would need to benefit from rehabilitation the most, take away far less than patients who are already able to locate, understand and apply health information. This in turn may lead to higher readmissions, higher health care costs and ultimately higher mortality for those patients with lower health literacy.

There are multiple solutions to this problem. Firstly, education in rehabilitation clinics could just assume that all patients have health literacy challenges. However, this could result in patients with adequate health literacy levels being uninterested and not taking away the maximum of knowledge they could have. Additionally, this form of rehabilitation care is not the most cost-efficient. A second approach may be to identify in which areas of health literacy patients face challenges and coach patients on an individual or group level with education more suited to their understanding. This has previously been shown to improve health outcomes in patients with cardiovascular disease with low health literacy [23]. Patient involvement in these studies appears to be limited.

While studies on how patients with various diseases conceptualize health literacy are available [24,25], studies on how cardiac rehabilitation inpatients identify the domains of health literacy they deem important for the purpose of cardiac rehabilitation are currently lacking from the literature. This has also been pointed out by the American Heart Association (AHA), that recommended high levels of patient involvement in care as well as scientific research [26]. In fact, many recommendations are congruent between the AHA and the NAP for HL in Germany. Both recommend a high level of patient activation and participation in all areas of the health care system.

Therefore, the aim of this study is to identify patient perceptions about the health literacy domains that are needed for successful rehabilitation of patients attending German cardiac rehabilitation clinics after an acute cardiac event. This has the potential to advance health literacy development in chronically ill populations by improving the understanding of the patient perspective. Examining this perspective has crucial implications as to how best design and deliver interventions in cardiac rehabilitation inpatients to address health literacy challenges.

2. Materials and Methods

2.1. Study Design

A non-experimental, qualitative focus group study was conducted in cardiac rehabilitation inpatients to elicit their views on which domains of health literacy were most important for a successful rehabilitation.

2.2. Interview Guide

The semi-structured interview guide was informed by the health literacy pathway model by Edwards and colleagues [25]. This model was adopted as a theoretical framework for the construct of health literacy to this study because it was specifically developed to explain health literacy in long-term health conditions. The model elaborates health literacy across five distinct stages: health knowledge, health literacy skills and practices, health literacy actions, production of informed options and informed decision-making. The interview guide was developed to cover all five stages of the model with 11 questions overall (see Supplementary Materials). Two stages (health literacy actions and informed-decision making) were discussed with the help of one scenario. Each scenario described a dilemma that patients could be confronted with after rehabilitation. The scenarios were designed to elicit required skills and domains of health literacy that were necessary to solve the dilemma, as perceived by the patients.

2.3. Setting

All interviews were held in the same rehabilitation clinic in Leichlingen, North Rhine-Westphalia, Germany. While Leichlingen is a more rural town, the catchment area of the clinic is the largest metropolitan area of Germany with a population of over 8 million people within a 50 km radius, encompassing not only big cities like Cologne (population: 1 million) or Duesseldorf (population: 600.000) but also very rural areas.

2.4. Recruitment

Since regular cardiac rehabilitation in Germany takes three weeks, patients were recruited in week two and the interviews were held in week three. The head physician at the clinic selected patients who matched the inclusion and exclusion criteria. A purposive sampling approach was adopted to ensure a diverse sample in terms of age, education, and migration background. Both male and female patients whose rehabilitation is paid for by the pension insurance fund "Rentenversicherung Rheinland" were eligible to be included. Because of the nature of this insurance fund, all patients were below the age of 65. Patients were not eligible to participate if they had no sufficient understanding of the German language and had other debilitating diseases, such as life-threatening cancer, dementia, or severe mental illnesses. Patients who were eligible were invited to a brief recruiting appointment, where they were told what to expect from the focus group interviews. After that, they had the opportunity to ask questions about the nature of the study. If they agreed to participate, they signed consent forms and were invited to a focus group interview in the following week. The patients were not incentivized for participating. Recruitment was arranged weekly on a rolling basis until theoretical saturation was reached, meaning that no new domains of health literacy could be identified in a preliminary analysis immediately after the interviews.

2.5. Procedure

The same two researchers (A.I. and L.L.) conducted all focus group interviews. The researchers are both experienced in conducting and analyzing qualitative research. The researchers were unknown to the patients prior to the interviews and were not involved in the care of patients thereafter. The main goal of the researchers was to allow every participant to speak their mind and to facilitate communication. To begin the conversation, patients were asked about their experiences in rehabilitation and the skills they feel they needed in rehabilitation and for navigating a healthy life after rehabilitation. To facilitate the conversation, the researchers asked the participants to identify skills that were necessary to handle the situations described in the scenarios.

All focus group discussions were audiotaped with the same voice recorder and with the permission of the participants. The audiotapes were turned on after the introduction round to ensure that no statements given could be traced back to any identifying information. After every focus group interview, the audiotape was transferred to a password protected computer and subsequently deleted from the voice recorder. A third-party transcription bureau performed the transcription of the audiotapes.

2.6. Analysis

The transcriptions were coded by two independent researchers (A.I. and L.L.) along an open coding scheme using qualitative content analysis by Mayring [27] via the software MAXQDA (VERBI GmbH, Berlin, Germany). Qualitative content analysis aims at classifying qualitative data into categories of similar connotation. Conflicts in coding were resolved by discussion among A.I., L.L., S.S.T., and M.R.

2.7. Ethical Considerations

The focus group interviews were carried out in accordance with the Declaration of Helsinki. The potential risk to focus group participants was reduced to a minimum by obtaining informed consent prior to the interview and by not discussing identifying information on the audio recordings. The University of Cologne ethics committee reviewed and approved the focus group protocols.

3. Results

Overall, 25 cardiac rehabilitation inpatients (20 male, five female) participated in the focus group interviews. Five patient focus group interviews were conducted. The patients ranged in age from 32 to 64 years with a mean of 55 years in female patients (age range: 46–63 years) and a mean of 52.4 years in male patients (age range: 32–64 years). The focus groups ranged in length from 45 to 100 min with a mean of 76 min. One hundred and ninety-seven single-spaced pages were included in the analysis.

The analysis of the focus group interviews resulted in the identification of five skills, that patients saw as the main domains of health literacy for cardiac rehabilitation: health-related knowledge, information-seeking, self-regulation, assumption of responsibility and communication/interactive skills. The results for each component of health literacy from the patients' perspective are presented with demonstrative quotes from the patients.

3.1. Identified Domains of Health Literacy

3.1.1. Knowledge

Our analysis showed that patients from all focus groups identified knowledge about cardiac events, illness, medication as well as healthy behaviors that will prevent future cardiac events as the most significant domain of health literacy for rehabilitation success. Knowledge was mentioned first in every single focus group interview, stressing the importance of having a solid understanding of disease and healthy living. Patients especially emphasized the need to get information suited to their needs, their own medical history and specifically, tailored to their level of understanding. Two patients noted:

"Knowledge about your condition and understanding is the utmost basis to take anything away from rehabilitation." (FG01-03, male patient, focus group 1)

"I should not have to go to medical school to understand my condition, but I should be able to understand, just for myself, what happened to me and where." (FG03-02, male patient, focus group 3)

3.1.2. Information-Seeking

While patients agreed that gathering and understanding health-related information was a crucial aspect of health literacy, they specified that identifying which sources for health information were reliable would be vital in this process. Most patients specifically experienced difficulties judging the dependability with information found on the internet and pointed out that learning about reliable sources would be an important step for rehabilitation and healthy living. Patients would often consult their primary care physician after finding information online.

"There are renowned websites, where you can certainly find information. [...] I think you need to be very careful, where you get your information." (FG01-05, male patient, focus group 1)

"[After searching online] I would ask my doctor, if the information are actually true. My doctor also said to me "Don't ask Dr. Google, ask me" (FG05-01, female patient, focus group 5)

"You probably can't trust everything you read online about your condition. But it can be difficult to judge which information are reliable" (FG04-02, male patient, focus group 4)

3.1.3. Self-Regulation

Patients agreed that forming intentions and upholding motivation after rehabilitation would be crucial to not be readmitted and therefore identified self-regulation an important aspect of health literacy. The term self-regulation encompasses the ability to form intentions, stay motivated and exert self-control. Despite identifying this component, some patients expressed doubts about their self-regulation skills in order to navigate a healthy lifestyle.

"I know myself—I always have good and strong intentions. I hope I can stick to them this time." (FG05-05, female patient, focus group 5)

"It is the inner couch potato that needs to be fought." (FG03-04, male patient, focus group 3)

"I think setting goals, devising plans and so forth are very important in the next few months. In the past, I would always say "I'll do it tomorrow", then "next week" and then you are lost. Hopefully, this [healthy living] will become a habit." (FG02-02, male patient, focus group 2)

3.1.4. Assumption of Responsibility

Most patients agreed that in order to care for one's health, one would first have to assume responsibility over one's health. Some patients admitted that before experiencing an acute cardiac event, they believed that health was likely the result of genetic advantages of some people or luck of the draw. Several patients reported that only after experiencing a "wake-up call", they now think that assuming responsibility over one's health is beneficial in making health-related decisions and for continued rehabilitation success.

> "All these risk factors, that I knew of deep down, I just ignored them. [...] Now I am extremely aware of my responsibility." (FG02-05, male patient, focus group 2)

> "[This is] what I meant–gaining consciousness. I have never even thought about my health before." (FG04-01, male patient, focus group 4)

> "Diet, exercise and smoking–these things are really up to myself. No one else. And now the doctor in the hospital said: "Don't look back", because it is up to me to move on and take control." (FG03-03, male patient, focus group 3)

3.1.5. Communication/Interactive Skills

Patients report that interactive skills with their health care providers and their social environment are crucial parts of health literacy. More specifically, patients agreed that communication with their health care providers and asking their social environment for support are an important aspect of health literacy and tremendously help rehabilitation success. While this skill overall was described by both male and female patients, the need for social support was more frequently mentioned by male patients.

> "I always think having my wife sit next to me [in rehabilitation], it would have double the effect." (FG01-03, male patient, focus group 1)

> "I never asked for help and always said "yes" to everything. [...] but sometimes I need help, too" (FG05-04, female patient, focus group 5)

> "I believe that the communication with your physician plays an important role and that you trust them with everything." (FG01-06, male patient, focus group 1)

4. Discussion

This qualitative study aimed at identifying and presenting components of health literacy for German cardiac rehabilitation inpatients from the patients' perspective. For this purpose, focus group interviews were carried out with patients from a German cardiac rehabilitation clinic. A thorough analysis of the collected data based on qualitative content analysis revealed that patients identified five domains of health literacy for rehabilitation success: knowledge about their health condition and healthy living (knowledge); being able to find and evaluate health-related information (information-seeking); being able to make plans and sticking to them (self-regulation); taking on responsibility over one's health (assumption of responsibility); and the ability to ask for and receive support (communication/interactive skills). Thus, patients agreed that in order to have rehabilitation success one would need to: (1) know about their condition and health in general, (2) to know where to look for and how to evaluate health information, (3) be able to make behavioral plans and uphold motivation to follow them, (4) take on the responsibility for one's health, and (5) have appropriate interactive skills to express needs for social support to their social environment as well as to express symptoms to their primary care physicians.

Many of those patient-identified domains have previously been included in various health literacy models. Knowledge has been included in virtually all health literacy definitions, including the comprehensive definition by Sørenson et al. [28] which comprises several different health literacy definitions in the literature.

Locating health-related information is also a very prominent component of health literacy models. In fact, the most used definition of health literacy states includes accessing and understanding health information [8]. The model by Nutbeam proposed that obtaining health information represents the base of functional health literacy, the lowest level of the stage model of health literacy [6].

Interactive skills, as defined by the patients in this study, can be compared to interactive health literacy as defined by Nutbeams stage model of health literacy [29]. According to this model, interactive health literacy refers to skills that can be used to stimulate self-help by communication, for example by more fruitful interactions with health care providers or the social environment.

Assumption of responsibility is not as prominent in health literacy models as knowledge or interactive skills, but a few definitions and models include the importance of people accepting responsibility over their own health, such as the health literacy definition by Kickbusch et al. [28] or the health literacy model by Rudinger [29]. In the latter, assumption of responsibility counts as an advanced psychosocial skill that in turn promotes better self-regulatory skills.

Finally, self-regulation has a long-standing history in research of health behavior on its own [30]. Previous research has found that while most people want to live a healthy lifestyle, many fail to form clear goals and strive for goal achievement. In the health literacy field, sufficient self-regulation has at times been listed as a component of health literacy [29], while other models propose that good self-regulation would be an outcome from sufficient health literacy [6,8]. To date, it is not generally agreed upon whether self-regulation is a part of health literacy or a consequence thereof.

Our results compare with longitudinal qualitative studies with patients with cardiovascular disease in Ireland that investigated improvements in health literacy after an outpatient cardiovascular risk reduction program that has similar content to German cardiac rehabilitation [31,32]. Patients in this study identified most improvements in control over their health and self-management, which are similar in meaning to assumption of responsibility and self-regulation identified in our study [32]. Furthermore, patients reported improved knowledge on their health condition as well as improvement with information-seeking.

Our study has several limitations that need to be addressed. First of all, even though it was intended to include patients from diverse backgrounds, self-selection bias cannot entirely be avoided. This means that patients who volunteered to participate in the focus group interviews were perhaps the patients who possess a certain degree of health literacy and had a good idea about what skills were necessary. Secondly, the researchers decided to conduct male and female interviews separately from each other after observing a high rate of refusal from female patients to participate in mixed focus groups. This could have multiple reasons, but the most likely reason seems to be that the portion of female patients is much lower than the portion of male patients, and that female patients did not want to disclose information in front of male patients. The researchers decided to add a female-only focus group interview, in which there were no refusals to participate. This further supports the notion of female patient refusal due to privacy reasons in an otherwise male dominated group. However, we cannot exclude that our results could have been slightly different in mixed groups due to greater heterogeneity.

Another limitation that needs to be addressed is the timing of the focus group interview. As described above, patients were recruited in week two of three and interviews were conducted in the final week of cardiac rehabilitation. Therefore, patients arguably were more knowledgeable as they would have been had interviews been conducted at the beginning of the rehabilitation. For future research, it would be worth-while to compare results from a more naïve sample to our results.

5. Conclusions

The integration of the qualitative results of this study into previous research demonstrates that the majority of domains identified by patients in cardiac rehabilitation are already part of health literacy definitions. It is interesting to observe that while many definitions of health literacy in the literature did not specifically include the patient perspective, the majority of domains are congruent with patient-identified domains. A key finding from this study is that patients included domains such as assumption of responsibility and self-regulation, which are not consistently included in health literacy models. These specific domains, in turn, have been included in other studies that have specifically asked patients for their insights. The identified domains of health literacy are currently not all sufficiently addressed in cardiac rehabilitation. An integration of these domains into cardiac rehabilitation should be considered as a focus on the integration of learned contents into daily life may be beneficial for patient outcomes.

On a broader level, the results of our study further the development of health literacy in chronic disease in general, as understanding health literacy from the patient perspective in chronically ill populations should be the first step in developing interventions and improving clinical care.

Supplementary Materials: The following are available online at https://www.mdpi.com/article/10.3390/ijerph19031300/s1, Semi-structured interview guide.

Author Contributions: M.R., W.M.-B. and S.S. were responsible for the conceptualization and funding acquisition of this project. A.I. and S.S. developed the semi-structured interview guide. W.M.-B. recruited the patients for the interviews. A.I. and L.L. conducted the interviews. A.I., L.L. and M.R. were responsible for data analysis. A.I. was responsible for the project administration. S.S. supervised the project. A.I. wrote the original draft, all authors gave reviews and edits. All authors have read and agreed to the published version of the manuscript.

Funding: This research was funded by refonet (www.refonet.de), the rehabilitation research network of Deutsche Rentenversicherung Rheinland, Germany (project number 14002).

Institutional Review Board Statement: The study was conducted according to the guidelines of the Declaration of Helsinki and approved by the Ethics Committee of the University Hospital of Cologne (protocol code 17-042; date of approval 15 November 2017).

Informed Consent Statement: Informed consent was obtained from all subjects involved in the study.

Data Availability Statement: The dataset used and/or analyzed during this study are available from the corresponding author upon reasonable request.

Acknowledgments: The authors would like to thank Burkhard Wild from refonet for his on-going support during the execution of this project.

Conflicts of Interest: The authors declare no conflict of interest.

References

1. World Health Organization Fact Sheet: Cardiovascular Diseases (CVDs). Available online: https://www.who.int/en/news-room/fact-sheets/detail/cardiovascular-diseases-(cvds) (accessed on 16 May 2021).
2. Wilkins, E.; Wilson, L.; Wickramasinghe, K.; Bhatnagar, P.; Leal, J.; Luengo-Fernandez, R.; Burns, R.; Rayner, M.; Townsend, N. *European Cardiovascular Disease Statistics 2017*; European Heart Network: Brussels, Belgium, 2017.
3. Virani, S.S.; Alonso, A.; Benjamin, E.J.; Bittencourt, M.S.; Callaway, C.W.; Carson, A.P.; Chamberlain, A.M.; Chang, A.R.; Cheng, S.; Delling, F.N.; et al. Heart Disease and Stroke Statistics—2020 Update: A Report from the American Heart Association. *Circulation* **2020**, *141*, e139–e596. [CrossRef] [PubMed]
4. Winkleby, M.A.; Jatulis, D.E.; Frank, E.; Fortmann, S.P. Socioeconomic status and health: How education, income, and occupation contribute to risk factors for cardiovascular disease. *Am. J. Public Health* **1992**, *82*, 816–820. [CrossRef] [PubMed]
5. Safeer, R.S.; Cooke, C.E.; Keenan, J. The impact of health literacy on cardiovascular disease. *Vasc. Health Risk Manag.* **2006**, *2*, 457–464. [CrossRef] [PubMed]
6. Nutbeam, D. Health literacy as a public health goal: A challenge for contemporary health education and communication strategies into the 21st century. *Health Promot. Int.* **2000**, *15*, 259–267. [CrossRef]
7. Nutbeam, D. The evolving concept of health literacy. *Soc. Sci. Med.* **2008**, *67*, 2072–2078. [CrossRef]
8. Sørensen, K.; Van den Broucke, S.; Fullam, J.; Doyle, G.; Pelikan, J.; Slonska, Z.; Brand, H.; (HLS-EU) Consortium Health Literacy Project European. Health literacy and public health: A systematic review and integration of definitions and models. *BMC Public Health* **2012**, *12*, 80. [CrossRef]
9. Scott, T.L.; Gazmararian, J.A.; Williams, M.V.; Baker, D.W. Health Literacy and Preventive Health Care Use Among Medicare Enrollees in a Managed Care Organization. *Med. Care* **2002**, *40*, 395–404. [CrossRef]
10. Kalichman, S.C.; Ramachandran, B.; Catz, S. Adherence to combination antiretroviral therapies in HIV patients of low health literacy. *J. Gen. Intern. Med.* **1999**, *14*, 267–273. [CrossRef]
11. Howard, D.H.; Gazmararian, J.; Parker, R.M. The impact of low health literacy on the medical costs of Medicare managed care enrollees. *Am. J. Med.* **2005**, *118*, 371–377. [CrossRef]

12. Berkman, N.D.; Sheridan, S.L.; Donahue, K.E.; Halpern, D.J.; Crotty, K. Low Health Literacy and Health Outcomes: An Updated Systematic Review. *Ann. Intern. Med.* **2011**, *155*, 97–107. [CrossRef]
13. Baker, D.W.; Parker, R.; Williams, M.V.; Clark, W.S. Health literacy and the risk of hospital admission. *J. Gen. Intern. Med.* **1998**, *13*, 791–798. [CrossRef] [PubMed]
14. Williams, M.V.; Baker, D.W.; Parker, R.M.; Nurss, J.R. Relationship of Functional Health Literacy to Patients' Knowledge of Their Chronic Disease. *Arch. Intern. Med.* **1998**, *158*, 166–172. [CrossRef] [PubMed]
15. Macabasco-O'Connell, A.; DeWalt, D.; Broucksou, K.A.; Hawk, V.; Baker, D.W.; Schillinger, D.; Ruo, B.; Bibbins-Domingo, K.; Holmes, G.M.; Erman, B.; et al. Relationship Between Literacy, Knowledge, Self-Care Behaviors, and Heart Failure-Related Quality of Life Among Patients with Heart Failure. *J. Gen. Intern. Med.* **2011**, *26*, 979–986. [CrossRef] [PubMed]
16. McNaughton, C.D.; Cawthon, C.; Kripalani, S.; Liu, D.; Storrow, A.B.; Roumie, C.L. Health Literacy and Mortality: A Cohort Study of Patients Hospitalized for Acute Heart Failure. *J. Am. Heart Assoc.* **2015**, *4*, 001799. [CrossRef] [PubMed]
17. Peterson, P.N. Health Literacy and Outcomes Among Patients with Heart Failure. *JAMA J. Am. Med. Assoc.* **2011**, *305*, 1695–1701. [CrossRef]
18. Karoff, M.; Held, K.; Bjarnason-Wehrens, B. Cardiac rehabilitation in Germany. *Eur. J. Cardiovasc. Prev. Rehabil.* **2007**, *14*, 18–27. [CrossRef]
19. Mittag, O.; Schramm, S.; Böhmen, S.; Hüppe, A.; Meyer, T.; Raspe, H. Medium-term effects of cardiac rehabilitation in Germany: Systematic review and meta-analysis of results from national and international trials. *Eur. J. Cardiovasc. Prev. Rehabil.* **2011**, *18*, 587–693. [CrossRef]
20. Bellmann, B.; Lin, T.; Greissinger, K.; Rottner, L.; Rillig, A.; Zimmerling, S. The Beneficial Effects of Cardiac Rehabilitation. *Cardiol. Ther.* **2020**, *9*, 35–44. [CrossRef]
21. Schaeffer, D.; Hurrelmann, K.; Bauer, U.; Kolpatzik, K. (Eds.) Nationaler Aktionsplan Gesundheitskompetenz. In *Die Gesundheitskompetenz in Deutschland Starken*; KomPart: Berlin, Germany, 2018.
22. Mattson, C.C.; Rawson, K.; Hughes, J.W.; Waechter, N.; Rosneck, J. Health literacy predicts cardiac knowledge gains in cardiac rehabilitation participants. *Heal. Educ. J.* **2014**, *74*, 96–102. [CrossRef]
23. Lee, T.W.; Lee, S.H.; Kim, H.H.; Kang, S.J. Effective Intervention Strategies to Improve Health Outcomes for Cardiovascular Disease Patients with Low Health Literacy Skills: A Systematic Review. *Asian Nurs. Res.* **2012**, *6*, 128–136. [CrossRef]
24. Jordan, J.E.; Buchbinder, R.; Osborne, R. Conceptualising health literacy from the patient perspective. *Patient Educ. Couns.* **2010**, *79*, 36–42. [CrossRef]
25. Edwards, M.; Wood, F.; Davies, M.; Edwards, A. The development of health literacy in patients with a long-term health condition: The health literacy pathway model. *BMC Public Health* **2012**, *12*, 130. [CrossRef]
26. Magnani, J.W.; Mujahid, M.S.; Aronow, H.D.; Cené, C.W.; Dickson, V.V.; Havranek, E.; Morgenstern, L.B.; Paasche-Orlow, M.K.; Pollak, A.; Willey, J.Z.; et al. Health Literacy and Cardiovascular Disease: Fundamental Relevance to Primary and Secondary Prevention: A Scientific Statement from the American Heart Association. *Circulation* **2018**, *138*, e48–e74. [CrossRef] [PubMed]
27. Mayring, P. *Qualitative Inhaltsanalyse—Grundlagen und Techniken [Qualitative Content Analysis—Basics and Techniques]*, 8th ed.; BeltzVerlag: Weinheim, Germany, 2003.
28. Kickbusch, I.; Wait, S.; Maag, D. Navigating health: The role of health literacy. In *London: Alliance for Health and the Future*; International Longevity Centre-UK: London, UK, 2006.
29. Lenartz, N.; Soellner, R.; Rudinger, G.G. Modellbildung und empirische Modellprüfung einer Schlüsselqualifikation für gesundes Leben. *DIE Z. für Erwachs.* **2014**, *2*, 29–32. [CrossRef]
30. De Ridder, D.T.D.; De Wit, J.B.F. (Eds.) Self-regulation in health behaviour: Concepts, theories, and central issues. In *Self-Regulation in Health Behaviour*; John Wiley & Sons: Chichester, UK, 2006; pp. 1–23.
31. McKenna, V.B.; Sixsmith, J.; Barry, M.M. A Qualitative Study of the Development of Health Literacy Capacities of Participants Attending a Community-Based Cardiovascular Health Programme. *Int. J. Environ. Res. Public Health* **2018**, *15*, 1157. [CrossRef] [PubMed]
32. McKenna, V.B.; Sixsmith, J.; Barry, M. Facilitators and Barriers to the Development of Health Literacy Capacities Over Time for Self-Management. *HLRP Health Lit. Res. Pract.* **2020**, *4*, e104–e118. [CrossRef]

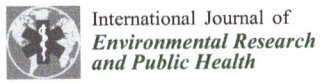

Article

Preferences and Experiences of People with Chronic Illness in Using Different Sources of Health Information: Results of a Mixed-Methods Study

Svea Gille [1,2,*], Lennert Griese [1] and Doris Schaeffer [1]

1 Interdisciplinary Centre for Health Literacy Research, School of Public Health, Bielefeld University, 33615 Bielefeld, Germany; lennert.griese@uni-bielefeld.de (L.G.); doris.schaeffer@uni-bielefeld.de (D.S.)
2 Department Public Health and Education, Hertie School, 10117 Berlin, Germany
* Correspondence: svea.gille@uni-bielefeld.de

Abstract: Background: People with chronic illness are particularly dependent on adequate health literacy (HL), but often report difficulties in accessing, understanding, appraising, and applying health information. To strengthen the HL of people with chronic illness, in-depth knowledge about how they deal with health information is crucial. Methods: To this end, quantitative data from the Second Health Literacy Survey Germany (HLS-GER 2) and qualitative data from seven focus group discussions were used to examine the interest in health information, preferred sources of information as well as experiences and challenges with information management among people with chronic illness. Results: The results show that people with chronic illness have a great interest in health information and use very different sources of health information, preferring personal information from physicians most. The results also point to several challenges in health information management that seem to be influenced by the illness duration as well as by the experiences made with the respective sources. Conclusions: Overall, the study provides important starting points for intervention development for the provision and communication of health-related information, but also to research on health information behavior and HL.

Keywords: health information sources; health literacy; focus groups; people with chronic illness; HLS-GER 2; Germany

Citation: Gille, S.; Griese, L.; Schaeffer, D. Preferences and Experiences of People with Chronic Illness in Using Different Sources of Health Information: Results of a Mixed-Methods Study. *Int. J. Environ. Res. Public Health* **2021**, *18*, 13185. https://doi.org/10.3390/ijerph182413185

Academic Editors: Marie-Luise Dierks, Jonas Lander and Melanie Hawkins

Received: 12 November 2021
Accepted: 10 December 2021
Published: 14 December 2021

Publisher's Note: MDPI stays neutral with regard to jurisdictional claims in published maps and institutional affiliations.

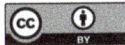

Copyright: © 2021 by the authors. Licensee MDPI, Basel, Switzerland. This article is an open access article distributed under the terms and conditions of the Creative Commons Attribution (CC BY) license (https://creativecommons.org/licenses/by/4.0/).

1. Introduction

Chronic diseases and enduring health problems constitute a major global challenge. They account for 71% of deaths worldwide and are the main determinant of the morbidity spectrum [1,2]. They are always coupled with a high demand for information, which is not uniform, but changes frequently over the course of illness, and becomes more extensive and multi-layered as the complexity of the medical condition increases [3–6].

For many years, people with chronic illness in Germany faced a lack when searching for information. Access to information was also inadequate. In the meantime, the situation has changed fundamentally. Triggered by digitalization, there is now an overload of information and information opportunities, also referred to in the discussion as 'information obesity' [7]. At the same time, the amount of misinformation and disinformation as well as advertising-supported and manipulated information has increased [8,9]. Consequently, new difficulties have arisen and information management—especially information accessing and appraising—has become a more complex and demanding task.

It is therefore not easy to meet the associated requirements, and this demands not only sufficient, easily accessible and comprehensible information, but also adequate health literacy [10]. In the context of chronic illness, health literacy can be understood as the motivation and ability to access, understand, appraise, and apply health-related information to cope with the challenges of living with chronic illness; to actively participate in the treatment, recovery, or preservation of health stability and the decisions necessary to do so; to navigate the healthcare system; and to cooperate constructively with healthcare professionals. Overall, it should aim at achieving an optimal management of the medical condition and the best possible treatment and health care [11,12]. However, available research shows that people with chronic illness often have low health literacy levels and face a host of problems in managing health-related information [13–17]. To comprehend these problems, it is necessary to gain a better understanding of the health information behavior of people with chronic illness, the significance of different information sources, and the experience gained with both.

Previous research on health information behavior in general has focused on different strands, such as the type and extend of information sought, the information needs and preferred sources as well as the personal and source-related characteristics affecting health information behavior [18–21]. In this context, especially the significance of individual information sources has been emphasized in the past: both quantitative and qualitative studies show that doctors particularly are the primary source of health information, but also that the Internet has become increasingly important [21–26].

In terms of chronic illness, research has shown that people with chronic illness are confronted with many, very different problems for which they need comprehensive information [5,27,28]. Similarly, studies show that information acquisition and management are an important part of coping with chronic illness, for which a lot of time and energy is spent [6,19]. When searching for health information, people with chronic illness use a wide range of information sources for different purposes [29–31], including various interpersonal sources, traditional, and new media, which are often used simultaneously [19,32]. Although the previously mentioned preferences for physicians as the most important source of health information have also been confirmed in the context of chronic illness [31,33], it must be assumed that the information behavior in the chronically ill is strongly influenced by several personal and contextual factors [34]. It is likely that health information behavior differs from stage to stage in the illness trajectory [35–37]. The same applies to information receptivity or absorption capacity, which also varies and is strongly dependent on the situation [10,37,38]. Moreover, the preferences for information sources and information needs are also strongly influenced by the illness situation (e.g., the progression of the chronic illness and/or therapy), the duration of illness, as well as by the experiences made with the respective sources [33,34,39,40].

However, to date, most of the results on health information behavior available in literature relate to selected diseases, such as cancer or diabetes (e.g., [18,30,41]), using either quantitative or qualitative data. There is a lack of studies, especially for Germany, combining both perspectives to provide insight into the preferences and motives for using different sources of information among people with chronic illness and which shed light on their information management. Therefore, the present article attempts to fill this research gap by analyzing: (1) the interest in health information and motivation for information management among people with chronic illness; (2) the sources used by people with chronic illness; and (3) their experiences with different sources of information and their information management, as well as the challenges they face in this context.

2. Materials and Methods

A mixed-methods approach was chosen to answer these questions. Data from the Second Health Literacy Survey Germany (HLS-GER 2) [42] as well as the results from seven focus group discussions [43] were used and analyzed. The HLS-GER 2 is an extended follow-up survey of the first German Health Literacy Survey (HLS-GER 1) [15] and was conducted within the framework of the international comparative study HLS_{19} of the M-POHL Network of the WHO Europe [44]. The HLS-GER 1 provided initial findings on health information management of the German population and formed the basis for focus group discussions [43], which presented first in-depth data among people with chronic illness. These findings were combined with new data on health information management of the German population provided by the HLS-GER 2 [42]. The aim of this combination was to complement the findings from the quantitative analysis with the experiences and challenges in health information management from the perspective of people with chronic illness to better understand their health information behavior.

The HLS-GER 2 involved a total of 2151 people aged 18 years and older living in Germany who participated in face-to-face interviews (PAPI) between December 2019 and January 2020. For measuring chronic illness, it was asked if respondents have any long-term illness or health problem, which has lasted or is expected to last for 6 months or more. Overall, 1086 of the respondents stated that they were affected by at least one chronic disease [42]. About one-third (30.1%) had one chronic disease, and 69.9% suffered from multiple chronic diseases. The average duration of illness was approx. 13 years (13.20; SD = 11.72). There were slightly more women (53.3%) than men (46.6%) with chronic conditions in the sample. On average, the respondents were 58.67 years old (SD = 16.63) (Table 1).

Table 1. Sample characteristics HLS-GER 2 (n = 1086) [1].

Variable	Proportion/Mean (SD)	N
Age [min, max: 18–92]	58.67 (16.63)	1080
18–29 years	7.3	79
30–45 years	15.3	165
46–64 years	36.1	390
65 years and older	41.3	446
Illness duration [min, max: 0–82]	13.20 (11.72)	1066
less than one year	2.4	26
1–5 years	28.6	305
6–10 years	11.3	121
>10 years	57.6	614
Number of chronic diseases [min, max: 1–12]		1086
one	30.1	327
more than one	69.9	759
Gender		1084
male	46.7	506
female	53.3	578

[1] Weighted sample based on the population structure of the German Microcensus 2018 adjusting for gender, age, population density, state, and education.

In addition to health literacy, the HLS-GER 2 also took a closer look at some aspects of health information behavior. Among other things, the questions covered interest in and motivation for dealing with health information, preferred sources of information, and experiences with these sources in understanding information (for more details see [42]). For the present analysis, the HLS-GER 2 findings were used and analyzed specifically for people with chronic illness. One main focus of the analysis is on stratification by duration of illness.

Furthermore, data were analyzed from a total of seven focus group discussions conducted between November 2017 and February 2018 on the perspectives and experiences of people with chronic illness in managing health information [43]. The focus groups were made up of five randomly composed patient groups (individuals with HIV/AIDS, tumor diseases, cardiovascular diseases, chronic pain, and rare chronic diseases). Contact was established through self-help facilities [45]. The members of two other focus group discussions were recruited by a survey institute and were individually assigned to a group. The participants in these focus groups were also chronically ill or were relatives of a chronically ill person (Table 2).

Each focus group consisted of four to nine discussants. A total of 41 people participated in the discussions, which were structured thematically and followed a guideline focusing on four thematic complexes derived from empirical findings on health information management of the German population [15]: (1) Understanding of health literacy; (2) significance and use of different health information sources as well as experiences made with health information management in different sources; (3) challenges in information management during the course of illness; (4) suggestions for improving health information and facilitating information management. The discussions lasted 90–120 min. Each participant consented to the discussions being recorded, transcribed, and anonymized. For the subsequent analysis, the data were sequenced and coded according to the topic. In addition, code trees were created. The codes, which were mainly derived from the data material (in vivo codes) [46], were then arranged in an organizational structure based on a first rough interpretation of the data. In a next step, the respective text segments were matched and then analyzed in detail. At the same time, the classification structure already developed was reviewed and modified where necessary.

Table 2. Characteristics of the focus group participants (n = 41).

Variable	Proportion/Mean (SD)	N
Focus group participants		41
FG1 AIDS		4
FG2 chronic pain		7
FG3 colon cancer		5
FG4 chronic ischemic heart disease		4
FG5 rare chronic illnesses		4
FG6 mixed group by survey institute		8
FG7 mixed group by survey institute		9
Age [min, max: 27–83]	58.34 (14.83)	38
Gender		41
male	56.1	23
female	43.9	18

3. Results

3.1. Interest in Health Information

Overall, people with chronic illness are highly interested in information on health and illness. According to the HLS-GER 2, more than 82% of the respondents with chronic conditions agreed with the statement that they wanted to know everything about their health. Only 18% could not identify with this statement [42]. A differentiated analysis according to the duration of chronic illness showed that interest in health information is lower in the first year following diagnosis, at 72.6%, but increases to up to 90.9% as the condition progresses. After having lived with the disease for more than 10 years, interest declines again, but is still higher than in the first year after diagnosis (Figure 1).

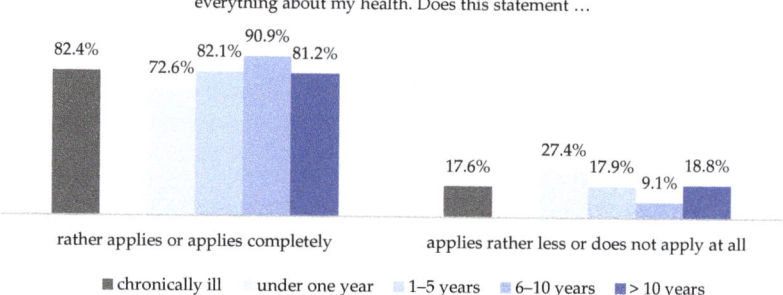

Figure 1. Interest in health information differentiated by duration of chronic disease (HLS-GER 2).

This tendency is also reflected by the focus groups, which also reported a greater interest in health information as the duration of illness increased. The participants emphasized that they experienced a crisis at the beginning of their illness and had to deal with the shock of the diagnosis, along with the resulting disruption of their previous reality (see also [47,48]). Therefore, their interest in extensive professional information was limited at this stage.

> "The patient is already ill and must first cope with the disease and is then bombarded with specialist information (.), which has nothing to do with the individual patient." (FG 4)

The last sentence is particularly noteworthy, because it shows that the capacity of people with chronic illness to absorb information at the time of diagnosis is limited. Moreover, the information received appears to be focused on specialist or medical textbook information that does not consider the patient's individual situation and the psychological and social stress of receiving a diagnosis.

Only when the shock of the diagnosis has lessened and there is hope of a return to normality, patients begin to take a greater and more active interest in information. At the same time, the desire for further information grows successively with an increase in the duration of the disease:

> "Yes definitely. Dealing (with health information) has become the central focus of my life. Every bit of information and every source is checked over and over." (FG 7)

Moreover, not only how often, but also in which manner people search information seems to change with longer illness duration:

> "I would say it has become more intense, more positive, much more targeted. So not taking in everything anymore, but really only targeted." (FG 2)

The quotes make clear that the management of health-related information is not only gaining in importance and scope, but is gradually becoming an integral part of life because every piece of information found, and every source of information used, is thoroughly and critically examined. The resulting difficulties for information management and especially for accessing and appraising information will be considered in the following.

3.2. Health Literacy among People with Chronic Illness

People with chronic illness are particularly dependent on health information and also on adequate health literacy, i.e., the ability to manage health information. However, the data of the HLS-GER 2 study show that almost two thirds (62.3%) of the people with chronic illness have difficulties with information management and thus show low health literacy levels. Especially appraising health information is particularly challenging. Overall, 76.4% of people with chronic illness have difficulties in this area. However, accessing information also poses challenges. More than half (51.8%) of the respondents with chronic illness report difficulties here [42]. This is also reflected in the focus groups, where the assessment of information is also seen as very challenging.

> "So, judging I sometimes find difficult because there is always this opinion and that opinion (...) That's why it is sometimes really hard to judge what's good for me and not and what I should do now." (FG 1)

As the quote shows, difficulties arise from the amount of different information, but also the different quality of information causes uncertainty and requires critical judgment.

> "I don't need to read this page any further, because it is all about selling me something. You have to be very careful." (FG 2)

Similar to the interest in health information being highest at 6–10 years of illness duration, accessing and appraising information is also most difficult at this stage. Overall, 60.8% of the people with a chronic illness lasting 6–10 years have problems finding appropriate information, and 85.1% consider it challenging to appraise the information they find. These values are significantly higher than those for chronically ill people with a shorter duration of illness. Of those who have been chronically ill for less than a year, 53.7% report difficulties in finding and 62.7% in appraising health information. Of those having a chronic disease for 1–5 years, 49.7% consider it challenging to find health information and 76.3% to appraise them.

3.3. Preferred Sources of Information

When asked which sources of information they prefer, people with chronic illness show a clear preference for information from doctors (Figure 2). For 80.4% of the respondents with chronic illness interviewed in the HLS-GER 2, primary care physicians are the most important source of health information, while just under half (47.5%) prefer medical specialists. The great importance of physicians as a source of information is also expressed in the focus groups. This is explained by the high level of trust placed in physicians. Information from physicians is predominantly regarded as credible, reliable and of high quality.

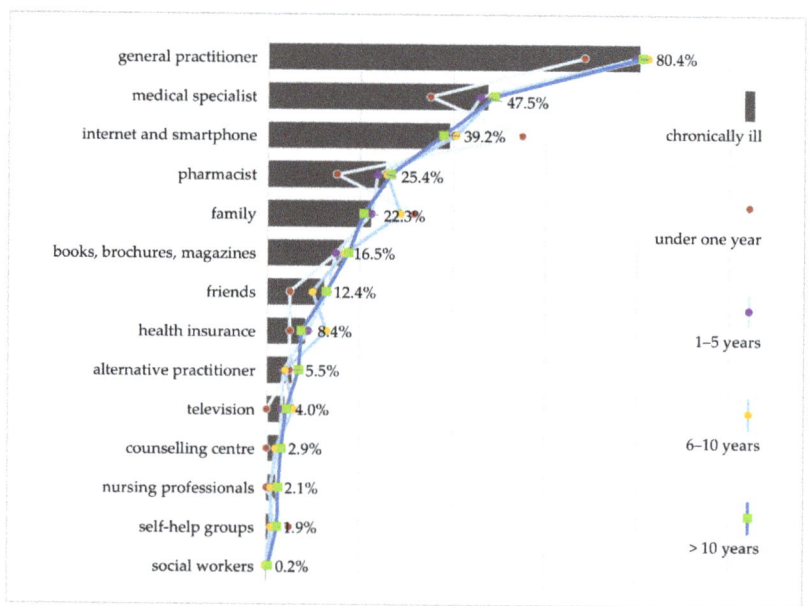

Figure 2. Preferred sources of information differentiated by duration of chronic disease (HLS-GER 2).

At 39.2%, the Internet ranks third in the hierarchy of preferred sources of information for people with chronic illness, behind general practitioners and specialists. According to the focus groups, it is mostly used to obtain an initial overview of the symptoms, effects, and treatment options.

> "So, I am very much googling and very often on Wikipedia. If a clinical picture comes up somewhere that affects not only me but also my family (...). When mom has a weird cough, I'm already looking, what could it be?" (FG 1)

At the same time, the Internet is used as a means of reassurance:

> "When I was diagnosed, when the doctor told me what I had, I got on the Internet and researched what it meant. She did tell me a few things (...), but then I got more detailed information from the Internet." (FG 5)

This quote shows that the Internet also serves as a supplementary source of information that allows patients to search for more in-depth or reassuring information before and after visiting the doctor. The search for structured and qualified information, as well as the need for emotional support and opportunities for exchange, are cited as further motives for using the Internet.

Pharmacies also play an important role in providing information. A quarter (25.4%) of people with chronic illness surveyed in the HLS-GER 2 used information provided by pharmacies. Pharmacists are the first point of contact for questions about the patient information leaflet, which more than half of the people with chronic illness surveyed in HLS-GER 2 (58.8%) found difficult to understand [42], as well as for questions about effects, tolerability, and interaction with other medications, and especially for complex medication regimes.

"If I am prescribed something new, because I receive medication from different doctors, then (...) the pharmacy is my point of contact to find out if the medications are all compatible (...) And I have a really competent pharmacy (...) that checks the medications against each other." (FG 2)

This quote shows that the role of the pharmacy as a hub of information is particularly valued. It bundles information obtained elsewhere and checks prescribed medications for compatibility or adverse side effects.

Approximately one-fifth (22.3%) of people with chronic illness prefer to obtain information from family members. The focus groups show that they pave the way for access to health information and are also important for people with chronic illness in further managing information, since they explain things that have been misunderstood and provide support in understanding information.

"Yes, then I show it to my sons, and they tell me what it means. I don't understand everything, and they explain it to me." (FG 2)

The family plays a particularly important role in classifying, assessing, and processing health information, and is perceived overall as a trustworthy and helpful complementary support for information management.

As with the interest in health information, individual sources of health information are assigned varying degrees of relevance depending on the illness duration (Figure 2). According to the HLS GER 2, doctors and pharmacists become more important the longer the illness lasts. During the first year, especially the Internet and family members seem to be the most important sources of information for people with chronic illness. It can be assumed that emotionally overcoming the acute crisis and the shock of diagnosis is the motivation behind the search for information, which makes detailed specialist information of secondary importance. According to the focus groups, sharing information among the family or searching online for the experiences of people with chronic illness is helpful to better understand their own situation, alleviate fears and overcome the shock of their diagnosis.

3.4. Experience in Searching for and Dealing with Health Information

People with chronic illness are usually very experienced in dealing with health information from the sources mentioned here. Four overarching themes emerge that are key in choosing these individual sources. These include *trust* in the source and the perceived competence, the time available and the comprehensibility of the information. If people with chronic illness are dissatisfied with any of these factors, they often continue to search for and use other sources of information.

3.4.1. Trust and Competence

Trust is a basic prerequisite for the use of certain information sources. Overall, physicians enjoy a high degree of trust, but do not always succeed in providing their patients with the information they desire. In the HLS-GER 2, 29.6% of people with chronic illness report significant difficulty in obtaining the exact information they need from their doctor [42]. Participants in the focus groups confirm this and emphasize how much this undermines their trust in competence because they believe trust is the most important prerequisite for a functioning doctor–patient relationship. People with rare chronic diseases especially, or those with symptoms that are difficult to diagnose, tell of numerous experiences where they received less than satisfactory information. This often leads to annoyance, confusion, uncertainty, and results in serious consequences for using health information sources:

"You start to search around when you feel uncertain and don't know what to do and reach a point where you just feel so alone, and that's when something has to happen. You either begin to look for other doctors or whatever." (FG 7)

Trust usually begins to erode when a patient starts to doubt the competence surrounding information, which is perceived to be unsatisfactory from a user perspective. This often leads to a search for further information, usually on the Internet, or a change of doctor is considered.

While physicians enjoy a high level of trust as sources of information, much of the information found on the Internet is regarded with skepticism. This skepticism results from the amount of contradictory and interest-driven information available on the Internet, which places high demands on information search and assessment. According to the HLS-GER 2, 83.5% of people with chronic illness consider it difficult or very difficult to assess the trustworthiness and reliability of digital information. A further 63.2% have difficulty in finding the exact information they are searching for on the Internet [42], which is also confirmed by the focus groups.

"When you search for such and such on the Internet, the first things that always appear are the worst things you could have, and that's more unsettling than it is reassuring. That's why it's better to go to the doctor." (FG 6)

This clearly shows that searching for information on the Internet is not only time-consuming, but also frustrating and unsettling due to the large amount of unreliable and low-quality information.

The family also plays an important role in this context. They are greatly trusted as a source of support and advice when uncertainty and confusion arise related to information management. To some extent, the family also assumes a protective function.

"My daughter always says: Stay away from the Internet, go to the doctor instead. If you Google, you'll be dead in six months." (FG 6)

As the quote shows, this also implies that it may not be advisable to use certain information sources.

The level of trust in individual sources of information fluctuates with an increase in the duration of an illness and the accumulation of experience with managing information and various information sources. Overall, the attitude toward information becomes more critical and the trustworthiness of individual sources of information is questioned more closely as a result. In the first year following their diagnosis, 69.1% of people with chronic illness find it difficult to assess the trustworthiness of digital information, in contrast to 89.5% of respondents with an illness lasting 6–10 years. Focus groups emphasize that this not only applies to digital information, but also to how they behave as patients.

"And then his (the physician's) statements need to be checked. And I do check them now but didn't ten years ago." (FG 5)

As this quote demonstrates, attitudes and actions regarding established and trusted sources of information (in this case doctors) change with an increase in the duration of illness.

3.4.2. Time

In addition to trust, the time available to manage information plays an important role. According to the HLS-GER 2, 49.4% of respondents with chronic illness state that obtaining enough consultation time is the most difficult aspect of interaction with their physicians [42].

"But that's just chop-chop: waiting three hours for five minutes, then you have a piece of paper in your hand with a medication and then you leave." (FG 2)

To address this, many patients develop targeted strategies to effectively use the narrow timeframe available.

"They don't have any time. That's why I (...) wrote down my questions beforehand, so I knew what to ask. But I still don't have the feeling that I know everything I should, because they just didn't take any time with me." (FG 6)

However, these strategies do not always produce the desired results for people with chronic illness. Some have shared their experiences concerning physicians who make ironic comments about their efforts and whose approaches are less than constructive. Actively seeking information is therefore often perceived as negative.

"And then you're considered the worst kind of patient if you've done your research beforehand! And oh brother, we've all gone through that at least once. When you already know a few things and go to the doctor—forget it, not a chance." (FG 7)

Experiences like these encourage people with chronic illness to adopt traditional, passive patient behavior and to forgo active participation, including requesting information. This also corresponds to the results of the HLS-GER 2, in which 34.7% of people with chronic illness assess communicating their personal views or ideas to their physician as (very) difficult. Nearly one-third (32.1%) find it difficult to participate in decisions that affect their own health [42].

According to the focus groups, frequently long waiting periods for an appointment and very brief consultation periods that leave little time for questions or further information limit the opportunity for more participation and co-production. These issues often lead to annoyance, which in turn leads to the search for information elsewhere.

The focus groups point out that a positive aspect of online searches is that they can take place any time and without an appointment. In addition, such searches are not limited to a certain timeframe and can be carried out until the desired information has been found. However, Internet searches can quickly become very time-consuming, since the information must be filtered out from a large number of search results. Searches also do not usually lead directly to the information sought.

"But then one page leads to another page and another and there's more and more information (...) and you continue reading and suddenly there are 1000 tabs open and at the end you're just confused." (FG 7)

This quote also shows that it is not only the abundance of information that makes searching difficult, but also the fragmentation of information or the lack of user-friendly guidance systems and navigation aids through digital space that causes disorientation.

Regarding the illness duration, the first year following the diagnosis is also particularly challenging here. As Figure 3 shows, people with chronic illness find it by far the most difficult during this phase to obtain sufficient consultation time with their physician.

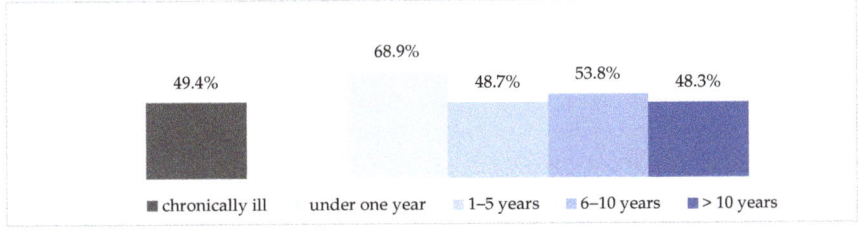

Figure 3. Difficulty in obtaining sufficient consultation time (HLS-GER 2).

3.4.3. Comprehensibility of Information and Communication

Communication that is easily comprehensible is another important criterion in choosing the medium of information. However, problems frequently arise here, as well. Almost half of the HLS-GER 2 respondents with chronic illness did not understand explanations given by a health professional at least once in the last 12 months. Difficulties in comprehension occur most frequently in communication with doctors. Overall, 31.4% report problems in understanding explanations by their specialists and 13.7% by their general practitioners (Figure 4). This is in line with the 47.2% of people with chronic illness who assess it as (very) difficult to understand the terms used by their doctors [42].

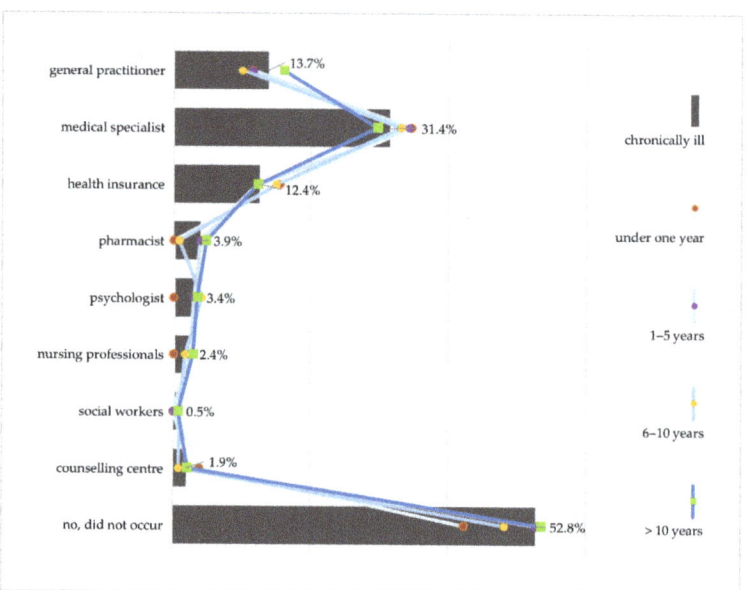

Figure 4. Difficulty in understanding explanations by healthcare providers differentiated by duration of chronic illness (HLS-GER 2).

Focus groups also frequently criticize the communication with physicians. Despite positive developments, focus group participants claim that doctors still express themselves too abstractly and use too many medical terms.

"I once had a doctor, an orthopedist. The receptionist was there during the examination. The doctor just rattled off something in Latin, went out and then the receptionist said: Okay, I'll translate for you, you probably didn't understand anything." (FG 7)

Some even suspect that this mode of communication is intentional to ensure patient compliance.

"We're not supposed to understand, that's why they also use the Latin medical terms. Patients are kept in the dark so they can't raise any objections or take matters into their own hands, which could be considered contra-productive (...)." (FG 3)

Taking the illness duration into consideration shows that difficulties in comprehension tend to decrease over time. While 57.7% report difficulties in understanding during the first year of diagnosis, this proportion is much lower at 46.4% among respondents with an illness of longer than 10 years. The results of the focus groups provide a possible explanation for this.

"When my doctor or a specialist now throws around a medical term, I immediately say: What does that mean? If I don't know something, I ask, but there are also people who are too afraid or shy to ask questions." (FG 6)

According to the focus groups, people with chronic illness grow into an active role as patients over time, ask more explicitly for comprehensible information, ask questions if they have not understood something correctly and want to be involved in decisions. At the same time, this is perceived as difficult because it requires a departure from traditional notions of the patient role, which, as previously mentioned, demands a great deal of effort because it is not supported by all physicians. This is the reason why focus groups advocate for more person-centered care, more sensitive communication, and a more perceptive style of interaction.

4. Discussion

The aim of the article was to generate in-depth knowledge about how people with chronic illness deal with information and information management. To this end, quantitative and qualitative data on information use were analyzed to examine interest in health information, preferred sources of information as well as experiences and challenges with information management.

The results show that people with chronic illness have a great interest in health information and are for the most part quite active in searching for and requesting information. However, this appears to be linked to the duration of chronic illness. In the first year after diagnosis, people with chronic illness usually find it difficult to deal with health and illness information, because they have to overcome the shock of the diagnosis and often find themselves in an acute crisis situation [48]. With an increase in the duration of illness, they become more interested in information, ask more specific and in-depth questions, and engage more intensively with illness and health information [48,49]. At the same time, they perceive information management to be more difficult and their health literacy is declining. This is surprising, because it could be assumed that a gain in competence would occur through the accumulation of experience. However, another interpretation is also possible. Precisely because people with chronic illness deal with information more intensively, they might assess the difficulties associated with information management more realistically and more critically—especially in terms of coping with the challenges associated with the abundance of information, such as finding the right information and being able to assess how reliable and trustworthy it is. This is not only critical for health information behavior, but also for disease management and care, as shown by studies on the effects of low health literacy and associated difficulties in information management [42,44]. This must be taken into consideration, as well as that the need for information varies depending on the stage of the disease and that not every time is the right time to provide it. As the results confirm, receptiveness to information is limited immediately following diagnosis and in times of crisis [48], yet information is often provided exactly during such periods. Therefore, it is important to support people with chronic illness through trajectory-oriented information management that takes into account the ever-changing need for new information during the course of the disease while remaining centered on the patient and on equal footing with them [10,11,49].

At the same time, the results also show that people with chronic illness consistently use very different sources of information, and prefer their information orally as opposed to in writing. This is often overlooked in the current discussion, which focuses primarily on written information and ways to improve it, and frequently targets a single source of information [50]. However, in our view, it is important to pay more attention to the mix and interplay of sources—especially from an intervention point of view, because according to our results, some sources of information, such as the Internet, serve especially to reassure patients who use it as a form of support.

The results show that physicians are the most important source of information; a number of other studies have also come to this conclusion [22,23,51]. This corresponds to the high status and social position doctors still enjoy in many countries, especially in Germany [52]. Both of these factors explain why, from the perspective of people with chronic illness, physicians are the first point of contact when seeking health information, and enjoy a high level of trust as a reliable and high-quality source of such information [25,31,34,53].

However, our analysis also points to the growing relevance of other sources of information in Germany—most notably the Internet [22,54–56]. A few years ago, the Internet was in fourth or fifth place on the list of popular information sources in Germany [15,56,57], but is now in second place after physicians [22,23] as a supplementary source of medical information, and becomes even more important when the trust between doctor and patient begins to erode. This is a curious finding, given the lagging development of digitalization in Germany [58,59].

As the focus group discussions specifically suggest, this is due in many cases to misgivings, confusion, and the resulting criticism of the communication and interaction with doctors, especially the lack of consultation time. Other studies confirm this finding [31,37,60]. Compared internationally, the number of physician consultations in Germany is much higher than in other countries, but also significantly shorter, which means that only a limited timeframe for in-depth information is available [61,62]. An adequate consultation period is especially important for people with chronic illness to communicate their wishes and views, and to participate actively and co-productively in their own treatment and care. According to the results of this study, however, a large number of people with chronic illness are unable to do so; this shows that the call for longer consultation periods and structural changes that has become louder over the years is still relevant [63,64]. This also applies to the communication with doctors. It has improved, as the results of this study show, but is relatively insignificant in everyday life, is usually from a purely medical point of view and is often incomprehensible, too complicated in terms of language, and too little geared to the problems and preferences of patients [42,65]. Improving the communication and interaction skills of physicians, as is currently being discussed in Germany [66], is therefore a high priority from the perspective of people with chronic illness.

In addition, as was repeatedly emphasized in the focus group discussions, the shift toward informed and critical patients is often met with rejection on the part of physicians. This often leads to a loss of trust and is the reason why people with chronic illness begin to 'shop around' and consult other sources of information—whether for reassurance or in the search for reliable information [49,60,67]. The Internet, but also the family, assume particular importance, especially during the initial stage of an illness. As other studies also show [31,67], both are a relevant source, especially in the search for emotional support and peer-to-peer exchanges. This underscores how important it is to improve the competences and skills of doctors.

However, using digital information is not easy. Finding the right health information among so much contradictory information on the Internet is difficult and time-consuming, as is distinguishing reliable information from the abundance of false information available. This is confirmed by the recent data on the population's digital health literacy [42,44,68–71]. Therefore, bundling tailored, evidence-based, comprehensible information on the Internet and creating information-related guidance systems is especially important for people with chronic illness and their individual information needs that constantly change over time. Initial efforts to this end, such as the creation of information portals, can already be observed in several countries such as Germany (www.gesund.bund.de, accessed on 13 December 2021), England (www.nhs.uk, accessed on 13 December 2021), Denmark (www.sundhed.dk, accessed on 13 December 2021) or Australia (www.healthdirect.gov.au, accessed on 13 December 2021). However, these services are usually not yet tailored to the specific needs of people with chronic illness and are not automatically available to users, but must be accessed independently. Improving this by shifting pull into push could give people with chronic illness the ability to face the challenges of personal responsibility and self-management that is expected of them at each stage of their disease to cope with their illness, as well as the difficulties that arise in managing the related information.

5. Limitations

There is a lack of findings that shed light on information management and the experience of using different health information sources from the perspective of people with chronic illness, especially in Germany. By using a mixed-methods approach, findings are now available based on an extensive database. However, there are also limitations; although the two surveys are closely linked, as they belong to a series of studies that build on each other starting in 2016 with the first German Health Literacy Survey (HLS-GER 1) [15], it must be taken into account that they are still two independent samples. In addition, the present study examines the importance of the duration of illness, but not the age of participants in regard to information use and information management. However, it can be assumed that age plays an important role, especially for the preference for digital information sources. A similar limitation must be made regarding other socio-demographic and socio-economic determinants that have already been found to be significant for information behavior as well as for health literacy in people with chronic illness [16,18]. This should also be taken into account when interpreting the results and should be examined in more detail in future analyses.

6. Conclusions

Overall, the results of the study provide important starting points for intervention development and illustrate that too little attention has been paid to the perspective of people with chronic illness. This applies not only to the provision and communication of health-related information but also to research on health information behavior and health literacy. More attention should be paid to the patient view in both of these cases. In order to support people with chronic illness in their health information management, the following starting points can be summarized from the previous results:

- Establish a trajectory-oriented information management that takes into account the ever-changing needs of people with chronic illness.
- Consider the mix of different information sources and, in addition to improving written information, pay particular attention to oral information and communication with health professionals.
- In doing so, foster the necessary structural changes and anchor skills and competencies required for information provision in the education and training of health care professionals.
- Establish special guidance systems and navigation aids for people with chronic illness that make it easier to find and use health information along the entire illness trajectory and thereby increasing health literacy.

Author Contributions: Conceptualization, S.G., L.G. and D.S. methodology, S.G., L.G. and D.S.; formal analysis, S.G.; writing—original draft preparation, S.G.; writing—review and editing, L.G. and D.S.; visualization, S.G.; supervision, D.S.; project administration, D.S.; funding acquisition, D.S. All authors have read and agreed to the published version of the manuscript.

Funding: This research was funded by the German Federal Ministry of Health, grant number: Kapitel 1504 Titel 54401, ZMV I 1-2518 004 (HLS-GER 2). The APC was funded by the Deutsche Forschungsgemeinschaft and the Open Access Publication Fund of Bielefeld University.

Institutional Review Board Statement: The study was conducted according to the guidelines of the Declaration of Helsinki, and approved by Ethics Committee of Bielefeld University (protocol code 2019–103-S on 14 April 2019).

Informed Consent Statement: Informed consent was obtained from all subjects involved in the study.

Data Availability Statement: All data relevant to the study are included in the article. For further questions regarding data availability, please contact the authors.

Acknowledgments: We acknowledge support for the publication costs by the Deutsche Forschungsgemeinschaft and the Open Access Publication Fund of Bielefeld University. We would like to thank Dominique Vogt for her support in preparing the manuscript.

Conflicts of Interest: The authors declare no conflict of interest. The funders had no role in the design of the study; in the collection, analyses, or interpretation of data; in the writing of the manuscript, or in the decision to publish the results.

References

1. World Health Organization. *Noncommunicable Diseases Country Profiles*; WHO: Geneva, Switzerland, 2018.
2. Eurostat. Personen mit Einem Lang Andauernden Gesundheitsproblem, Nach Geschlecht, Alter und Erwerbsstatus: Europäische Gesundheitsstatistiken. Available online: https://ec.europa.eu/eurostat/databrowser/view/hlth_silc_04/default/table?lang=de (accessed on 8 November 2021).
3. Hyman, R.B.; Corbin, J. (Eds.) *Chronic Illness*; Springer: New York, NY, USA, 2001.
4. Schaeffer, D. (Ed.) *Bewältigung Chronischer Erkrankungen im Lebenslauf*; Huber: Bern, Switzerland, 2009.
5. Corbin, J.M.; Strauss, A.L.; Hildenbrand, A. *Weiterleben Lernen: Verlauf und Bewältigung Chronischer Krankheit*, 3rd ed.; Huber: Bern, Switzerland, 2010.
6. Schaeffer, D.; Haslbeck, J. Bewältigung chronischer Krankheit. In *Soziologie von Gesundheit und Krankheit*; Richter, M., Hurrelmann, K., Eds.; Springer Fachmedien: Wiesbaden, Germany, 2016; pp. 243–256.
7. Whitworth, A. *Information Obesity*; Chandos Publishing: Oxford, UK, 2009.
8. Okan, O.; Bollweg, T.M.; Berens, E.-M.; Hurrelmann, K.; Bauer, U.; Schaeffer, D. Coronavirus-Related Health Literacy: A Cross-Sectional Study in Adults during the COVID-19 Infodemic in Germany. *Int. J. Environ. Res. Public Health* **2020**, *17*, 5503. [CrossRef] [PubMed]
9. World Health Organization. Infodemic management: A key component of the COVID-19 global response. *Wkly. Epidemiol. Rec.* **2020**, *95*, 145–148.
10. Schaeffer, D. Chronische Krankheit und Health Literacy. In *Health Literacy: Forschungsstand und Perspektiven*, 1st ed.; Schaeffer, D., Pelikan, J.M., Eds.; Hogrefe: Bern, Switzerland, 2017; pp. 53–70.
11. Schaeffer, D.; Schmidt-Kaehler, S.; Dierks, M.-L.; Ewers, M.; Vogt, D. *Strategiepapier #2 zu den Empfehlungen des Nationalen Aktionsplans. Gesundheitskompetenz in die Versorgung von Menschen mit Chronischer Erkrankung Integrieren*; Nationaler Aktionsplan Gesundheitskompetenz: Berlin, Germany, 2019.
12. Sørensen, K.; van den Broucke, S.; Fullam, J.; Doyle, G.; Pelikan, J.; Slonska, Z.; Brand, H. Health literacy and public health: A systematic review and integration of definitions and models. *BMC Public Health* **2012**, *12*, 80. [CrossRef] [PubMed]
13. Rademakers, J.; Heijmans, M. Beyond Reading and Understanding: Health Literacy as the Capacity to Act. *Int. J. Environ. Res. Public Health* **2018**, *15*, 1676. [CrossRef] [PubMed]
14. Rowlands, G.; Protheroe, P.; Saboga-Nunes, L.; van den Broucke, S.; Levin-Zamir, D.; Okan, O. Health literacy and chronic conditions: A life course perspective. In *International Handbook of Health Literacy. Research, Practice and Policy across the Life-Span*; Okan, O., Bauer, U., Levin-Zamir, D., Pinheiro, P., Sørensen, K., Eds.; The Policy Press: Bristol, UK, 2019; pp. 183–197.
15. Schaeffer, D.; Vogt, D.; Berens, E.M.; Hurrelmann, K. *Gesundheitskompetenz der Bevölkerung in Deutschland—Ergebnisbericht*; Universität Bielefeld: Bielefeld, Germany, 2016.
16. Schaeffer, D.; Griese, L.; Berens, E.-M. Gesundheitskompetenz von Menschen mit chronischer Erkrankung in Deutschland. *Gesundheitswesen* **2020**, *82*, 836–843. [CrossRef]
17. Sørensen, K.; Pelikan, J.M.; Röthlin, F.; Ganahl, K.; Slonska, Z.; Doyle, G.; Fullam, J.; Kondilis, B.; Agrafiotis, D.; Uiters, E.; et al. Health literacy in Europe: Comparative results of the European health literacy survey (HLS-EU). *Eur. J. Public Health* **2015**, *25*, 1053–1058. [CrossRef]
18. Mirzaei, A.; Aslani, P.; Luca, E.J.; Schneider, C.R. Predictors of Health Information-Seeking Behavior: Systematic Literature Review and Network Analysis. *J. Med. Internet Res.* **2021**, *23*, e21680. [CrossRef]
19. Lambert, S.D.; Loiselle, C.G. Health information seeking behavior. *Qual. Health Res.* **2007**, *17*, 1006–1019. [CrossRef]
20. Clarke, M.A.; Moore, J.L.; Steege, L.M.; Koopman, R.J.; Belden, J.L.; Canfield, S.M.; Meadows, S.E.; Elliott, S.G.; Kim, M.S. Health information needs, sources, and barriers of primary care patients to achieve patient-centered care: A literature review. *J. Health Inform.* **2016**, *22*, 992–1016. [CrossRef]
21. Ramsey, I.; Corsini, N.; Peters, M.D.J.; Eckert, M. A rapid review of consumer health information needs and preferences. *Patient Educ. Couns.* **2017**, *100*, 1634–1642. [CrossRef]
22. Baumann, E.; Czerwinski, F.; Rosset, M.; Seelig, M.; Suhr, R. Wie informieren sich die Menschen in Deutschland zum Thema Gesundheit? Erkenntnisse aus der ersten Welle von HINTS Germany. *Bundesgesundheitsblatt Gesundh. Gesundh.* **2020**, *63*, 1151–1160. [CrossRef]
23. Hurrelmann, K.; Klinger, J.; Schaeffer, D. *Gesundheitskompetenz der Bevölkerung in Deutschland: Vergleich der Erhebungen 2014 und 2020*; Universität Bielefeld, Interdisziplinäres Zentrum für Gesundheitskompetenzforschung: Bielefeld, Germany, 2020.
24. Zimmerman, M.S.; Shaw, G. Health information seeking behaviour: A concept analysis. *Health Inf. Libr. J.* **2020**, *37*, 173–191. [CrossRef] [PubMed]
25. Schaeffer, D.; Dierks, M.L. Patientenberatung in Deutschland. In *Lehrbuch Patientenberatung*, 2nd ed.; Schaeffer, D., Schmidt-Kaehler, S., Eds.; Huber: Bern, Switzerland, 2012; pp. 159–183.
26. Jacobs, W.; Amuta, A.O.; Jeon, K.C. Health information seeking in the digital age: An analysis of health information seeking behavior among US adults. *Cogent Soc. Sci.* **2017**, *3*, 1302785. [CrossRef]

27. Corbin, J.; Strauss, A. *Unending Work and Care: Managing Chronic Illness at Home*; Jossey-Bass: San Francisco, CA, USA, 1988.
28. Haslbeck, J. *Medikamente und Chronische Krankheit. Selbstmanagementerfordernisse im Krankheitsverlauf aus Sicht der Erkrankten*; Huber: Bern, Switzerland, 2010.
29. Engqvist Boman, L.; Sandelin, K.; Wengström, Y.; Silén, C. Patients' learning and understanding during their breast cancer trajectory. *Patient Educ. Couns.* **2017**, *100*, 795–804. [CrossRef]
30. Longo, D.R.; Ge, B.; Radina, M.E.; Greiner, A.; Williams, C.D.; Longo, G.S.; Mouzon, D.M.; Natale-Pereira, A.; Salas-Lopez, D. Understanding breast-cancer patients' perceptions: Health information-seeking behaviour and passive information receipt. *J. Healthc. Commun.* **2009**, *2*, 184–206. [CrossRef]
31. Todd, L.; Hoffman-Goetz, L. A qualitative study of cancer information seeking among English-as-a-second-Language older Chinese immigrant women to canada: Sources, barriers, and strategies. *J. Cancer Educ.* **2011**, *26*, 333–340. [CrossRef] [PubMed]
32. Nagler, R.H.; Gray, S.W.; Romantan, A.; Kelly, B.J.; DeMichele, A.; Armstrong, K.; Schwartz, J.S.; Hornik, R.C. Differences in information seeking among breast, prostate, and colorectal cancer patients: Results from a population-based survey. *Patient Educ. Couns.* **2010**, *81* (Suppl. 1), S54–S62. [CrossRef]
33. Kalantzi, S.; Kostagiolas, P.; Kechagias, G.; Niakas, D.; Makrilakis, K. Information seeking behavior of patients with diabetes mellitus: A cross sectional study in an outpatient clinic of a university-affiliated hospital in Athens, Greece. *BMC Res. Notes* **2015**, *8*, 48. [CrossRef]
34. O'Leary, K.A.; Estabrooks, C.A.; Olson, K.; Cumming, C. Information acquisition for women facing surgical treatment for breast cancer: Influencing factors and selected outcomes. *Patient Educ. Couns.* **2007**, *69*, 5–19. [CrossRef] [PubMed]
35. Schaeffer, D.; Moers, M. Bewältigung chronischer Krankheiten—Herausforderungen für die Pflege. In *Handbuch Pflegewissenschaft*; Schaffer, D., Wingenfeld, K., Eds.; Juventa: Weinheim, Germany, 2014; pp. 329–363.
36. Chen, A.T. The Relationship between Health Management and Information Behavior over Time: A Study of the Illness Journeys of People Living with Fibromyalgia. *J. Med. Internet Res.* **2016**, *18*, e26. [CrossRef] [PubMed]
37. Hambrock, U. *Die Suche nach Gesundheitsinformationen: Patientenperspektiven und Marktüberblick*; Bertelsmann Stiftung: Gütersloh, Germany, 2018.
38. Baumann, E.; Hastall, M.R. Nutzung von Gesundheitsinformationen. In *Handbuch Gesundheitskommunikation*; Hurrelmann, K., Baumann, E., Eds.; Huber: Bern, Switzerland, 2014; pp. 451–466.
39. Zare-Farashbandi, F.; Lalazaryan, A.; Rahimi, A.; Hasssanzadeh, A. The Effect of Contextual Factors on Health Information–Seeking Behavior of Isfahan Diabetic Patients. *J. Hosp. Librariansh.* **2016**, *16*, 1–13. [CrossRef]
40. Lui, C.-W.; Col, J.R.; Donald, M.; Dower, J.; Boyle, F.M. Health and social correlates of Internet use for diabetes information: Findings from Australia's Living with Diabetes Study. *Aust. J. Prim. Health* **2015**, *21*, 327–333. [CrossRef] [PubMed]
41. Kuske, S.; Schiereck, T.; Grobosch, S.; Paduch, A.; Droste, S.; Halbach, S.; Icks, A. Diabetes-related information-seeking behaviour: A systematic review. *Syst. Rev.* **2017**, *6*, 212. [CrossRef] [PubMed]
42. Schaeffer, D.; Berens, E.-M.; Gille, S.; Griese, L.; Klinger, J.; de Sombre, S.; Vogt, D.; Hurrelmann, K. *Gesundheitskompetenz der Bevölkerung in Deutschland vor und während der Corona Pandemie: Ergebnisse des HLS-GER 2*; Universität Bielefeld, Interdisziplinäres Zentrum für Gesundheitskompetenzforschung: Bielefeld, Germany, 2021.
43. Schaeffer, D.; Vogt, D.; Gille, S. *Gesundheitskompetenz-Perspektive und Erfahrungen von Menschen mit Chronischer Erkrankung*; Universität Bielefeld: Bielefeld, Germany, 2019.
44. The HLS19 Consortium of the WHO Action Network M-POHL. *International Report on the Methodology, Results, and Recommendations of the European Health Literacy Population Survey 2019–2021 (HLS19) of M-POHL*; Austrian National Public Health Institute: Vienna, Austria, 2021.
45. Dierks, M.-L.; Kofahl, C. Die Rolle der gemeinschaftlichen Selbsthilfe in der Weiterentwicklung der Gesundheitskompetenz der Bevölkerung. *Bundesgesundheitsblatt Gesundh. Gesundh.* **2019**, *62*, 17–25. [CrossRef]
46. Flick, U. *Qualitative Sozialforschung: Eine Einführung*, 8th ed.; Rowohlt Taschenbuch: Reinbek bei Hamburg, Germany, 2007.
47. Bury, M. Chronic illness as biographical disruption. *Sociol. Health Illn.* **1982**, *4*, 167–182. [CrossRef]
48. Schaeffer, D.; Moers, M. Abschied von der Patientenrolle? Bewältigungshandeln im Verlauf chronischer Krankheit. In *Bewältigung chronischer Krankheit im Lebenslauf*, 1st ed.; Schaeffer, D., Ed.; Huber: Bern, Switzerland, 2009; pp. 111–139.
49. Newton, P.; Asimakopoulou, K.; Scambler, S. Information seeking and use amongst people living with type 2 diabetes: An information continuum. *Int. J. Health Promot. Educ.* **2012**, *50*, 92–99. [CrossRef]
50. Albrecht, M.; Mühlhauser, I.; Steckelberg, A. Evidenzbasierte Gesundheitsinformation. In *Handbuch Gesundheitskommunikation*; Hurrelmann, K., Baumann, E., Eds.; Huber: Bern, Switzerland, 2014; pp. 142–158.
51. Oedekoven, M.; Herrmann, W.J.; Ernsting, C.; Schnitzer, S.; Kanzler, M.; Kuhlmey, A.; Gellert, P. Patients' health literacy in relation to the preference for a general practitioner as the source of health information. *BMC Fam. Pract.* **2019**, *20*, 94. [CrossRef]
52. Ebner, C.; Rohrbach-Schmidt, D. *Berufliches Ansehen in Deutschland für die Klassifikation der Berufe 2010: Beschreibung der Methodischen Vorgehensweise, erste Deskriptive Ergebnisse und Güte der Messung*; Bundesinstitut für Berufsbildung: Bonn, Germany, 2019.
53. Stiftung Gesundheitswissen. *Statussymbol Gesundheit. Wie sich der soziale Status auf Prävention und Gesundheit Auswirken Kann: Gesundheitsbericht 2020 der Stiftung Gesundheitswissen*; Stiftung Gesundheitswissen: Berlin, Germany, 2020.
54. Link, E.; Baumann, E. Nutzung von Gesundheitsinformationen im Internet: Personenbezogene und motivationale Einflussfaktoren. *Bundesgesundheitsblatt Gesundh. Gesundh.* **2020**, *63*, 681–689. [CrossRef]

55. Robert Koch-Institut. *Kommunikation und Information im Gesundheitswesen aus Sicht der Bevölkerung. Patientensicherheit und informierte Entscheidung (KomPaS): Sachbericht*; Robert Koch-Institut: Berlin, Germany, 2019.
56. Marstedt, G. *Das Internet: Auch Ihr Ratgeber für Gesundheitsfragen? Bevölkerungsumfrage zur Suche von Gesundheitsinformationen im Internet und zur Reaktion der Ärzte*; Bertelsmann Stiftung: Gütersloh, Germany, 2018.
57. Baumann, E.; Czerwinski, F. Erst mal Doktor Google fragen? Nutzung Neuer Medien zur Information und zum Austausch über Gesundheitsthemen. In *Gesundheitsmonitor 2015: Bürgerorientierung im Gesundheitswesen*; Böcken, J., Braun, B., Meierjürgen, R., Eds.; Bertelsmann Stiftung: Gütersloh, Germany, 2015; pp. 57–79.
58. Thiel, R.; Deimel, L.; Schmidtmann, D.; Piesche, K.; Hüsing, T.; Rennoch, J.; Stroetmann, V.; Stroetmann, K. *#SmartHealthSystems: Digitalisierungsstrategien im Internationalen Vergleich*; Bertelsmann Stiftung: Gütersloh, Germany, 2018.
59. Schmidt-Kaehler, S.; Dadaczynski, K.; Gille, S.; Okan, O.; Schellinger, A.; Weigand, M.; Schaeffer, D. Gesundheitskompetenz: Deutschland in der digitalen Aufholjagd Einführung technologischer Innovationen greift zu kurz. *Gesundheitswesen* **2021**, *83*, 327–332. [CrossRef] [PubMed]
60. Lee, K.; Hoti, K.; Hughes, J.D.; Emmerton, L. Dr Google and the consumer: A qualitative study exploring the navigational needs and online health information-seeking behaviors of consumers with chronic health conditions. *J. Med. Internet Res.* **2014**, *16*, e262. [CrossRef]
61. Irving, G.; Neves, A.L.; Dambha-Miller, H.; Oishi, A.; Tagashira, H.; Verho, A.; Holden, J. International variations in primary care physician consultation time: A systematic review of 67 countries. *BMJ Open* **2017**, *7*, e017902. [CrossRef] [PubMed]
62. OECD. *Health at a Glance 2019*; OECD Publishing: Paris, France, 2019.
63. Sachverständigenrat zur Begutachtung der Entwicklung im Gesundheitswesen. *Koordination und Integration-Gesundheitsversorgung in einer Gesellschaft des Längeren Lebens. Sondergutachten 2009*; SVR: Baden-Baden, Germany, 2009.
64. Cartwright, J.; Magee, J. *Information for People Living with Conditions that Affect their Appearance: Report I. The Views and Experiences of Patients and the Health Professionals Involved in Their Care—A Qualitative Study*; Picker Institute Europe: Oxford, UK, 2006.
65. Hannawa, A.F.; Rothenfluh, F.B. Arzt-Patient-Interaktion. In *Handbuch Gesundheitskommunikation*; Hurrelmann, K., Baumann, E., Eds.; Huber: Bern, Switzerland, 2014; pp. 110–128.
66. Hinding, B.; Brünahl, C.A.; Buggenhagen, H.; Gronewold, N.; Hollinderbäumer, A.; Reschke, K.; Schultz, J.-H.; Jünger, J. Pilot implementation of the national longitudinal communication curriculum: Experiences from four German faculties. *GMS J. Med. Educ.* **2021**, *38*, Doc52.
67. Ayers, S.L.; Kronenfeld, J.J. Chronic illness and health-seeking information on the Internet. *Health* **2007**, *11*, 327–347. [CrossRef] [PubMed]
68. Griebler, R.; Straßmayr, C.; Mikšová, D.; Link, T.; Nowak, P. die Arbeitsgruppe Gesundheitskompetenz-Messung der ÖPGK. *Gesundheitskompetenz in Österreich: Ergebnisse der Österreichischen Gesundheitskompetenzerhebung HLS19-AT*; Bundesministerium für Soziales, Gesundheit, Pflege und Konsumentenschutz: Wien, Austria, 2021.
69. De Gani, S.M.; Jaks, R.; Bieri, U.; Kocher, J.P. *Health Literacy Survey Schweiz 2019–2021: Schlussbericht im Auftrag des Bundesamtes für Gesundheit BAG*; Careum Stiftung: Zürich, Switzerland, 2021.
70. Shiferaw, K.B.; Tilahun, B.C.; Endehabtu, B.F.; Gullslett, M.K.; Mengiste, S.A. E-health literacy and associated factors among chronic patients in a low-income country: A cross-sectional survey. *BMC Med. Inform. Decis. Mak.* **2020**, *20*, 181. [CrossRef]
71. Schaeffer, D.; Gille, S.; Berens, E.-M.; Griese, L.; Klinger, J.; Vogt, D.; Hurrelmann, K. Digitale Gesundheitskompetenz der Bevölkerung in Deutschland: Ergebnisse des HLS-GER 2. *Gesundheitswesen* **2021**, in press.

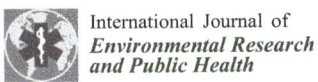

Article

Use of the English Health Literacy Questionnaire (HLQ) with Health Science University Students in Nepal: A Validity Testing Study

Shyam Sundar Budhathoki [1,2,*,†], Melanie Hawkins [3,†], Gerald Elsworth [3], Michael T. Fahey [4,5], Jeevan Thapa [6], Sandeepa Karki [7], Lila Bahadur Basnet [8], Paras K. Pokharel [9] and Richard H. Osborne [3]

1. Department of Primary Care and Public Health, School of Public Health, Imperial College London, St. Mary's Campus, London W2 1PG, UK
2. Nepalese Society of Community Medicine, Lalitpur 44700, Nepal
3. Centre for Global Health and Equity, School of Health Sciences, Swinburne University of Technology, Melbourne, VIC 3122, Australia; melaniehawkins@swin.edu.au (M.H.); gelsworth@swin.edu.au (G.E.); rosborne@swin.edu.au (R.H.O.)
4. Department of Health Sciences and Biostatistics, School of Health Sciences, Swinburne University of Technology, Melbourne, VIC 3122, Australia; mt_fahey@hotmail.com
5. Department of Biostatistics and Clinical Trials, Peter MacCallum Cancer Centre, Melbourne, VIC 3000, Australia
6. Department of Community Health Sciences, Patan Academy of Health Sciences, Lalitpur 44700, Nepal; linktojeevan@gmail.com
7. Department of Health Services, Epidemiology and Disease Control Division, Ministry of Health and Population, Kathmandu 44600, Nepal; sandeepakarki07@gmail.com
8. Department of Health Services, Curative Service Division, Ministry of Health and Population, Kathmandu 44600, Nepal; drlbbasnet@gmail.com
9. School of Public Health and Community Medicine, B.P. Koirala Institute of Health Sciences, Dharan 56700, Nepal; paras.k.pokharel@gmail.com
* Correspondence: s.budhathoki19@imperial.ac.uk
† These authors contributed equally to this work.

Abstract: Research evidence shows that health literacy development is a key factor influencing non-communicable diseases care and patient outcomes. Healthcare professionals with strong health literacy skills are essential for providing quality care. We aimed to report the validation testing of the Health Literacy Questionnaire (HLQ) among health professional students in Nepal. A cross-sectional study was conducted with 419 health sciences students using the HLQ in Nepal. Validation testing and reporting were conducted using five sources outlined by 'the 2014 Standards for Educational and Psychological Testing'. The average difficulty was lowest (17.4%) for Scale 4. *Social support for health*, and highest (51.9%) for Scale 6. *Ability to actively engage with healthcare providers*. One factor Confirmatory Factor Analysis (CFA) model showed a good fit for Scale 2, Scale 7 and Scale 9 and a reasonable fit for Scale 3 and Scale 4. The restricted nine-factor CFA model showed a satisfactory level of fit. The use of HLQ is seen to be meaningful in Nepal and warrants translation into native Nepali and other dominant local languages with careful consideration of cultural appropriateness using cognitive interviews.

Keywords: health literacy development; health literacy questionnaire (HLQ); health literacy measurement; non-native English users; Nepal; Standards for Educational and Psychological Testing; university students; validation study

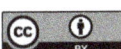

1. Introduction

Health literacy is a multidimensional concept that encompasses an individual's, a family's or a community's knowledge, confidence and comfort (which accumulate through daily activities, social interactions and across generations) to access, understand, appraise, remember and use information about health and healthcare [1]. Health literacy responsiveness describes the way in which policies, services, environments and providers make health information and healthcare available and accessible to people with different health literacy strengths, needs and preferences [2]. Environments, including clinical environments, enable health literacy development to increase the knowledge, confidence and comfort of individuals and communities to manage their health and make a healthy choice the easy choice [1]. In the past 20 years, health literacy research has been largely correlational, where causal links are difficult to determine between health literacy and specific health behaviours or health outcomes [3]. However, recent longitudinal and intervention research is providing increasing evidence that health literacy is a determinant of health outcomes [4–8]. These studies are predominantly from upper-middle- and high-income countries. Hence, there is a dearth of evidence from low-income countries about health literacy and health outcomes. In countries where health systems are under-resourced, an in-depth and nuanced understanding of the local health literacy strengths, needs and preferences of communities using a multidimensional health literacy questionnaire could be an effective way of matching needs to resources to maximize the utilization of available healthcare resources for improving population health outcomes. In an age of technology and swift exchange of information via digital platforms, it can be challenging for people to manage the quantity of information (and misinformation) and understand and use the information for immediate decision making and future wellbeing. The health literacy responsiveness of healthcare services and providers to local needs is of the utmost importance to facilitate people's access to and understanding of health information and to support their capacity to use information and services effectively to make appropriate health decisions [2,9–11].

Understanding the health literacy strengths, needs and preferences of individuals, communities and populations has proven useful to support healthcare providers to respond to the needs of the people they serve [12–14]. Recently, research has expanded to include measurement of the health literacy of healthcare professionals and of students of the healthcare professions in efforts to increase their awareness and knowledge of health literacy [15–17]. If healthcare professionals themselves have health literacy needs, then this can hinder their abilities to support their patients. In an era that has a strong focus on patient-centred care, it becomes critical that healthcare professionals understand and can detect, accommodate and respond appropriately to the health literacy diversity of their communities [18–20]. The measurement of the health literacy strengths, needs and preferences of students studying the health professions enables early support for students' own health literacy and helps to identify and address gaps in the curriculum for their health literacy training for their future roles as healthcare professionals [15,21]. There is a growing consensus that health sciences education curricula should not only focus on producing graduates that are able to identify people with low health literacy but also equip them with skills to engage with their patients in a fair and equitable manner [22]. Interprofessional education in health sciences is considered a potential mechanism for improving the health literacy of students [23].

The World Health Organization (WHO) Shanghai Declaration holds health literacy as one of the three pillars of health promotion to achieve sustainable health development by 2030 [24], and several countries have now incorporated health literacy into national health policy [25]. A challenge for health literacy-related policy is the generation of health literacy data that provide clear evidence on what stakeholders need to do in order to enact and deliver on health policies that improve health. Evidence is generated from specific instruments to measure health literacy and these range from tests of functional health literacy (reading, numeracy and comprehension) developed for clinical purposes [26–28] to self-report instruments that measure the multidimensional nature of the construct of health literacy [29,30].

Research about the properties of instruments is important to help researchers and policymakers understand which instruments are useful for intended decision-making purposes (e.g., community health initiatives, and national policy). Assumptions underlying the use of a measurement instrument in contexts that are different from that in which it was developed include that the instrument will measure the same construct in the same way across contexts, despite cultural, linguistic or other differences [31].

Nepal is classified amongst the least developed countries by the United Nations. The life expectancy at birth in Nepal is 68 years. The country's population is 26.4 million, with 83% living in rural areas. One-fourth of the population lives below the poverty line and the adult literacy rate is 66%; however, the literacy rate in females is lower, at 57%. The doctor to population ratio in Nepal is 0.37/1000 people (as low as 0.008 in rural areas and 1.5/1000 people in the capital city). Individuals bear 55% of total healthcare expenditure as out-of-pocket payments [32]. About two-thirds of healthcare in the acute sector is provided by private hospitals. While Nepal still faces a burden of infectious diseases, it is struggling with inadequate basic hygiene and sanitation, the burden of non-communicable diseases (NCDs) is also on the rise. Health science students will increasingly find themselves needing to provide and communicate information to patients about health conditions that show no visible signs or symptoms until well established. Challenges associated with the prevention and control of NCDs can be numerous and health literacy development is now a recognized factor influencing NCD outcomes [1].

There is little research about health literacy in Nepal and there is a dearth of literature about the health literacy needs of the people of Nepal [33]. Even though Nepali is the official spoken language for all 125 ethnic groups in Nepal, there are 123 spoken languages registered in Nepal [32]. Health sciences education is conducted completely in English, which is the academic language used in all universities in Nepal. These students are likely to work in both community health and clinical settings after graduating from their university studies. The professional working language amongst doctors in Nepal is also English.

Rationale

The Health Literacy Questionnaire (HLQ) was developed by Osborne et al. in Australia using a validity-driven approach [30,34]. The nine domains of the HLQ are designed to measure the experiences people have when they engage in understanding, accessing and using health information and health services. In its development context, the HLQ was found to have strong construct validity, reliability and acceptability to clients and clinicians [30,35] and confirmatory factor analysis (CFA) has found that the items and scales in HLQ translations tend to behave in comparable ways to the English-language HLQ [36–39], even among disparate groups in low-resource settings [40–42]. HLQ data are used in pre-post evaluations and to develop profiles of health literacy strengths and needs to describe the health literacy of individuals and whole populations [12,43]. These health literacy profiles can be used within the Ophelia (Optimising Health Literacy and Access) process to inform community co-design initiatives to build interventions that are fit for purpose and appropriate to specific health literacy needs in specific contexts [4,12,15,30,37,44–48]. Although the HLQ has been translated to Nepali, this study used the original English HLQ for assessing the health literacy of the health science students [30] because English is the official language of instruction in health sciences education and for communication between professionals in universities in Nepal.

This paper reports validity evidence from a secondary analysis of data collected from Nepalese university health science students [15]. This paper aims to evaluate the validity of the data from the English HLQ for the purpose of assessing the health literacy strengths and needs of a population of health science students in a university in Nepal.

2. Materials and Methods

2.1. The Study Setting and the Population

This study was conducted on university students enrolled for undergraduate and postgraduate studies at the largest health sciences university in Nepal. The university offers education through a community-based curriculum and students enrolled are from Nepal and India. All students enrolled at the university with undergraduate and postgraduate health sciences degrees were eligible for recruitment in the study. Any students taking courses/training that did not lead to a university degree were excluded.

2.2. The Health Literacy Questionnaire (HLQ)

The HLQ is a tool with strong psychometric properties [30] that was developed in Australia through consultation with community members, health practitioners and policymakers. The HLQ is widely used around the world and has undergone psychometric evaluation in a variety of contexts, including in university student settings [49].

There are 44 items across nine scales in the HLQ with each scale measuring a distinct element of health literacy construct, both conceptually and psychometrically [30]. The scales are:

1. Feeling understood and supported by healthcare providers (4 items);
2. Having sufficient information to manage my health (4 items);
3. Actively managing my health (5 items);
4. Social support for health (5 items);
5. Appraisal of health information (5 items);
6. Ability to actively engage with healthcare providers (5 items);
7. Navigating the healthcare system (6 items);
8. Ability to find good health information (5 items);
9. Understanding health information well enough to know what to do (5 items).

The HLQ measures the scores in a 4-point Likert-type response (Strongly disagree, Disagree, Agree, and Strongly agree) for the first five scales, later referred to as Part 1 scales. There is a 5-point response for the latter four scales, where the items ask about the difficulty in undertaking a task (ranging from Cannot do to Very easy), later referred to as Part 2 scales. Measurement with the HLQ results in 9 scale scores that form profiles of health literacy strengths and needs.

In this study, HLQ data will be interpreted according to the item intents of the 44 HLQ items and the high and low descriptors of the nine HLQ domains [30,47]. The HLQ scores will be used to create profiles of health literacy strengths and needs of the health science students to inform the development of health literacy initiatives.

2.3. Theoretical Framework

Questionnaire adaptation and translation methods usually include validity testing methods to confirm or refute conceptual and measurement equivalence across languages and cultures [47]. Validation is defined by the 2014 Standards for Educational and Psychological Testing (the Standards) as the *process* of ' ... accumulating relevant evidence to provide a sound scientific basis for the proposed score interpretations' [50]. Validity is the extent to which evidence and the theory of the construct being measured support the proposed interpretation and use of an instrument's scores [51,52]. Validity testing is akin to hypothesis testing: first, state the proposed interpretation and use of scores (an interpretive argument); then, evaluate existing evidence or collect new evidence to determine the extent to which the evidence supports the interpretive argument [47,53]. The Standards describes the need for evidence-based on five sources: test content; the response processes of respondents and users; the internal structure of the measurement instrument; relations to other variables; and the consequences of testing (as related to a source of invalidities such as construct under-representation or construct-irrelevant variance) [51]. These five sources of evidence rely on qualitative and quantitative research methods to generate evidence to establish if and how respondents understand and engage with the content and concepts of an instrument; the extent to which item inter-relationships conform to the intended construct; the patterns of relationships of scores to other variables as predicted by the intended construct; and the extent to which the intended consequences of testing are realized (and if there are unintended consequences of testing, as related to validity) [47,51,52]. It is argued that the use of contemporary validity testing frameworks improves the transparency of the evaluation of validity evidence, which supports other potential users of the measurement instrument [31].

2.4. Sampling and Data Collection

A total of 700 students who were contactable through email and Facebook messages were invited to the study between February and July 2015. Details on sampling and recruitment can be found in a previously published paper [15]. All participants provided their informed consent before they participated in the study. Ethical approval for this research was obtained from the Human Participants Ethics Committee (2013/010790) of the University of Auckland and the Institutional Review Committee (IRC430/014) at the B. P. Koirala Institute of Health Sciences. A licence to administer the HLQ was obtained from Deakin University, Australia.

This validation paper is a part of a published research study that explains the data collection process in detail [15]. The decision to use an online version of HLQ was supported by a study at the same university that showed that 92% of the students accessed the internet every day [54].

Cognitive interviews (pre-testing) were conducted using the English HLQ among 10 university students and 5 researchers (including student educators) in order to explore if the English HLQ required a linguistic or cultural adaptation. Information about the comprehensibility of the questions, students' understanding of questions and their reasons for selecting their responses was collected. The interviews were recorded after taking informed consent.

2.5. Data Analysis

Descriptive statistics and plots were used to examine the demographic characteristics of the sample and, for each item, to examine the extent of missing data, the presence of floor or ceiling effects, and the HLQ item distributions.

Initially, nine separate single-factor CFA models based on the items hypothesized to measure each of the HLQ scales were fitted to the data without any additional residual correlations (RCs) among the items. Following this, a highly restricted nine-factor CFA model with neither residual correlations (RCs) among items nor cross-loading (XLs) of items across scales was fitted to the data. Modification indices associated with models were used to improve the model fit by adding RCs or XLs according to the following strategy:

1. Identify a single RC to add for each scale based on the greatest standardized expected parameter change (SEPC) associated with each of the single-factor CFA models in the case that the model did not fit according to the overall chi-square test.
2. Fit modified nine-factor CFA model, allowing correlations among factors and with both (a) the RCs identified in step 1 added and (b) the single XLs from the restricted nine-factor CFA model having largest SEPC for items 32 and 36.
3. Identify a single XL to add based on the greatest SEPC reported for the CFA model in step 2 and refit a new unrestricted nine-factor CFA model including this XL.
4. Repeat step 3 adding a single XL iteratively to the new modified CFA model until model fit is achieved (CFI ≥ 0.95 and RMSEA ≤ 0.05).
5. Remove any standardized target loadings (TLs), XLs or RCs that are close to zero (TLs ≤ 0.10, RCs ≤ 0.05 in absolute value) from the final model.

All CFA models were fitted using the weighted least squares mean and variance adjusted (WLSMV) estimator for ordinal data available in Mplus version 8.4. Goodness of fit was reported using the overall model chi-square test, the comparative fit index (CFI), the Tucker–Lewis index (TLI), and the root mean square error of approximation (RMSEA).

2.5.1. Test Content

Evidence for the development of the content of the HLQ items has been thoroughly investigated in previous studies [30,55]. In this study, item difficulty was investigated as an indicator of the extent to which respondents understood the content of each item. For each item of the HLQ, the difficulty level was measured, which describes how easy or difficult it is for the respondents to score high. The difficulty level for Part 1 of the HLQ (Scales 1–5) was calculated as the fraction of *'disagree/strongly disagree'* responses as against *'agree/strongly agree'*. The difficulty level for Part 2 of the questionnaire (Scales 6–9) was calculated as the fraction responding *'cannot do or always difficult/usually difficult/sometimes difficult'* against *'usually easy/always easy'*.

2.5.2. The Response Processes of Respondents and Users

Cognitive interviews with students and staff which examined the extent to which respondents engaged with the concepts and meanings of the English-language items (i.e., evidence-based on response processes), according to the item intent descriptions provided by the HLQ developers, were analysed using thematic analysis. Information was collected on the comprehensibility of the questions, students' understanding of questions and reasons for selecting their responses.

2.5.3. The Internal Structure of the Measurement Instrument

Evidence based on the internal structure of the items and scales was examined through a series of nine single-factor confirmatory factor analysis (CFA) models to investigate scale homogeneity followed by a nine-factor CFA model to confirm that the hypothesized nine-scale structure of the HLQ was a good fit to the data and investigate, by exploring possible cross-loadings, whether each item was clearly associated with its hypothesized scale. The CFA models were also used to investigate if the data collected in Nepal can be compared with previous studies reporting factor structure for the HLQ [30,36,41] applied to this Nepalese population.

2.5.4. Relations to Other Variables

The evidence for the relationship with the personal and sociodemographic characteristics of the students are published elsewhere in 2019 [15]. In this paper, we present an overview of the findings to the report as per 'the Standards'. Cronbach's alpha was calculated for each of the one-factor models.

2.5.5. The Consequences of Testing

Discussions with university students and staff were used to investigate the consequences of measurement with the HLQ—that is, to understand if the results of the study reflected health literacy strengths and needs, as perceived by the health sciences students and staff, and if the resulting health literacy profiles indicated areas in which meaningful, implementable, and useful actions for health literacy development could be undertaken.

Discussions were held separately with students and teaching staff to examine the key findings of the study. The focus of the discussions was on the HLQ scales with higher and lower scores, as suggested by the participants. The discussions aimed to gather views about the relevance and implications of the results for the study population.

3. Results

Cognitive testing and cultural adaptation revealed that all items of the HLQ were understood well by the students and no changes were required.

A total of 419 students participated in the study. Over two-thirds of the participants (68.3%) were between 15 and 19 years and over half of the participants were male students (55.8%). About 62% of the participants had one parent who had completed university education. A huge proportion of students were enrolled in an undergraduate course, with 61% of the participants studying medicine. The socio-demographic characteristics of the study population along with the overall results of the study were published previously [15].

The Standards' five sources of evidence framework was used to report the results of the validity testing process.

3.1. Evidence Based on the Content of the HLQ Items and Scales

The difficulty level for each HLQ item was assessed quantitatively for the survey respondents. For Part 1, the lowest average difficulty level was 17.4% for Scale 4. *Social support for health* and the highest difficulty level was 30.4% for Scale 2. *Having sufficient information to manage my health*. At the item level, the lowest difficulty level observed was 6.9% for the item *I feel I have good information about* ... and the highest difficulty level was 41.3% for the item *I have all of the information I need* ... Both these extremes were part of Scale 2. Having sufficient information to manage my health (Table 1).

Table 1. Difficulty level and psychometric properties of English HLQ among students in Nepal (Part 1 Scales 1–5).

Scale/item	n	Difficulty Level (%)	Average Item Difficulty (%)	One-Factor CFA			Nine-Factor CFA (Unrestricted)	
				Factor Loadings	R^2	Cronbach's Alpha	Factor Loadings	R^2
Part 1: Scales 1–5: How strongly you disagree or agree with the following statements (strongly disagree/disagree/disagree/agree/strongly agree)								
1. Feeling understood and supported by healthcare providers								
I have at least one healthcare provider ...	419	20.1		0.750	0.562		0.713	0.508
I have at least one healthcare provider ...	419	24.8	21.5	0.851	0.724	0.797	0.799	0.638
I have the healthcare providers I need to help me ...	419	18.6		0.709	0.503		0.224	0.658
I can rely on at least one ...	419	22.4		0.790	0.624		0.889	0.791
Model fit (one-factor CFA) chi square = 55.839, p-value = 0, CFI = 0.971, TLI = 0.913, RMSEA = 0.253, SRMR = 0.033								
2. Having sufficient information to manage my health								
I feel I have good information about ...	419	6.9		0.581	0.337		0.647	0.418
I have enough information to help me ...	419	32.0	30.2	0.817	0.668	0.794	0.879	0.772
I am sure I have all the information I need ...	419	40.8		0.838	0.702		0.823	0.677
I have all of the information I need ...	419	41.3		0.886	0.785		0.829	0.687
Model fit (one-factor CFA) chi square = 1.924, p-value = 0.382, CFI = 1, TLI = 1, RMSEA = 0, SRMR = 0.007								
3. Actively managing my health								
I spend quite a lot of time actively ...	419	33.4		0.699	0.488		0.639	0.408
I make plans for what I need to do ...	419	22.4		0.810	0.657		0.792	0.627
Despite other things in my life, I make time to ...	419	17.9	22.4	0.781	0.610	0.786	0.714	0.509
I set my own goals ...	419	18.6		0.654	0.427		0.740	0.547
There are things that I do regularly ...	419	19.8		0.735	0.540		0.773	0.598
Model fit (one-factor CFA) chi square = 11.446, p-value = 0.043, CFI = 0.996, TLI = 0.992, RMSEA = 0.055, SRMR = 0.017								
4. Social support for health								
I can get access to several people ...	419	12.7		0.764	0.584		0.730	0.532
When I feel ill, the people ...	419	25.3		0.541	0.292		0.613	0.375
If I need help, I have plenty of ...	419	21.5	17.4	0.797	0.635	0.767	0.804	0.646
I have at least one person who can come to ...	419	19.1		0.676	0.457		0.612	0.375
I have strong support from family ...	419	8.6		0.749	0.561		0.677	0.459
Model fit (one-factor CFA) chi square = 15.692, p-value = 0.008, CFI = 0.992, TLI = 0.985, RMSEA = 0.071, SRMR = 0.02								
5. Appraisal of health information								
I compare health information ...	419	18.4		0.681	0.464		0.622	0.387
When I see new information about health ...	419	27.9		0.710	0.504		0.622	0.386
I always compare health information ...	419	21.0	22.6	0.730	0.532	0.738	0.650	0.422
I know how to find out if the health information I receive ... *	419	19.6		0.605	0.366		-	-
I ask healthcare providers about ...	419	26.0		0.629	0.396		0.877	0.769
Model fit (one-factor CFA) chi square = 43.957, p-value = 0, CFI = 0.962, TLI = 0.923, RMSEA = 0.136, SRMR = 0.038								

* target loadings dropped in unrestricted nine-factor CFA.

For Part 2, the lowest average difficulty level was 39.9% for Scale 9. *Understand health information well enough to know what to do* and the highest difficulty level was 51.9% for Scale 6. *Ability to actively engage with healthcare providers*. At the item level, the lowest difficulty level observed was 34.1% for the item *Confidently fill in medical forms* ... from Scale 9. *Understand health information well enough to know what to do* and the highest difficulty level was 58.0% for the item *Make sure that healthcare providers . . .* from Scale 6. *Ability to actively engage with health care providers* (Table 2).

Table 2. Difficulty level and psychometric properties of English HLQ among students in Nepal (Part 2, Scales 6–9).

Scale/Item	n	Difficulty Level (%)	Average Item Difficulty (%)	One-Factor CFA			Nine-Factor CFA (Unrestricted)	
				Factor Loadings	R^2	Standardized Cronbach's Alpha	Factor Loadings	R^2
Part 2: Scales 6–9: How easy or difficult the following tasks are for you to do now (cannot do or always difficult/usually difficult/sometimes difficult/usually easy/always easy)								
6. Ability to actively engage with health care providers								
Make sure that healthcare providers . . .	419	58.0		0.748	0.560		0.762	0.580
Feel able to discuss your health . . .	419	48.9		0.840	0.705		0.824	0.680
Have good discussions about . . .	419	48.9	51.9	0.856	0.733	0.881	0.906	0.649
Discuss things with healthcare . . .	419	52.3		0.847	0.718		0.866	0.750
Ask healthcare providers questions . . .	419	51.6		0.815	0.664		0.315	0.698
Model fit (one-factor CFA) chi square = 36.357, p-value = 0, CFI = 0.992, TLI = 0.983, RMSEA = 0.122, SRMR = 0.018								
7. Navigating the health care system								
Find the right . . .	419	52.0		0.589	0.347		0.606	0.368
Get to see the healthcare providers you . . . *	419	50.8		0.695	0.484		-	-
Decide which healthcare provider . . .	419	49.9	49.6	0.824	0.680	0.841	0.799	0.639
Make sure you find the right place . . .	419	45.1		0.821	0.675		0.865	0.748
Find out what healthcare services you are . . .	419	43.0		0.784	0.614		0.275	0.659
Work out what is the best . . . *	419	56.6		0.713	0.508		-	-
Model fit (one-factor CFA) chi square = 14.696, p-value = 0.099, CFI = 0.998, TLI = 0.996, RMSEA = 0.039, SRMR = 0.015								
8. Ability to find good health information								
Find information about . . .	419	47.0		0.674	0.455		0.690	0.477
Find health information from several different . . .	419	55.4		0.798	0.637		0.783	0.612
Get information about health so you . . .	419	57.3	50.0	0.804	0.646	0.839	0.798	0.637
Get health information in . . . *	419	38.0		0.765	0.586		-	-
Get health information . . .	419	52.3		0.795	0.632		0.820	0.672
Model fit (one-factor CFA) chi square = 32.792, p-value = 0, CFI = 0.988, TLI = 0.976, RMSEA = 0.115, SRMR = 0.023								
9. Understand health information well enough to know what to do								
Confidently fill in medical forms . . .	419	34.1		0.662	0.438		0.738	0.545
Accurately follow instructions . . .	419	50.6		0.600	0.360		0.685	0.469
Read and understand . . .	419	35.1	39.9	0.732	0.536	0.823	0.784	0.614
Read and understand all the . . .	419	39.6		0.738	0.545		0.744	0.554
Understand what healthcare providers . . .	419	40.1		0.738	0.545		0.824	0.679
Model fit (one-factor CFA) chi square = 9.986, p-value = 0.0756, CFI = 0.993, TLI = 0.985, RMSEA = 0.049, SRMR = 0.018								
Model fit (nine-factor CFA) chi square = 1684.947, p-value = 0.0000, CFI = 0.959, TLI = 0.955, RMSEA = 0.048, SRMR = 0.049								

* target loadings dropped in unrestricted nine-factor CFA.

3.2. Evidence Based on the Response Processes of HLQ Respondents

In-depth cognitive interviews were conducted with 10 students and 5 teaching staff in order to assess the extent to which respondents engaged with the English language items as intended by the HLQ developers. This was essential because the native language of the study population was not English, but rather the population uses English as an academic and professional language. No changes were deemed necessary.

3.3. Evidence Based on the Internal Structure of the HLQ

For the restricted nine-factor CFA model, the values indicate satisfactory level of fit (chi-square = 1993, df = 866, p-value < 0.0001, CFI = 0.945, TLI = 0.939 and RMSEA = 0.056)

Following the data analysis protocol outlined in Section 2.5, modification indices, in particular, the SEPC, were used to seek improvements to the highly restricted model, yielding a modified model with a chi-square = 1684.947, and p-value < 0.0001 was obtained. Other indices of goodness of fit obtained were CFI = 0.959, TLI = 0.955 and RMSEA = 0.048, indicating a good model fit. The factor loadings, R square and the model parameters for this model are shown in Tables 1 and 2.

The modified model had four target loadings dropped (item: I know how to find out if the health information I receive . . . from Scale 5; items: Get to see the healthcare providers . . . and Work out what is the best . . . from Scale 7; and item: Get health information in . . . from Scale 8). There were four residual correlations and eight item cross-loadings in the final model. However, the cross-loading of the item I always compare health information . . . was dropped, and the remaining seven item cross-loadings of Scales 4, 6, 8 and 9 are presented separately in Table 3.

Table 3. Cross-loadings of items in different factors obtained through unrestricted nine-factor CFA.

Scale/Item	n	Nine-Factor CFA (Unrestricted)	
		Factor Loadings	R^2
4. Social support for health			
I know how to find out if the health information I receive is . . .	419	0.846	0.715
I have the healthcare providers I need to help me . . .	419	0.63	0.658
6. Ability to actively engage with healthcare providers			
Get to see the healthcare providers you . . .	419	0.779	0.608
8. Ability to find good health information			
Work out what is the best . . .	419	0.742	0.551
9. Understand health information well enough to know what to do			
Get health information in . . .	419	0.852	0.726
Ask healthcare providers questions . . .	419	0.547	0.698
Find out what healthcare services you are . . .	419	0.561	0.659

The one-factor CFA model showed good fit for three Scales: 2. *Having sufficient information to manage my health* (CFI = 1, TLI = 1, RMSEA = 0), 7. *Navigating the health care system* (CFI = 0.998, TLI = 0.996, RMSEA = 0.039) and 9. *Understand health information well enough to know what to do* (CFI = 0.993, TLI = 0.985, RMSEA = 0.049). There was a reasonable fit seen for Scale 3. *Actively managing my health* (CFI = 0.996, TLI = 0.992, RMSEA = 0.055) and Scale 4. *Social support for health* (CFI = 0.992, TLI = 0.985, RMSEA = 0.071) (Tables 1 and 2).

3.4. Evidence Based on the Relationships of the Scores to Other Variables

The results of the association of personal and sociodemographic characteristics of the study population are published in a 2019 paper [15]. In summary, male students had higher scores on Scales 2. *Having sufficient information to manage my health*, 6. *Ability to actively engage with healthcare providers*, and 8. *Ability to find good health information* compared to female students. Older students (≥ 20 y of age) had higher for Scales 1. *Feeling understood by my healthcare providers*, and 2. *Having sufficient information to manage my health* than students who were less than 20 y of age. Participants whose parents had attained a university level of education had higher scores on Scale 7. *Navigate the healthcare system* compared with students whose parents did not attain a university education. Postgraduate students scored higher on Scales 1. *Feeling understood by my healthcare providers*, 2. *Having sufficient information to manage my health* and 7. *Able to navigate the healthcare system* compared to undergraduate students.

Cronbach's alpha scores were of an acceptable or good level of reliability for most items (α = 0.6 or higher), except for three: *I have the healthcare providers I need to help me . . .* (α = 0.224) from Scale 1, *Ask healthcare providers questions . . .* (α = 0.315) from Scale 6, and *Find out what healthcare services you are . . .* (α = 0.275) from Scale 7.

3.5. Evidence Based on Validity and the Consequences of Measurement Using the HLQ

For Part 1, the highest score was found for Scale 4. Social support for health and lowest score in Scale 1. Having sufficient information to manage their health. For Part 2, the highest score was found for Scale 9. Understanding health information well enough to know what to do and the lowest score on Scale 6. Ability to actively engage with healthcare providers. The discussions in both the student and teaching staff groups separately came to the agreement that the overall results are convincing and realistically reflect their individually perceived health literacy strengths and needs of the population. As suggested by the participants, the potential health literacy development initiative to support students to access health information was to digitize the central library resources. For improving active engagement with healthcare providers, the participants suggested conducting workshops to engage students with the healthcare providers, who are usually their teachers and clinical supervisors.

4. Discussion

This validity testing paper reports the first-ever use of HLQ in a Nepali population. This study is unique in another way in that it reports the use of the English HLQ in a Nepali speaking population who use English as their academic and professional language. Additionally, this paper presents the study methods and results according to the five sources of validity evidence from the Standards for Educational and Psychological Testing [48], which gives a clear framework in which to describe what the data mean for score interpretation and use and enable the evidence to tell a story about the HLQ in the Nepali context.

The five sources of evidence are best employed prospectively to gather information about the interpretation and use of data generated by a new questionnaire or of data generated by a questionnaire in a new context [55]. This study used a questionnaire in a new context. The HLQ is a questionnaire that is well established in the field of health literacy measurement [56]. Having a tool that generates valid multidimensional health literacy data is an opportunity to promote the assessment of health literacy strengths, needs and preferences of patients and communities. However, the HLQ had not previously been used in Nepal, in English, with a largely Nepali-speaking population. The study population was health sciences students who will graduate to work as clinicians and healthcare professionals in Nepal and around the world, who are likely to mostly use English as their professional language. The validity of the interpretation and use of HLQ data in this context was unknown. Investigations were required into all aspects of the questionnaire, including potential consequences of using the data for making decisions about initiatives to develop the health literacy of the health sciences students who are the future healthcare professionals. The use of HLQ has shown that Nepalese health sciences students have good information about health but may not have adequate skills to take care of their health. This could be because they have limited skills for using health knowledge to make healthcare decisions. They also express difficulty in engaging in discussion with their healthcare providers who are their teachers in medical school [15]. This could be at least partly explained to be an influence of the existing social hierarchy that places doctors, teachers and professionals at a higher social level in Nepali culture than students.

As a collectivistic society, the sense of social support would generally be expected to be higher than reported in [15]. This opens up opportunities for future studies to consider the role of interprofessional education to support improved health literacy of health science students because Nepalese health sciences education also incorporates the multidisciplinary education of medical, dental and nursing students in the curriculum [57].

Given the very restricted model, its fit is comparable to the fit of other psychometric analyses of the English-language HLQ [30]. The satisfactory model fit seen in this paper may not only apply to the health sciences students and could possibly be generalizable to healthcare professionals who use English as an academic and professional language. However, given the large number of parameters (236) estimated in our sample of 419 observations, we acknowledge that out-of-sample performance needs further investigation.

When measurements are undertaken, it implies some action will take place [58], and these actions need to be appropriate, meaningful, and useful for the target population. Health professionals must understand and address their own health literacy strengths, needs and preferences because this may enable professionals to more quickly recognize their patients' health literacy strengths, needs and preferences and to engage their patients in meaningful discussions to co-design appropriate health actions or interventions.

Given that the HLQ was developed in a Western context, it is important to establish that the content of the HLQ's items is meaningful in the Nepalese context. The synthesis of the investigations in this study reveals that the content and meaning of the English HLQ items are appropriate for the study population (content and response processes investigations), that the items and scales function in the same way within each scale and between scales in this population as they do in the population in the HLQ development study (investigations into internal structure and relations to other variables) [30], and that the results of the study resonate with and are meaningful to the members of the study population, which indicates that the data are likely to be useful for informing health literacy development initiatives to support health sciences students in Nepal now and into their futures.

With the increasing incidence of NCDs around the world, the responsibility of creating medical environments that support the prevention and control of these conditions will fall to the health professionals of the future, as well as clinical researchers, managers and policymakers [59]. Harnessing the health literacy strengths and understanding and responding to the health literacy needs of diverse populations will be essential components of healthcare delivery [1]. Early training in health literacy will be an asset to all students of health sciences and medical disciplines, as will be understanding their own health literacy strengths and needs [60].

5. Conclusions

The health literacy development implications of the HLQ validity testing in this study is twofold: first is the potential for using the English HLQ among health professionals, not only students, in Nepal; and second is the potential for using the English HLQ among health professionals from non-English-speaking countries who work in English-speaking countries around the world. The analyses suggest that the nine HLQ constructs appear to be potentially meaningful for use in Nepal. However, having HLQ translated into Nepali and a few dominant languages for specific community populations within Nepal is a useful next step. Given the societal and cultural differences between high-income English-speaking countries, where the communities are more individualistic, and Nepal where the community is more collective, careful consideration of the cultural appropriateness through cognitive interviews is still essential.

Author Contributions: Conceptualization, S.S.B., M.H., S.K., L.B.B., P.K.P. and R.H.O.; methodology, S.S.B., M.H., G.E., M.T.F., J.T. and R.H.O.; formal analysis, S.S.B., M.H., G.E., M.T.F., J.T. and R.H.O.; data curation, S.S.B., M.T.F., J.T., S.K., L.B.B. and P.K.P.; writing—original draft preparation, S.S.B., M.H., S.K., L.B.B. and P.K.P.; writing—review and editing, S.S.B., M.H., G.E., M.T.F., J.T., S.K., L.B.B., P.K.P. and R.H.O. All authors have read and agreed to the published version of the manuscript.

Funding: This research received no external funding. RHO was funded in part through a National Health and Medical Research Council (NHMRC) of Australia Principal Research Fellowship (APP1155125).

Institutional Review Board Statement: The study was conducted following the Declaration of Helsinki and approved by the Human Participants Ethics Committee (2013/010790) of the University of Auckland and the Institutional Review Committee (IRC430/014) at the B. P. Koirala Institute of Health Sciences. A licence to administer the HLQ was obtained from Deakin University, Australia.

Informed Consent Statement: Informed consent was obtained from all subjects involved in the study.

Data Availability Statement: The data presented in this study are available on request from the corresponding author.

Conflicts of Interest: The authors declare no conflict of interest.

References

1. World Health Organization. *Health Literacy Development for the Prevention and Control of Noncommunicable Diseases*; Final Report of the GCM/NCD Member State-Led Global Working Group on Health Education and Health Literacy for NCDs; WHO: Geneva, Switzerland, 2022; in press.
2. Dodson, S.; Good, S.; Osborne, R.H. *Health Literacy Toolkit for Low and Middle-Income Countries: A Series of Information Sheets to Empower Communities and Strengthen Health Systems*; World Health Organisation, Regional Office for South East Asia: New Delhi, India, 2015.
3. Walters, R.; Leslie, S.J.; Polson, R.; Cusack, T.; Gorely, T. Establishing the Efficacy of Interventions to Improve Health Literacy and Health Behaviours: A Systematic Review. *BMC Public Health* **2020**, *20*, 1040. [CrossRef]
4. Beauchamp, A.; Mohebbi, M.; Cooper, A.; Pridmore, V.; Livingston, P.; Scanlon, M.; Davis, M.; O'Hara, J.; Osborne, R. The Impact of Translated Reminder Letters and Phone Calls on Mammography Screening Booking Rates: Two Randomised Controlled Trials. *PLoS ONE* **2020**, *15*, e0226610. [CrossRef]
5. Friis, K.; Aaby, A.; Lasgaard, M.; Pedersen, M.H.; Osborne, R.H.; Maindal, H.T. Low Health Literacy and Mortality in Individuals with Cardiovascular Disease, Chronic Obstructive Pulmonary Disease, Diabetes, and Mental Illness: A 6-Year Population-Based Follow-Up Study. *Int. J. Environ. Res. Public Health* **2020**, *17*, 9399. [CrossRef]
6. Griva, K.; Yoong, R.K.L.; Nandakumar, M.; Rajeswari, M.; Khoo, E.Y.H.; Lee, V.Y.W.; Kang, A.W.C.; Osborne, R.H.; Brini, S.; Newman, S.P. Associations between Health Literacy and Health Care Utilization and Mortality in Patients with Coexisting Diabetes and End-stage Renal Disease: A Prospective Cohort Study. *Br. J. Health Psychol.* **2020**, *25*, 405–427. [CrossRef]
7. Paasche-Orlow, M.K.; Wolf, M.S. The Causal Pathways to Linking Health Literacy to Health Outcomes. *Am. J. Health Behav.* **2007**, *31*, S19–S26. [CrossRef]
8. Mantwill, S.; Monestel-Umaña, S.; Schulz, P.J. The Relationship between Health Literacy and Health Disparities: A Systematic Review. *PLoS ONE* **2015**, *10*, e0145455. [CrossRef]
9. Nutbeam, D. The Evolving Concept of Health Literacy. *Soc. Sci. Med.* **2008**, *67*, 2072–2078. [CrossRef] [PubMed]
10. Laing, R.; Thompson, S.C.; Elmer, S.; Rasiah, R.L. Fostering Health Literacy Responsiveness in a Remote Primary Health Care Setting: A Pilot Study. *Int. J. Environ. Res. Public Health* **2020**, *17*, 2730. [CrossRef] [PubMed]
11. Brach, C.; Keller, D.; Hernandez, L.M.; Baur, C.; Parker, R.; Dreyer, B.; Schyve, P.; Lemerise, A.J.; Schillinger, D. *Ten Attributes of Health Literate Health Care Organizations*; National Academy of Medicine: Washington, DC, USA, 2012.
12. Anwar, W.A.; Mostafa, N.S.; Hakim, S.A.; Sos, D.G.; Abozaid, D.A.; Osborne, R.H. Health Literacy Strengths and Limitations among Rural Fishing Communities in Egypt Using the Health Literacy Questionnaire (HLQ). *PLoS ONE* **2020**, *15*, e0235550. [CrossRef] [PubMed]
13. Boateng, M.A.; Agyei-Baffour, P.; Angel, S.; Asare, O.; Prempeh, B.; Enemark, U. Co-Creation and Prototyping of An Intervention Focusing on Health Literacy in Management of Malaria at Community-Level in Ghana. *Res. Involv. Engagem.* **2021**, *7*, 55. [CrossRef] [PubMed]
14. Aaby, A.; Beauchamp, A.; O'Hara, J.; Maindal, H.T. Large Diversity in Danish Health Literacy Profiles: Perspectives for Care of Long-Term Illness and Multimorbidity. *Eur. J. Public Health* **2020**, *30*, 75–80. [CrossRef] [PubMed]
15. Budhathoki, S.S.; Pokharel, P.K.; Jha, N.; Moselen, E.; Dixon, R.; Bhattachan, M.; Osborne, R.H. Health Literacy of Future Healthcare Professionals: A Cross-Sectional Study among Health Sciences Students in Nepal. *Int. Health* **2019**, *11*, 15–23. [CrossRef] [PubMed]
16. Johnson, A. Health Literacy: How Nurses Can Make a Difference. *Aust. J. Adv. Nurs.* **2015**, *33*, 20–27.
17. The University of Auckland. Exploring Health Literacy in Tertiary Students: An International Study. Available online: https://www.fmhs.auckland.ac.nz/en/faculty/health-literacy-project.html (accessed on 21 August 2020).
18. Greaney, M.L.; Wallington, S.F.; Rampa, S.; Vigliotti, V.S.; Cummings, C.A. Assessing Health Professionals' Perception of Health Literacy in Rhode Island Community Health Centers: A Qualitative Study. *BMC Public Health* **2020**, *20*, 1289. [CrossRef]
19. Coelho, R. Perceptions and Knowledge of Health Literacy among Healthcare Providers in a Community Based Cancer Centre. *J. Med. Imaging Radiat. Sci.* **2018**, *49*, S11–S12. [CrossRef]
20. Batterham, R.W.; Hawkins, M.; Collins, P.A.; Buchbinder, R.; Osborne, R.H. Health Literacy: Applying Current Concepts to Improve Health Services and Reduce Health Inequalities. *Public Health* **2016**, *132*, 3–12. [CrossRef]
21. Mullan, J.; Burns, P.; Weston, K.; Mclennan, P.; Rich, W.; Crowther, S.; Mansfield, K.; Dixon, R.; Moselen, E.; Osborne, R.H. Health Literacy amongst Health Professional University Student: A Study Using the Health Literacy Questionnaire. *Educ. Sci.* **2017**, *7*, 54. [CrossRef]
22. Coleman, C.A.; Hudson, S.; Maine, L.L. Health Literacy Practices and Educational Competencies for Health Professionals: A Consensus Study. *J. Health Commun.* **2013**, *18*, 82–102. [CrossRef]
23. Ulbrich, S.; Campbell, J.; Dyer, C.; Gregory, G.; Hudson, S. Interprofessional Education on Health Literacy: Session Development, Implementation, and Evaluation. *Ann. Behav. Sci. Med. Educ.* **2013**, *19*, 3–7. [CrossRef]

24. World Health Organisation. In Proceedings of the 9th Global Conference on Health Promotion, Shanghai, China, 21–24 November 2016. Available online: http://www.who.int/healthpromotion/conferences/9gchp/en/ (accessed on 17 August 2020).
25. Trezona, A.; Rowlands, G.; Nutbeam, D. Progress in Implementing National Policies and Strategies for Health Literacy—What Have We Learned so Far? *Int. J. Environ. Res. Public Health* **2018**, *15*, 1554. [CrossRef]
26. Parker, R.M.; Baker, D.W.; Williams, M.V.; Nurss, J.R. The Test of Functional Health Literacy in Adults. *J. Gen. Intern. Med.* **1995**, *10*, 537–541. [CrossRef] [PubMed]
27. Weiss, B.D.; Mays, M.Z.; Martz, W.; Castro, K.M.; Dewalt, D.A.; Pignone, M.P.; Mockbee, J.; Hale, F.A. Quick Assessment of Literacy in Primary Care: The Newest Vital Sign. *Ann. Fam. Med.* **2005**, *3*, 514–522. [CrossRef] [PubMed]
28. Arozullah, A.M.; Yarnold, P.R.; Bennett, C.L.; Soltysik, R.C.; Wolf, M.S.; Ferreira, R.M.; Lee, S.-Y.D.; Costello, S.; Shakir, A.; Denwood, C.; et al. Development and Validation of a Short-Form, Rapid Estimate of Adult Literacy in Medicine. *Med. Care* **2007**, *45*, 1026–1033. [CrossRef] [PubMed]
29. Sørensen, K.; Van den Broucke, S.; Pelikan, J.M.; Fullam, J.; Doyle, G.; Slonska, Z.; Kondilis, B.; Stoffels, V.; Osborne, R.H.; Brand, H. Measuring Health Literacy in Populations: Illuminating the Design and Development Process of the European Health Literacy Survey Questionnaire (HLS-EU-Q). *BMC Public Health* **2013**, *13*, 948. [CrossRef] [PubMed]
30. Osborne, R.H.; Batterham, R.W.; Elsworth, G.R.; Hawkins, M.; Buchbinder, R. The Grounded Psychometric Development and Initial Validation of the Health Literacy Questionnaire (HLQ). *BMC Public Health* **2013**, *13*, 658. [CrossRef]
31. Hawkins, M.; Elsworth, G.R.; Hoban, E.; Osborne, R.H. Questionnaire Validation Practice within a Theoretical Framework: A Systematic Descriptive Literature Review of Health Literacy Assessments. *BMJ Open* **2020**, *10*, e035974. [CrossRef]
32. Central Bureau of Statistics. *National Population and Housing Census 2011 (National Report)*; National Planning Commission: Kathmandu, Nepal, 2012.
33. Budhathoki, S.S.; Pokharel, P.K.; Good, S.; Limbu, S.; Bhattachan, M.; Osborne, R.H. The Potential of Health Literacy to Address the Health Related UN Sustainable Development Goal 3 (SDG3) in Nepal: A Rapid Review. *BMC Health Serv. Res.* **2017**, *17*, 237. [CrossRef]
34. Buchbinder, R.; Batterham, R.; Elsworth, G.; Dionne, C.E.; Irvin, E.; Osborne, R.H. A Validity-Driven Approach to the Understanding of the Personal and Societal Burden of Low Back Pain: Development of a Conceptual and Measurement Model. *Arthritis Res. Ther.* **2011**, *13*, R152. [CrossRef]
35. Elsworth, G.R.; Beauchamp, A.; Osborne, R.H. Measuring Health Literacy in Community Agencies: A Bayesian Study of the Factor Structure and Measurement Invariance of the Health Literacy Questionnaire (HLQ). *BMC Health Serv. Res.* **2016**, *16*, 508. [CrossRef]
36. Maindal, H.T.; Kayser, L.; Norgaard, O.; Bo, A.; Ellsworth, G.; Osborne, R. Cultural Adaptation and Validation of the Health Literacy Questionnaire (HLQ): Robust Nine-Dimension Danish Language Confirmatory Factor Model. *Springerplus* **2016**, *5*, 1232. [CrossRef] [PubMed]
37. Kolarčik, P.; Čepová, E.; Madarasová Gecková, A.; Tavel, P.; Osborne, R. Validation of Slovak Version of Health Literacy Questionnaire. *Eur. J. Public Health* **2015**, *25*, 2015. [CrossRef]
38. Nolte, S.; Osborne, R.H.; Dwinger, S.; Elsworth, G.R.; Conrad, M.L.; Rose, M.; Härter, M.; Dirmaier, J.; Zill, J.M. German Translation, Cultural Adaptation, and Validation of the Health Literacy Questionnaire (HLQ). *PLoS ONE* **2017**, *12*, e0172340. [CrossRef] [PubMed]
39. Wahl, A.K.; Hermansen, Å.; Osborne, R.H.; Larsen, M.H. A Validation Study of the Norwegian Version of the Health Literacy Questionnaire: A Robust Nine-Dimension Factor Model. *Scand. J. Public Health* **2021**, *49*, 471–478. [CrossRef] [PubMed]
40. Mbada, C.E.; Johnson, O.E.; Oyewole, O.O.; Adejube, O.J.; Fatoye, C.; Idowu, O.A.; Odeyemi, R.V.; Akinirinbola, K.B.; Ganiyu, D.; Fatoye, F. Cultural Adaptation and Psychometric Evaluation of the Yoruba Version of the Health Literacy Questionnaire. *Ann. Ig.* **2022**, *34*, 54–69. [CrossRef] [PubMed]
41. Saleem, M.; Steadman, K.J.; Osborne, R.H.; La Caze, A. Translating and Validating the Health Literacy Questionnaire into Urdu: A Robust Nine-Dimension Confirmatory Factor Model. *Health Promot. Int.* **2021**, *36*, 1219–1230. [CrossRef]
42. Boateng, M.A.; Agyei-Baffour, P.; Angel, S.; Enemark, U. Translation, Cultural Adaptation and Psychometric Properties of the Ghanaian Language (Akan; Asante Twi) Version of the Health Literacy Questionnaire. *BMC Health Serv. Res.* **2020**, *20*, 1064. [CrossRef]
43. Beauchamp, A.; Buchbinder, R.; Dodson, S.; Batterham, R.W.; Elsworth, G.R.; McPhee, C.; Sparkes, L.; Hawkins, M.; Osborne, R.H. Distribution of Health Literacy Strengths and Weaknesses across Socio-Demographic Groups: A Cross-Sectional Survey Using the Health Literacy Questionnaire (HLQ). *BMC Public Health* **2015**, *15*, 678. [CrossRef]
44. Bakker, M.M.; Putrik, P.; Rademakers, J.; van de Laar, M.; Vonkeman, H.; Kok, M.R.; Voorneveld-Nieuwenhuis, H.; Ramiro, S.; de Wit, M.; Buchbinder, R.; et al. Addressing Health Literacy Needs in Rheumatology—Which Patient Health Literacy Profiles Need the Attention of Health Professionals? *Arthritis Care Res.* **2020**, *73*, 100–109. [CrossRef] [PubMed]
45. Bo, A.; Friis, K.; Osborne, R.H.; Maindal, H.T. National Indicators of Health Literacy: Ability to Understand Health Information and to Engage Actively with Healthcare Providers -a Population- Based Survey among Danish Adults. *BMC Public Health* **2014**, *14*, 1095. [CrossRef]
46. Debussche, X.; Lenclume, V.; Balcou-Debussche, M.; Alakian, D.; Sokolowsky, C.; Ballet, D.; Elsworth, G.R.; Osborne, R.H.; Huiart, L. Characterisation of Health Literacy Strengths and Weaknesses among People at Metabolic and Cardiovascular Risk: Validity Testing of the Health Literacy Questionnaire. *SAGE Open Med.* **2018**, *6*, 2050312118801125. [CrossRef]

47. Hawkins, M.; Cheng, C.; Elsworth, G.R.; Osborne, R.H. Translation Method Is Validity Evidence for Construct Equivalence: Analysis of Secondary Data Routinely Collected during Translations of the Health Literacy Questionnaire (HLQ). *BMC Med. Res. Methodol.* **2020**, *20*, 130. [CrossRef]
48. Beauchamp, A.; Batterham, R.W.; Dodson, S.; Astbury, B.; Elsworth, G.R.; McPhee, C.; Jacobson, J.; Buchbinder, R.; Osborne, R.H. Systematic Development and Implementation of Interventions to OPtimise Health Literacy and Access (Ophelia). *BMC Public Health* **2017**, *17*, 230. [CrossRef] [PubMed]
49. Kühn, L.; Bachert, P.; Hildebrand, C.; Kunkel, J.; Reitermayer, J.; Wäsche, H.; Woll, A. Health Literacy Among University Students: A Systematic Review of Cross-Sectional Studies. *Front. Public Health* **2022**, *9*, 680999. [CrossRef]
50. American Educational Research Association; American Psychological Association Joint Committee on Standards for Educational and Psychological Testing (US). *Standards for Educational and Psychological Testing*; National Council on Measurement in Education American Educational Research Association: Washington, DC, USA, 1985.
51. National Council on Measurement in Education American Educational Research Association. *Standards for Educational & Psychological Testing*; National Council on Measurement in Education American Educational Research Association: Washington, DC, USA, 2014.
52. Hawkins, M.; Elsworth, G.R.; Osborne, R.H. Application of Validity Theory and Methodology to Patient-Reported Outcome Measures (PROMs): Building an Argument for Validity. *Qual. Life Res.* **2018**, *27*, 1695–1710. [CrossRef] [PubMed]
53. Kane, M.T. Validity as the Evaluation of the Claims Based on Test Scores. *Assess. Educ. Princ. Policy Pract.* **2016**, *23*, 309–311. [CrossRef]
54. Pokharel, P.K.; Budhathoki, S.S.; Pokharel, H.P. Electronic Health Literacy Skills among Medical and Dental Interns at B P Koirala Institute of Health Sciences. *J. Nepal Health Res. Counc.* **2016**, *14*, 159–164. [PubMed]
55. Hawkins, M.; Elsworth, G.R.; Nolte, S.; Osborne, R.H. Validity Arguments for Patient-Reported Outcomes: Justifying the Intended Interpretation and Use of Data. *J. Patient Rep. Outcomes* **2021**, *5*, 64. [CrossRef]
56. Slatyer, S.; Toye, C.; Burton, E.; Jacinto, A.F.; Hill, K.D. Measurement Properties of Self-Report Instruments to Assess Health Literacy in Older Adults: A Systematic Review. *Disabil. Rehabil.* **2020**, 1–17. [CrossRef]
57. Pokharel, P.K.; Budhathoki, S.S.; Upadhyay, M.P. Teaching District Concept of BP Koirala Institute of Health Sciences: An Inter-Disciplinary Community Based Medical Education and Health Service Delivery Model in Rural Nepal. *Kathmandu Univ. Med. J.* **2016**, *55*, 293–297.
58. Messick, S. Foundations of Validity: Meaning and Consequences in Psychological Assessment. *ETS Res. Rep. Ser.* **1993**, *1993*, i–18. [CrossRef]
59. Debussche, X. Addressing Health Literacy Responsiveness in Diabetes. *Diabetes Epidemiol. Manag.* **2021**, *4*, 100033. [CrossRef]
60. Coleman, C.A.; Fromer, A. A Health Literacy Training Intervention for Physicians and Other Health Professionals. *Fam. Med.* **2015**, *47*, 388–392. [CrossRef] [PubMed]

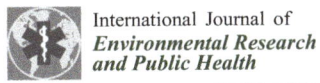

Article

Patients' Health Literacy in Rehabilitation: Comparison between the Estimation of Patients and Health Care Professionals

Mona Voigt-Barbarowicz [1,*], Günter Dietz [2], Nicole Renken [2], Ruben Schmöger [1] and Anna Levke Brütt [1]

[1] Junior Research Group for Rehabilitation Sciences, Department of Health Services Research, University of Oldenburg, 26129 Oldenburg, Germany; ruben.schmoeger@uni-oldenburg.de (R.S.); anna.levke.bruett@uol.de (A.L.B.)
[2] Clinic for Orthopedic and Rheumatological Rehabilitation, Rehabilitation Centre Bad Zwischenahn, 26160 Bad Zwischenahn, Germany; g.dietz@rehazentrum-am-meer.de (G.D.); n.renken@rehazentrum-am-meer.de (N.R.)
* Correspondence: mona.voigt-barbarowicz@uol.de

Abstract: The term health literacy (HL) comprises the handling of health information and disease-specific and generic self-management skills, especially relevant for patients with chronic conditions. Health care professionals (HCPs) should correctly identify patients' communication needs and their HL levels. Therefore, the aims of the study were (1) to determine inpatient medical rehabilitation patients' HL based on self-assessment, (2) to evaluate changes from admission to discharge, (3) to identify HCPs estimation of patients' HL, and (4) to compare the estimated patient HL by patients and HCPs. A combined cross-sectional and longitudinal study was conducted in an orthopedic rehabilitation center in Germany. The multidimensional Health Literacy Questionnaire (HLQ) was filled in by patients (admission, discharge). An adapted version was administered to HCPs ($n = 32$) in order to assess HL of individual patients. Data from 287 patients were used for the longitudinal analysis, and comparison was based on $n = 278$ cases with at least two HL estimations. The results showed a significant increase in HL in five of nine scales with small effect sizes. Moreover, HCPs mostly provided higher scores than patients, and agreement was poor to fair. Differences between the HL estimation might lead to communication problems, and communication training could be useful.

Keywords: HCP; rehabilitants; agreement; HLQ; intraclass correlation (ICC); physicians; physiotherapists; social workers; nurses; orthopedic

1. Introduction

Health literacy (HL) is defined as "the degree to which individuals can obtain, process, understand, and communicate about health-related information needed to make informed health decisions" (p. 16) [1]. These HL skills enable a person to make health-related decisions. Low HL is a public health challenge throughout Europe [2]; previous research showed that almost 50% of adults in eight European countries have problematic or insufficient HL [3]. Approximately 54% of the German population cannot obtain, understand, and use relevant health information for their health choices [4]. Low HL of persons is associated with higher health care costs and poorer health outcomes [5–9]. Among other underprivileged groups, persons with chronic diseases are characterized by a lower level of HL than the general population [10,11].

HL is relevant in all health care sectors, but it is particularly relevant in medical rehabilitation. Medical rehabilitation is particularly important to make rehabilitants experts in their own chronic illnesses and thus positively influence the course [12]. In Germany, medical rehabilitation is characterized by several special features compared to other countries. This form of rehabilitation is predominantly carried out on an inpatient basis in clinics far from the patient's home, and the duration of rehabilitation is three weeks. Only approximately every seventh rehabilitation is based on outpatient treatment. In general, rehabilitation aims to help people with chronic diseases, disabled people, and people at risk of disability continue living as independently as possible and support a return to work. Medical rehabilitation can be further subdivided into specialist areas, such as orthopedic, neurological, or psychosomatic rehabilitation. In orthopedic rehabilitation, diseases and restrictions of the musculoskeletal system caused by chronic conditions, degenerative diseases, tumors, or accidents are treated. Other distinguishing features include specialization according to indications and the interdisciplinary composition of the rehabilitation team (e.g., physicians, physiotherapists, social workers, nurses, or psychologists) [13].

Especially for patients with chronic diseases and multimorbidity, professional conversations place high demands on those concerned since complex issues have to be discussed [14,15]. Therefore, health care professionals (HCPs) need to be able to adequately estimate the level of HL of their patients and adapt conversations or interventions to them to optimize their effects. Brief communication trainings for HCPs focusing on clear communication skills and HL principles can already improve patient–HCP communication [16–18]. Voigt-Barbarowicz and Brütt [19] described in their systematic review that HCPs had difficulty determining patients' HL adequately. The current state of studies highlighted that most frequently, the estimation of patient HL by physicians was investigated, and other HCP groups, such as nurses, were only considered in one study. Physiotherapists or social workers did not participate in any study.

Furthermore, all studies were conducted in hospital-based care or primary care settings. There are no studies examining the agreement between patients and various HCPs, such as physicians, nurses, physiotherapists, or social workers, in estimating patients' HL in a rehabilitation setting. In addition, methodological limitations apply, as one-dimensional questionnaires were predominantly used to assess patients' HL levels.

Therefore, the overall purpose of this study is to supplement the findings of previous research by examining HL levels as estimated by patients and HCPs. Specific aims of the study are (1) to determine inpatient medical rehabilitation patients' HL based on self-assessment at admission, (2) to evaluate changes in patients' self-assessed HL from admission to discharge, (3) to identify HCPs estimation of patients' HL, and (4) to compare the estimated patient HL by patients and rehabilitation HCPs.

2. Materials and Methods

2.1. Study Design and Setting

A combined cross-sectional (HCP) and longitudinal (patient) study were conducted from September to December 2020 at a rehabilitation clinic in Germany. The study was presented to patients at admission. After consent was obtained, the patients could fill in the questionnaires immediately on location. HCPs completed the questionnaires in their meeting room after patient contact.

2.2. Sampling and Participants

The research team handled the recruitment of patients and HCPs in a clinic for orthopedic and rheumatological rehabilitation. Patients with the following indications were treated in orthopedic rehabilitation: diseases and restrictions of the musculoskeletal system caused by chronic conditions, degenerative diseases, tumors, or accidents. Patients might have additional diagnoses (e.g., a cognitive/psychiatric disorder). Inpatients were included in the study if they were of working age (up to 67 years), were at least 18 years old, and had rehabilitation financed by the German Pension Insurance (especially DRV Oldenburg-Bremen, DRV Braunschweig-Hannover, DRV Bund). Patients were excluded if they could not understand the provided questionnaire although supported by a research assistant—these concerned inpatients with language difficulties. Employees from four HCP groups (physicians, nurses, physiotherapists, social workers) were also recruited for the study.

2.3. Measures

2.3.1. Health Literacy

For this study, we chose a multidimensional and well-validated instrument [20–22], the Health Literacy Questionnaire (HLQ) [23], to measure patients' HL levels by patients. The HLQ was developed using a "validity driven" approach. The multidimensional measurement is used for surveys, needs assessment, evaluation, and outcomes assessment as well as for informing service improvement and the development of interventions. The HLQ is available upon request [23]. This questionnaire has been tested in various studies and used in many areas, e.g., for population health surveys [24] or the evaluation of health programs [25]. The HLQ comprises 44 items in nine distinct scales:

1. Feeling understood and supported by health care providers (four items)
   (Sample question: "I have at least one healthcare provider who ... ");
2. Having sufficient information to manage my health (four items)
   (Sample question: "I am sure I have all the information I ... ");
3. Actively managing my health (five items)
   (Sample question: "I spend quite a lot of time actively managing ... ");
4. Social support for health (five items)
   (Sample question: "I can get access to several people who ... ");
5. Appraisal of health information (five items)
   (Sample question: "When I see new information about health, I ... ");
6. Ability to actively engage with health care providers (five items)
   (Sample question: "Make sure that healthcare providers understand ... ");
7. Navigating the health care system (six items)
   (Sample question: "Decide which healthcare provider you need ... ");
8. Ability to find good health information (five items)
   (Sample question: "Find health information from several ... ");
9. Understanding health information well enough to know what to do (five items)
   (Sample question: "Confidently fill medical forms in the correct ... ").

Each scale measures an independent domain of HL. The first five scales contain items with responses ranging from one (strongly disagree) to four (strongly agree). The scales six to nine include items with five responses: 1 = cannot do or always difficult, 2 = usually difficult, 3 = sometimes difficult, 4 = usually easy, and 5 = always easy. A higher score indicates greater ability or more support. There is no total score for the HLQ, and it is recommended to calculate the scores for each scale as the mean average of the items within that scale. In different settings, the HLQ demonstrated Cronbach's alpha > 0.8 for most scales [23].

In this study, the German version of the HLQ (HLQ-G) was used, which was provided by the questionnaire developers, and a license agreement was concluded. This measurement was translated and culturally adapted to the German context, and the psychometric properties of the HLQ-G were ensured. A nine-factor model replication of the English version was achieved with fit indices and psychometric properties similar to the original HLQ. Cronbach's alpha was at least 0.77 for all scales [20].

2.3.2. Patients Survey

Patients estimated their HL with a paper-based version of the HLQ-G at two measurement points (T0 and T1), based on 44 items representing all 9 scales. In addition, items regarding age, gender, nationality, living situation, education level, employment status, doctor contacts, diseases, and disability were assessed at T0.

2.3.3. HCPs Survey

HCPs were asked to complete the HLQ-G about their patient from their perceptions of their HL status. Therefore, the items were adapted to the wording of the HCPs. For example, "I feel I have good information ... " to "I feel **my patient** has good information ... ". In other studies, HLQ was also completed by patients and HCPs [21]. In our study,

HCPs estimated patients' HL using only 4 scales (scales 2, 3, 6, 9) [22] and a total of 19 items (abbreviated HLQ-4HCP in the following). The scales focused on having sufficient information (scale 2), actively managing my health (scale 3), engaging with health care professionals (scale 6), and understanding and reading health information (scale 9) because these are important for the rehabilitation process. HCPs could influence these domains in a short time of stay. A selection of scales shortened the questionnaire and made it easier to use in everyday clinical practice. Furthermore, items regarding age, gender, nationality, professional group, and work experience were assessed once at the beginning of the study. Completing the demographic items was voluntary, so HCPs who did not complete the demographics questionnaire could also estimate patients' HL in the study.

2.4. Data Collection

Study participation (HCPs and patients) was voluntary, and written informed consent was obtained. HCPs were informed before the study started. Patients were sent a short information leaflet before admission to the rehabilitation clinic. The patients were informed in detail about the study in the rehabilitation clinic at admission (T0), and the T0 questionnaire was administered. Five days before their discharge (T1), patients received the T1 questionnaire and were asked to complete and submit it in a sealable envelope before discharge. Patients were usually hospitalized for at least three weeks. Patients were surveyed at two points to determine changes in assessment during a rehabilitation stay. The time between T0 and T1 was at least 16 days. The patients had the opportunity to complete the T1 questionnaire from day 16 (until discharge). After patient informed consent, four HCPs from different professional groups (physicians, nurses, physiotherapists, social workers in each patient) were asked to estimate their patients' HL by the HLQ-4HCPs after a detailed initial interview.

The matching process between patients and HCP estimation was as follows: Patient questionnaires were prepared with ID codes. A code list, including ID and name, was available in the clinic. HCPs indicated patients' names on their estimation. To match data, names were replaced by ID codes, and the respective data were deleted from the code list. Therefore, data were anonymized after matching.

2.5. Data Analysis

The HLQ-G scale scores and demographic data were analyzed descriptively using SPSS (version 27) [26]. According to the HLQ handbook, missing data by patients and HCPs were imputed using the expectation-maximization algorithm. From scales with 4 to 5 items, missing data were imputed only if no more than two questions were missing. From scales with 6 items, missing data were imputed only if no more than three questions were missing within the scale. If there were more missing data, a scale score was not calculated for that individual scale. For demographic data no further imputations were conducted since missing data for each variable were below 5%.

Descriptive statistics were used to analyze demographic data and HLQ data (of patients and estimations by HCPs). Primary inferential statistical analysis was performed using calculations of measures of correlation and by testing for differences in means in dependent and independent samples. The statistical significance level was set at $p < 0.05$, and the Bonferroni method was used to adjust the p-values for pairwise comparisons ($p < 0.05/9 = 0.0055$; corrected for 9 pairwise comparisons). Cohen's [26] measures described the effect size. To measure the agreement between patients' HL and HCPs, estimation of their patients' HL at T0 intraclass correlation (ICC 2, k (average measure), two-way random, absolute agreement) was calculated and reported by Cicchetti (1994) guidelines. The guidelines for interpretation for ICC interrater agreement measure are as follows: less than 0.40—poor agreement; between 0.40 and 0.59—fair agreement; between 0.60 and 0.74—good agreement; and between 0.75 and 1.00—excellent agreement [27].

2.6. Ethical Considerations and Trial Registration

The study protocol was submitted to the Ethics Committee of the Medical Faculty of Oldenburg (number: 2020-034) for counseling and is in accordance with the Declaration of Helsinki in its current version (World Medical Association (WMA, Ferney-Voltaire, France, 2013). The works council of the rehabilitation center and the German pension insurance also gave their consent to the study. Written informed consent was obtained based on current data protection regulations. Data security was approved by all institutions involved in data collection. The code list is stored separately from the research data.

The study has been registered in the German Clinical Trials Register (DRKS) (registration number: DRKS00021071).

3. Results

3.1. Sample Characteristics

The demographic characteristics of the patients are shown in Table 1. A total of 361 patients by T0 and 287 patients by T1 participated. Data from 287 patients were used for the analysis. Patients were mostly 50–59 years old (48.8%); 62.0% were female ($n = 178$); 90.9% indicated German as their mother tongue. The highest level of education was a General Certificate of Secondary Education (GCSE) or equivalent (53.3%), followed by A-level education (41.8%). More than half (53.7%) had full-time jobs and had no work experience (75.3%) in the health care sector. A majority reported having joint replacement surgery (34.3%), spine surgery (17.8%), and wear and tear diseases (11.9%) prior to rehabilitation. Almost half (45.1%) had two or more (chronic) conditions.

Table 1. Demographic characteristics of patients.

Demographic and Health Characteristics	Total $n = 287$
Age, n (%)	
Until 29 years	4 (1.4)
30–39 years	15 (5.2)
40–49 years	32 (11.1)
50–59 years	140 (48.8)
60 years and older	95 (33.1)
Prefer not to answer	1 (0.3)
Gender, n (%)	
Women	178 (62.0)
Men	109 (38.0)
Live alone, n (%)	
Alone	55 (19.2)
Not alone	224 (78.0)
Prefer not to answer	8 (2.8)
Nationality, n (%)	
German	273 (95.1)
Other	6 (2.1)
Prefer not to answer	8 (2.8)
Mother tongue, n (%)	
German	261 (90.9)
Other languages	17 (5.9)
Prefer not to answer	9 (3.1)
Language skills in German	
very good	3 (17.6)
good	12 (70.6)
medium	2 (11.8)

Table 1. *Cont.*

Demographic and Health Characteristics	Total n = 287
Education, n (%)	
A-level or higher	120 (41.8)
GCSE or equivalent	153 (53.3)
No Qualification	5 (1.7)
Prefer not to answer	9 (3.1)
Reasons for rehabilitation, n (%)	
Joint replacement surgery (e.g., hip, knee)	135 (34.3)
Spine surgery (e.g., intervertebral disc)	70 (17.8)
Wear disease (e.g., arthrosis)	47 (11.9)
Functional disorders of the musculoskeletal system	46 (11.7)
Chronic back pain	38 (9.7)
Bone fracture, muscle-tendon rupture, capsular ligament injury	21 (5.4)
Other diseases	35 (9.0)
1 (chronic) disease	215 (54.9)
≥2 (chronic) diseases	177 (45.1)
Status of disability	
No severe disability	250 (87.1)
Severe disability (≥50%)	35 (12.2)
Not sure	2 (0.7)

A total of 32 HCPs (13 physicians, 6 physiotherapists, 4 social workers, 3 nurses, 6 HCPs without sociodemographic data) were recruited. Across the patient encounters by T0 (n = 361), HCPs had to assess several patients. Most HCPs were 50–59 years old (30.8%); 46.2% of HCPs were female (n = 12). HCPs graduated an average of 21.7 (SD 13.7) years and worked an average of 8.9 (SD 8.2) years in the current rehabilitation center, with a maximum of 26 years.

3.2. Estimations by Patients and HCPs

Figure 1 gives an overview of the estimations by patients and HCPs. Completed T0 (response rate: 99.8%) and T1 (response rate: 79.5%) questionnaires by patients (n = 287) were used to describe the level of patient HL. Estimations completed by patients and HCPs (n = 278; response rate: 76.8%) were used to analyze HCPs' and patients' estimation of patients' HL and compare the estimation of the patient's HL by rehabilitation HCPs. The response of the HCPs was as follows: complete data from n = 126 estimation by one HCP, n = 112 estimation of two HCPs, n = 35 estimations by three HCPs, and n = 5 estimations by all HCPs were available. Only 3.3% of the patients (n = 12) required assistance to complete the questionnaire.

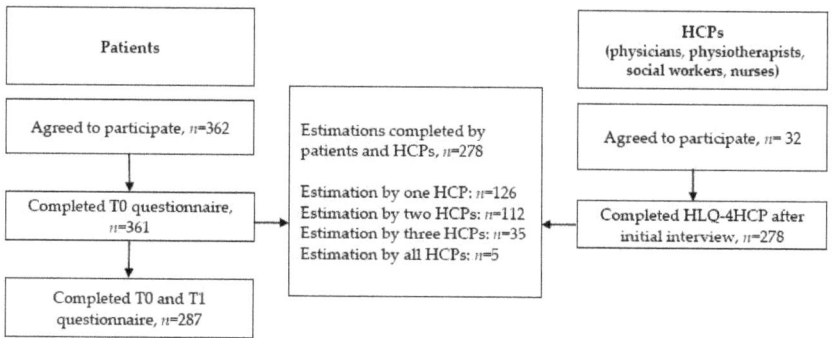

Figure 1. Estimations by patients and HCPs.

3.3. Self-Assessment of Patients' HL Level

Mean scores for each HLQ scale by the patient (T0 and T1) are displayed in Table 2. For scales 1 to 5, the score range is 1 to 4, and higher scores indicate greater agreement; and for scales 6 to 9, the score range is 1 to 5, with higher scores indicating less difficulty. The mean scores for the four HLQ scales by HCPs were also calculated. Due to the different scoring of the HLQ, of the scales 1–5 (range 1–4), scale 1, *"Feeling understood and supported by health care providers"*, had the highest mean scores (mean = 3.15, SD 0.47 at T0, mean = 3.18, SD 0.46 at T1), and the lowest overall was seen in scale 5, *"Appraisal of health information"* (mean = 2.86, SD 0.48 at T0, mean = 2.89, SD 0.50 at T1), self-assessed by patients. Of the scales 6–9 (range 1–5), scale 6, *"Ability to actively engage with health care providers"*, had the highest mean scores (mean = 3.84, SD 0.57 at T0, mean = 3.92, SD 0.56 at T1), and the lowest mean scores were seen in scale 7, *"Navigating the health care system"* (mean = 3.68, SD 0.56 at T0, mean = 3.79, SD 0.58 at T1), self-assessed by patients.

Table 2. Patients (T0, T1)—Health Literacy Questionnaire (HLQ) scale scores and *t*-tests for dependent samples; HCPs (T0)—Health Literacy Questionnaire (HLQ) scale scores.

HLQ Scale	Mean (SD) (95% CI), Patients T0 (n = 287) [a]	Mean (SD) (95% CI), Patients T1 (n = 287) [b]	p-Value *	Cohens d **	Mean (SD) (95% CI), Physicians (n = 176)	Mean (SD) (95% CI), Physio-Therapists (n = 141)	Mean (SD) (95% CI), Social Workers (n = 113) [c]	Mean (SD) (95% CI]), Nurses (n = 45) [d]
			Range 1 (lowest)–4 (highest)					
1. Feeling understood and supported by health care providers	3.15 (0.47) (3.09, 3.20)	3.18 (0.46) (3.12, 3.23)	0.261					
2. Having sufficient information to manage my health	2.85 (0.50) (2.80, 2.91)	3.02 (0.48) (2.96, 3.08)	0.000	−0.35	2.82 (0.61) (2.73, 2.91)	2.73 (0.60) (2.63, 2.83)	2.93 (0.61) (2.82, 3.05)	3.24 (0.46) (3.09, 3.38)
3. Actively managing my health	2.95 (0.44) (2.90, 3.00)	3.07 (0.42) (3.02, 3.12)	0.000	−0.28	2.73 (0.69) (2.63, 2.83)	2.90 (0.54) (2.81, 2.99)	2.76 (0.54) (2.66, 2.86)	3.18 (0.45) (3.03, 3.32)
4. Social support for health	3.06 (0.50) (3.00, 3.11)	3.10 (0.49) (3.04, 3.15)	0.082					
5. Appraisal of health information	2.86 (0.48) (2.80, 2.91)	2.89 (0.50) (2.83, 2.95)	0.113					
			Range 1 (lowest)–5 (highest)					
6. Ability to actively engage with health care providers	3.84 (0.57) (3.77, 3.90)	3.92 (0.56) (3.86, 3.99)	0.003	−0.14	4.04 (0.61) (3.95, 4.13)	4.05 (0.52) (3.96, 4.13)	4.18 (0.72) (4.04, 4.31)	4.46 (0.53) (4.30, 4.62)
7. Navigating the health care system	3.68 (0.56) (3.62, 3.75)	3.79 (0.58) (3.72, 3.86)	0.000	−0.19				
8. Ability to find good health information	3.79 (0.56) (3.72, 3.85)	3.89 (0.55) (3.82, 3.95)	0.000	−0.18				
9. Understanding health information well enough to know what to do	3.83 (0.55) (3.77, 3.89)	3.89 (0.55) (3.83, 3.96)	0.011		4.04 (0.58) (3.95, 4.13)	4.30 (0.58) (4.20, 4.40)	4.01 (0.72) (3.87, 4.14)	4.37 (0.57) (4.20, 4.54)

[a] Missing data, patients T0: Scale 1 = 1, scale 6 = 1, scale 7 = 1, scale 8 = 1, scale 9 = 1; [b] Missing data, patients T1: Scale 2 = 1, scale 5 = 2, scale 6 = 3, scale 7 = 4, scale 8 = 3, scale 9 = 3. [c] Missing data, Social workers: Scale 3 = 1; [d] Missing data, nurses: Scale 2 = 4, scale 3 = 4, scale 6 = 1, scale 9 = 1. * Bonferroni correction: $p < 0.0055$; ** Cohen (1988): <0.5—small effect size; 0.5–0.8—medium effect size; > 0.8—large effect size.

Regarding the estimation by patients at two points in time (T0 and T1), there was a statistically significant group difference for scale 2, *"Having sufficient information to manage my health"* ($p < 0.0055$, d = −0.35); scale 3, *"Actively managing my health"*; scale 6, *"Ability to actively engage with health care providers"* ($p < 0.0055$, d = −0.28); scale 7, *"Navigating the health care system*: ($p < 0.0055$, d = −0.14); and scale 8, *"Ability to find good health information"* ($p < 0.0055$, d = −0.18).

3.4. HCPs Estimation of Patients' HL Level

The patients' self-assessed HL levels (T0) compared with the HCP estimation (T0) can be described as follows: The physicians (total estimations $n = 176$) showed higher mean scores on scale 6, *"Ability to actively engage with health care providers"* (mean = 4.04, SD 0.61), and scale 9, *"Understanding health information well enough to know what to do"* (mean = 4.04, SD 0.58), than the patients. The physiotherapists (total estimations $n = 141$) also presented higher mean scores on scale 6, *"Ability to actively engage with health care providers"* (mean = 4.05, SD 0.52), and scale 9, *"Understanding health information well enough to know what to do"* (mean = 4.30, SD 0.58), than the patients. The social workers (total estimations $n = 113$) demonstrated a higher scale score in three scales (scale 2, *"Having sufficient information to manage my health"* (mean = 2.93, SD 0.61); scale 6, *"Ability to actively engage with health care providers"* (mean = 4.18, SD 0.72); and scale 9, *"Understanding health information well"* (mean = 4.01, SD 0.72) than patients' self-assessment. Nurses (total estimations $n = 45$) showed a higher mean score in all scales estimated (scale 2, *"Having sufficient information to manage my health"* (mean = 3.24, SD 0.46); scale 3, *"Actively managing my health"* (mean = 3.18, SD 0.45); scale 6, *"Ability to actively engage with health care providers"* (mean = 4.46, SD 0.53); and scale 9, *"Understanding health information well enough to know what to do"* (mean = 4.37, SD 0.57)). Group differences were not tested for significance.

3.5. HL Agreement

The intraclass coefficient of agreement was computed to estimate the level of agreement between patient HL levels by patients and HCPs' predicted level of patient HL levels measured by the HLQ (scale 2, 3, 6, 9).

In identifying specific groups of HCPs, the results demonstrated poor to fair agreement and could be described as follows: The best agreement between HCPs and patients' overall estimation of patients' HL level was found at scale 3, and the lowest overall agreement was found at scale 6. The results of scale 3, *"Actively managing my health"*, stated fair agreement between physiotherapists' (ICC = 0.45), social workers' (ICC = 0.44), and nurses' perceptions of patients' HL and patients' self-assessment of their HL level.

Physicians' and patients' estimations of patients' HL levels showed fair agreement in scale 9, *"Understanding health information well enough to know what to do"* (ICC = 0.44).

In three scales, social workers and patients had a fair level of agreement (scale 2, *"Having sufficient information to manage my health"*, ICC = 0.47; scale 3, *"Actively managing my health"*, ICC = 0.44; and scale 9 *"Understanding health information well enough to know what to do"*, ICC = 0.56) regarding the estimation of patients' HL levels. Scale 6, *"Ability to actively engage with health care providers"* (ICC = 0.31), had poor agreement (see Table 3).

Table 3. Intraclass coefficient (ICC) of HCPs' and patients' estimation of patients' HL.

		ICC *			
	HLQ Scale	Physicians ($n = 176$)	Physiotherapists ($n = 141$)	Social Workers ($n = 113$)	Nurses ($n = 45$)
Patients	2. Having sufficient information to manage my health	0.21	0.20	0.47	0.10
	3. Actively managing my health	0.27	0.45	0.44	0.40
	6. Ability to actively engage with health care providers	0.21	0.02	0.31	0.16
	9. Understanding health information well enough to know what to do	0.44	0.16	0.56	0.27

* Cicchetti (1994): Less than 0.40—poor agreement; between 0.40 and 0.59—fair agreement; between 0.60 and 0.74—good agreement; between 0.75 and 1.00—excellent agreement.

4. Discussion

This study aimed to determine inpatient medical rehabilitation patients' HL based on self-assessment, evaluate changes from admission to discharge, identify rehabilitation HCPs estimation of patients' HL, and compare the estimated patient HL by patients and HCPs.

Compared to other studies, HL levels at admission were quite similar. A significant increase in HL with small effect sizes was shown in five (scale 2, "*Having sufficient information to manage my health*"; scale 3, "*Actively managing my health*"; scale 6, "*Ability to actively engage with health care providers*"; and scale 7, "*Navigating the health care system*") out of the nine HLQ scales. These are especially the scales that focused on the rehabilitation process, and these domains improved after three weeks of rehabilitation stay. Whether these changes are caused by interventions, communication, or the fact that patients were in a rehabilitation clinic needs to be researched in further studies. Moreover, these domains (e.g., "*Ability to actively engage with health care providers*") can be improved in the short term because they do not directly change reading and writing skills (individual skills). Nonetheless, the maintenance of these changes needs to be determined. Other longitudinal studies related to individuals with chronic obstructive pulmonary disease have shown that on scale 3, the main scores decreased after 6 and 12 months [28]. Scales 1, 4, 5, 8, and 9 did not significantly differ between T0 and T1. Although effects do not seem to last for 6 or 12 months, our study shows that there are short-term effects of medical rehabilitation with regard to health literacy. Strategies to perpetuate these effects are needed and should be integrated into after care.

The findings demonstrated higher mean scores estimated by HCPs than patients on most scales. In particular, the mean scores by scale 6, "*Ability to actively engage with health care providers*", and scale 9, "*Understanding health information well enough to know what to do*", were higher by all HCPs' assessment than by patients' self-assessment. The results of the intraclass coefficient indicated poor to fair agreement between patients' and HCPs' estimation of patients' HL. Our findings for setting rehabilitation are consistent with the previous literature, which showed poor agreement between patients' and HCPs' (especially physicians) estimation of patients' HL [21,29–35]. HCPs tended to overestimate patients' HL. Different perspectives between patients and HCPs in estimating the HL of patients may not be because HCPs do not know how they identify patients' HL levels. After all, they have different perceptions or expectations of HL than patients. For example, scale 6, "*Ability to actively engage with health care providers*", could be easier for HCPs to estimate, as an impression can be gained through brief communication with the patient. On the other hand, "*Social support for health*" (scale 4) may be more difficult to estimate by HCPs in rehabilitation, as they do not have an accurate overview of the social background of patients in rehabilitation.

Social workers had fair agreement on three out of four scales, and all other HCPs had fair agreement on only one scale. All other estimations were in poor agreement. Reasons for a better agreement but lower scale scores could be that the social workers had focused contact, which enables enough time to identify and adapt to patients' communication needs during the initial interview. A quiet conversation environment and as few sources of irritation as possible are helpful in this context. Different estimation results between the HCPs could also be due to different training statuses and working experiences [36,37]. The different assessments of HCPs for individual patients should also be discussed within the team, so it is also useful to improve communication within a caring team.

To enhance patients' disease knowledge, their ability to self-manage, and adherence to health care recommendations, awareness of the importance of HL may be integrated into clinical practice by the HCP rehabilitation team [38,39]. HCPs should intervene to improve HL because patients with chronic disease often use rehabilitation programs and can benefit from them.

4.1. Implications for Practice and Research

Differences in HL estimation in patients and HCPs may lead to communication problems. On-the-job training for HCPs could be useful [40]. This training should focus on identifying the needs of patients with low HL and include strategies to promote communication between HCPs and patients. For example, the "teach-back" [41] or "chunk and check" [42] methods can be used. With these methods [41,42], HCPs check patients' understanding by asking them to reproduce in their own words what was explained to them by the health care professional [43]. HL communication training for HCPs in hospital settings was developed and successfully tested in several countries and diverse settings [17,18,44,45]. The results showed that this training subjectively improved HCP knowledge about HL, understanding HL needs, awareness of their jargon, self-efficacy, and adaptations in patient interactions [44,46]. Other effects of the differences in HL estimation in patients and HCPs should be addressed in further research.

4.2. Strengths and Limitations

A strength of the study is that a multidimensional instrument, the HLQ [23], was used to assess patients' HL according to patients and HCPs to reflect different domains of HL. In addition, the research questions were answered through the participation of different HCP groups in an unresearched setting, the rehabilitation setting. In contrast, previous studies [18] have provided new findings on different professional groups. In addition, there were high response rates among patients (response rates T0: 99.8%; T1: 79.5%) and HCPs (overall response rate: 76.8%). However, we conducted the study only in one center focused on orthopedic and rheumatological rehabilitation. Therefore, a homogeneous patient group can be assumed, which does not reflect the diversity of patients in rehabilitation. Another limitation of the study is that only a small number of HCPs was recruited, posing a risk of identification. Additionally, no exact number of patients estimated per HCP can be given because HL estimation of HCPs was anonymized. Furthermore, to avoid multiple testing, data of the comparison of patients (T0) and HCP HLQ scale scores were not tested for statistical significance.

5. Conclusions

This study provides preliminary evidence on the patients' and HCPs' estimation of rehabilitation patients' HL and their agreement. The results reveal that patients' and HCPs' estimation of patients' HL often dissents. Communication training could help to improve communication between patients and HCPs. Rehabilitation is particularly linked to HL [39], and the topic of HL should be given higher awareness in the rehabilitation process to improve patients' HL, including patients with chronic diseases.

Author Contributions: Conceptualization, M.V.-B., G.D., N.R. and A.L.B.; methodology, M.V.-B. and A.L.B.; software, M.V.-B. and R.S.; formal analysis, M.V.-B.; data curation, M.V.-B. and R.S.; writing—original draft preparation, M.V.-B.; writing—review and editing, G.D., N.R., R.S. and A.L.B.; visualization, M.V.-B.; supervision, A.L.B.; project administration, M.V.-B. and A.L.B.; funding acquisition, A.L.B. All authors have read and agreed to the published version of the manuscript.

Funding: This research received no external funding, but the junior research group is funded by the German pension insurance (Deutsche Rentenversicherung Oldenburg-Bremen).

Institutional Review Board Statement: The study was conducted according to the guidelines of the Declaration of Helsinki and approved by the Ethics Committee of the Medical Faculty of Oldenburg.

Informed Consent Statement: Informed consent was obtained from all subjects involved in the study.

Data Availability Statement: The data presented in this study are available on request from the corresponding author.

Acknowledgments: The authors thank the participating rehabilitation center, all employees, as well as all patients for participating in this study.

Conflicts of Interest: The authors declare no conflict of interest.

References

1. Berkman, N.D.; Davis, T.C.; McCormack, L. Health literacy: What is it? *J. Health Commun.* **2010**, *15*, 9–19. [CrossRef] [PubMed]
2. Baccolini, V.; Rosso, A.; Di Paolo, C.; Isonne, C.; Salerno, C.; Migliara, G.; Prencipe, G.P.; Massimi, A.; Marzuillo, C.; De Vito, C.; et al. What is the Prevalence of Low Health Literacy in European Union Member States? A Systematic Review and Meta-analysis. *J. Gen. Intern. Med.* **2021**, *36*, 753–761. [CrossRef] [PubMed]
3. Sørensen, K.; Pelikan, J.M.; Röthlin, F.; Ganahl, K.; Slonska, Z.; Doyle, G.; Fullam, J.; Kondilis, B.; Agrafiotis, D.; Uiters, E.; et al. Health literacy in Europe: Comparative results of the European health literacy survey (HLS-EU). *Eur. J. Public Health* **2015**, *25*, 1053–1058. [CrossRef] [PubMed]
4. Schaeffer, D.; Berens, E.M.; Vogt, D. Health Literacy in the German Population. *Dtsch. Arztebl. Int.* **2017**, *114*, 53–60. [CrossRef] [PubMed]
5. Sheridan, S.L.; Halpern, D.J.; Viera, A.J.; Berkman, N.D.; Donahue, K.E.; Crotty, K. Interventions for individuals with low health literacy: A systematic review. *J. Health Commun.* **2011**, *16* (Suppl. 3), 30–54. [CrossRef] [PubMed]
6. Brach, C.; Keller, D.; Hernandez, L.M.; Baur, C.; Parker, R.; Dreyer, B.; Schyve, P.; Lemerise, A.J.; Schillinger, D. Ten Attributes of Health Literate Health Care Organizations. *NAM Perspect.* **2012**. [CrossRef]
7. Schillinger, D.; Grumbach, K.; Piette, J.; Wang, F.; Osmond, D.; Daher, C.; Palacios, J.; Sullivan, G.D.; Bindman, A.B. Association of health literacy with diabetes outcomes. *JAMA* **2002**, *288*, 475–482. [CrossRef] [PubMed]
8. Cajita, M.I.; Cajita, T.R.; Han, H.R. Health Literacy and Heart Failure: A Systematic Review. *J. Cardiovasc. Nurs.* **2016**, *31*, 121–130. [CrossRef] [PubMed]
9. Baker, D.W.; Parker, R.M.; Clark, W.S. Health literacy and the risk of hospital admission. *J. Gen. Intern. Med.* **1998**, *13*, 791–798. [CrossRef] [PubMed]
10. Schaeffer, D.; Vogt, D.; Berens, E.M.; Hurrelmann, K. *Gesundheitskompetenz der Bevölkerung in Deutschland: Ergebnisbericht*; Universität Bielefeld: Bielefeld, Germany, 2017.
11. Hasseler, M. Menschen mit geistigen und mehrfachen Behinderungen als vulnerable Bevölkerungsgruppe in gesundheitlicher Versorgung. *Dtsch. Med. Wochenschr.* **2014**, *139*, 2030–2034. [CrossRef] [PubMed]
12. Bitzer, E.M.; Dierks, M.L.; Heine, W.; Becker, P.; Vogel, H.; Beckmann, U.; Butsch, R.; Dörning, H.; Brüggemann, S. Empowerment and health literacy in medical rehabilitation—recommendations for strengthening patient education. *Rehabilitation* **2009**, *48*, 202–210. [CrossRef] [PubMed]
13. Mittag, O.; Welti, F. Medizinische Rehabilitation im europäischen Vergleich und Auswirkungen des europäischen Rechts auf die deutsche Rehabilitation. *Bundesgesundheitsblatt Gesundh. Gesundh.* **2017**, *60*, 378–385. [CrossRef] [PubMed]
14. Ernstmann, N.; Bauer, U.; Berens, E.-M.; Bitzer, E.M.; Bollweg, T.M.; Danner, M.; Dehn-Hindenberg, A.; Dierks, M.L.; Farin, E.; Grobosch, S.; et al. DNVF Memorandum Gesundheitskompetenz (Teil 1)—Hintergrund, Relevanz, Gegenstand und Fragestellungen in der Versorgungsforschung. *Gesundheitswesen* **2020**, *82*, e77–e93. [CrossRef] [PubMed]
15. Schmidt, E.; Schöpf, A.C.; Farin, E. What is competent communication behaviour of patients in physician consultations?—Chronically-ill patients answer in focus groups. *Psychol. Health Med.* **2017**, *22*, 987–1000. [CrossRef]
16. Schillinger, D.; Bindman, A.; Wang, F.; Stewart, A.; Piette, J. Functional health literacy and the quality of physician–patient communication among diabetes patients. *Patient Educ. Couns.* **2004**, *52*, 315–323. [CrossRef]
17. Allenbaugh, J.; Spagnoletti, C.L.; Rack, L.; Rubio, D.; Corbelli, J. Health Literacy and Clear Bedside Communication: A Curricular Intervention for Internal Medicine Physicians and Medicine Nurses. *MedEdPORTAL* **2019**, *15*, 10795. [CrossRef]

18. Tavakoly Sany, S.B.; Behzhad, F.; Ferns, G.; Peyman, N. Communication skills training for physicians improves health literacy and medical outcomes among patients with hypertension: A randomized controlled trial. *BMC Health Serv. Res.* **2020**, *20*, 60. [CrossRef]
19. Voigt-Barbarowicz, M.; Brütt, A.L. The Agreement between Patients' and Healthcare Professionals' Assessment of Patients' Health Literacy-A Systematic Review. *Int. J. Environ. Res. Public Health* **2020**, *17*, 2372. [CrossRef]
20. Nolte, S.; Osborne, R.H.; Dwinger, S.; Elsworth, G.R.; Conrad, M.L.; Rose, M.; Härter, M.; Dirmaier, J.; Zill, J.M. German translation, cultural adaptation, and validation of the Health Literacy Questionnaire (HLQ). *PLoS ONE* **2017**, *12*, e0172340. [CrossRef]
21. Hawkins, M.; Gill, S.D.; Batterham, R.; Elsworth, G.R.; Osborne, R.H. The Health Literacy Questionnaire (HLQ) at the patient-clinician interface: A qualitative study of what patients and clinicians mean by their HLQ scores. *BMC Health Serv. Res.* **2017**, *17*, 309. [CrossRef]
22. Maindal, H.T.; Kayser, L.; Norgaard, O.; Bo, A.; Elsworth, G.R.; Osborne, R.H. Cultural adaptation and validation of the Health Literacy Questionnaire (HLQ): Robust nine-dimension Danish language confirmatory factor model. *Springerplus* **2016**, *5*, 1232. [CrossRef] [PubMed]
23. Osborne, R.H.; Batterham, R.W.; Elsworth, G.R.; Hawkins, M.; Buchbinder, R. The grounded psychometric development and initial validation of HLQ. *BMC Public Health* **2013**, *13*, 658. [CrossRef] [PubMed]
24. Bo, A.; Friis, K.; Osborne, R.H.; Maindal, T.H. National indicators of health literacy: Ability to understand health information and to engage actively with healthcare providers—A population based survey among Danish adults. *BMC Public Health* **2014**, *14*, 1095. Available online: http://www.biomedcentral.com/1471-2458/14/1095 (accessed on 17 January 2022). [CrossRef] [PubMed]
25. Faruqi, N.; Stocks, N.; Spooner, C.; El Haddad, N.; Harris, M.F. Research protocol: Management of obesity in patients with low health literacy in primary health care. *BMC Obes.* **2015**, *2*, 5. [CrossRef] [PubMed]
26. IBM Corp. *IBM SPSS Statistics for Windows, Version 27.0*; IBM Corp: Armonk, NY, USA, 2020.
27. Cicchetti, D.V. Guidelines, criteria, and rules of thumb for evaluating normed and standardized assessment instruments in psychology. *Psychol. Assess.* **1994**, *6*, 284–290. [CrossRef]
28. Lindskrog, S.; Christensen, K.B.; Osborne, R.H.; Vingtoft, S.; Phanareth, K.; Kayser, L. Relationship Between Patient-Reported Outcome Measures and the Severity of Chronic Obstructive Pulmonary Disease in the Context of an Innovative Digitally Supported 24-Hour Service: Longitudinal Study. *J. Med. Internet. Res.* **2019**, *21*, e10924. [CrossRef]
29. Bass, P.F., III; Wilson, J.F.; Griffith, C.H.; Barnett, D.R. Residents' Ability to Identify Patients with Poor literacy Skills. *Acad. Med.* **2002**, *77*, 1030–1041. [CrossRef]
30. Dickens, C.; Lambert, B.L.; Cromwell, T.; Piano, M.R. Nurse overestimation of patients' health literacy. *J. Health Commun.* **2013**, *18* (Suppl. 1), 62–69. [CrossRef]
31. Kelly, P.A.; Haidet, P. Physician overestimation of patient literacy: A potential source of health care disparities. *Patient Educ. Couns.* **2007**, *66*, 119–122. [CrossRef]
32. Lindau, S.T.; Basu, A.; Leitsch, S.A. Health Literacy as a Predictor of Follow-Up After an Abnormal Pap Smear. *J. Gen. Intern. Med.* **2006**, *21*, 829–834. [CrossRef]
33. Rogers, E.D.; Wallace, L.S.; Weiss, B.D. Misperceptions of Medical Understanding in low. *Cancer Control* **2006**, *13*, 225–229. [CrossRef] [PubMed]
34. Storms, H.; Aertgeerts, B.; Vandenabeele, F.; Claes, N. General practitioners' predictions of their own patients´ health literacy. *BMJ Open* **2019**, *9*, e029357. [CrossRef] [PubMed]
35. Zawilinski, L.L.; Kirkpatrick, H.; Pawlaczyk, B.; Yarlagadda, H. Actual and perceived patient health literacy: How accurate are residents' predictions? *Int. J. Psychiatry Med.* **2019**, *54*, 290–295. [CrossRef] [PubMed]
36. Toronto, C.E.; Weatherford, B.J. Health Literacy Education in Health Professions Schools: An Integrative Review. *Nurs. Educ.* **2015**, *54*, 669–676. [CrossRef]
37. Saunders, C.; Palesy, D.; Lewis, J. Systematic Review and Conceptual Framework for Health Literacy Training in Health Professions Education. *Health Prof. Edu.* **2019**, *5*, 13–29. [CrossRef]
38. Sadeghi, S.; Brooks, D.; Goldstein, R.S. Patients' and providers' perceptions of the impact of health literacy on communication in pulmonary rehabilitation. *Chron. Respir. Dis.* **2013**, *10*, 65–76. [CrossRef] [PubMed]
39. Levasseur, M.; Carrier, A. Do rehabilitation professionals need to consider their clients' health literacy for effective practice? *Clin. Rehabil.* **2010**, *24*, 756–765. [CrossRef]
40. Coleman, C. Teaching health care professionals about health literacy: A review of the literature. *Nurs. Outlook* **2011**, *59*, 70–78. [CrossRef]
41. Brega, A.G.; Barnard, J.; Mabachi, N.M.; Weiss, B.D.; DeWalt, D.A.; Brach, C.; Cifuentes, M.; Albright, K.; West, D.R. *Use the Teach-Back Method: Tool 5*; AHRQ Health Literacy Universal Precautions Toolkit: Rockville, MD, USA, 2015.
42. Schmidt-Kaehler, S.; Vogt, D.; Berens, E.M.; Horn, A.; Schaeffer, D. *Gesundheitskompetenz: Verständlich Informieren und Beraten. Material-und Methodensammlung zur Verbraucher-und Patientenberatung für Zielgruppen mit Geringer Gesundheitskompetenz*; Bielefeld University: Bielefeld, Germany, 2017.
43. Kountz, D.S. Strategies for improving low health literacy. *Postgrad. Med.* **2009**, *121*, 171–177. [CrossRef] [PubMed]
44. Kaper, M.S.; Winter, A.F.; Bevilacqua, R.; Giammarchi, C.; McCusker, A.; Sixsmith, J.; Koot, J.A.R.; Reijneveld, S.A. Positive Outcomes of a Comprehensive Health Literacy Communication Training for Health Professionals in Three European Countries: A Multi-centre Pre-post Intervention Study. *Int. J. Environ. Res. Public Health* **2019**, *16*, 20. [CrossRef] [PubMed]

45. Kaper, M.S.; Reijneveld, S.A.; van Es, F.D.; de Zeeuw, J.; Almansa, J.; Koot, J.A.R.; de Winter, A.F. Effectiveness of a Comprehensive Health Literacy Consultation Skills Training for Undergraduate Medical Students: A Randomized Controlled Trial. *Int. J. Environ. Res. Public Health* **2019**, *17*, 81. [CrossRef] [PubMed]
46. Kripalani, S.; Weiss, B.D. Teaching about health literacy and clear communication. *J. Gen. Intern. Med.* **2006**, *21*, 888–890. [CrossRef] [PubMed]

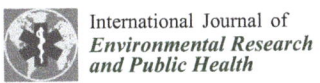

Article

Health Literacy-Sensitive Counselling on Early Childhood Allergy Prevention: Results of a Qualitative Study on German Midwives' Perspectives

Julia von Sommoggy [1,*], Eva-Maria Grepmeier [2] and Janina Curbach [3]

1. Medical Sociology, Department of Epidemiology and Preventive Medicine, University of Regensburg, 93051 Regensburg, Germany
2. Medical Faculty, Institute of Social Medicine & Health Systems Research, Otto von Guericke University Magdeburg, 39120 Magdeburg, Germany; eva-maria.grepmeier@med.ovgu.de
3. Department of Business Studies, Ostbayerische Technische Hochschule Regensburg, 93053 Regensburg, Germany; janina.curbach@oth-regensburg.de
* Correspondence: julia.sommoggy@ukr.de

Abstract: In Germany, midwives are involved in extensive antenatal and postnatal care. As health professionals, they can play a key role in strengthening health literacy (HL) of parents on how to prevent chronic allergic diseases in their children. The objective of this study is to explore midwives' perspectives regarding HL-sensitive counselling in early childhood allergy prevention (ECAP). Twenty-four qualitative semi-structured interviews were conducted with midwives, and data were analyzed using qualitative content analysis. Only a small number of study participants were aware of HL as a concept. However, most of these use screening and counselling strategies which consider individual information needs and which support parental HL. HL sensitivity in counselling is largely based on the midwives' "gut feelings" and counselling experience, rather than on formal education. The midwives were largely aware of evidence-based ECAP recommendations; however, allergy prevention was not seen as a stand-alone topic but as part of their general counselling on infant feeding and hygiene. They found parents to be more open to receiving complex prevention information during antenatal counselling. In order to strengthen midwives' roles in HL-sensitive ECAP counselling, their formal education should provide them with explicit HL knowledge and counselling skills. ECAP should be an inherent part of antenatal care.

Keywords: health literacy; allergy prevention; health professionals; qualitative methods; midwives

Citation: von Sommoggy, J.; Grepmeier, E.-M.; Curbach, J. Health Literacy-Sensitive Counselling on Early Childhood Allergy Prevention: Results of a Qualitative Study on German Midwives' Perspectives. *Int. J. Environ. Res. Public Health* **2022**, *19*, 4182. https://doi.org/10.3390/ijerph19074182

Academic Editors: Marie-Luise Dierks, Jonas Lander and Melanie Hawkins

Received: 31 January 2022
Accepted: 29 March 2022
Published: 31 March 2022

Publisher's Note: MDPI stays neutral with regard to jurisdictional claims in published maps and institutional affiliations.

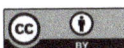

Copyright: © 2022 by the authors. Licensee MDPI, Basel, Switzerland. This article is an open access article distributed under the terms and conditions of the Creative Commons Attribution (CC BY) license (https://creativecommons.org/licenses/by/4.0/).

1. Introduction

Health literacy (HL) enables people to make informed health-related decisions to take care of their own health. It is defined as "knowledge, motivation and competencies related to the process of accessing, understanding, appraising and applying health-related information within the healthcare, disease prevention and health promotion setting" [1,2]. A low level of HL is associated with poor health-related knowledge and comprehension, infrequent use of preventive healthcare services, and, especially in older people, poor overall health status and high mortality [3,4]. When it comes to prevention, a higher level of HL is positively associated with health-promoting behavior [5]. It is helpful for patients to understand the connection between health behavior now and health outcomes later, as this encourages them to adhere to prevention recommendations. This is especially challenging when prevention and health outcomes are temporally distant, which is the case for most chronic diseases, e.g., heart conditions or diabetes mellitus. Another example is the prevention of allergies, which will be the focus of this article.

Allergies are chronic diseases which can have a major impact on quality of life [6]. Asthma, eczema, but also allergic rhinitis can present a significant risk to personal well-being [7]. Since the 1990s, an increase in the prevalence of allergic diseases has been observed internationally [8,9]. Allergic diseases are now recognized as a significant public health concern in many developed countries. Research on allergies indicates the importance of early childhood allergy prevention (ECAP), since health-related behaviors in the first three years of life can help prevent allergic conditions [10]. Based on current scientific evidence, exclusive breastfeeding for the first few months, the introduction of solid food after four months, and early exposure to allergens while breastfeeding seem to prevent or lessen the risk of allergies in later life [11]. However, providing advice on allergy prevention is challenging as evidence on risk factors for childhood allergy tends to change quickly due to the high level of research activity in this field [12]. For example, while former guidelines recommended avoidance of allergens (e.g., nuts) and delayed introduction of some solid foods, the current guidelines emphasize that parents do not need to take any specific preventive action regarding their child's diet [12]. In addition, new myths have emerged from misleading stories in the news and social media, and from product marketers taking advantage of uncertainty [13–15].

Although challenging, counselling parents on allergy prevention is important in order to reduce the occurrence of this chronic condition. Health professionals are an important source of information for mothers regarding health-related behaviors [16,17]. Moreover, research has shown that preventive counselling by health professionals can be effective in improving patients' HL and preventive health behavior, e.g., with respect to smoking cessation or increasing physical activity [18–22]. With regard to the effectiveness of HL-sensitive preventive counselling, a clinical trial conducted by Gharachourlo et al. showed that by counselling in an HL-sensitive way on routine pregnancy care and on modifying lifestyles, healthy lifestyles could be increased in the intervention group [16]. Thus, advice from health professionals may also help prevent chronic allergic conditions [17]. Patients' HL and health outcomes can be enhanced if health professionals engage in HL-sensitive care, i.e., they take the HL of patients into account when counselling and healthcare settings (private practices, clinical settings) create a shame-free environment for patients with low HL [23,24]. Applying HL counselling techniques, e.g., using simple language and visuals, can help support parents with any level of HL to better understand the information provided [25–27]. Thus, HL in general, including that of mothers caring for young children, is not only an individual trait; it is strongly influenced by the healthcare system individuals have to navigate [28].

Enhancing the HL of parents as caregivers is important as research has shown that low parental HL has adverse impacts on child health outcomes [29]. For example, a study by DeWalt et al. on asthma shows that children whose parents had a low level of HL reported more severe asthma symptoms, were more likely to miss school, and were hospitalized more frequently [30]. Another study by Stafford et al. shows a correlation between low HL and maternal intention to exclusively breastfeed [31]. Since breastfeeding is a major contributing factor to the prevention of allergies in later life, mothers' HL is an important aspect to be addressed in the promotion of allergy prevention [12].

In the German healthcare system, statutory health insurance provides expectant and new mothers with extensive midwife care before, during, and after birth—similar to family nurses in other countries. Midwives provide voluntary antenatal courses advising on childbirth and parenthood, which are offered to pregnant women and their partners. These courses inform participants about breastfeeding and infant care [32] and therefore cover aspects that are also relevant for ECAP [33]. After birth, mothers are entitled to two home visits per day for the first ten days. Thereafter, they can have an additional 16 midwife visits during the first 12 weeks, and eight more up until the end of the ninth month [34]. Data from Bavaria (one of the German federal states this study focuses on) show that 65% (antenatal) and 94.9% (postnatal) of mothers make use of this service [35]. A Czech study showed that pregnant women's long-term prenatal contact with a midwife was associated with higher HL, suggesting a positive effect of midwives' interaction with mothers [36]. Due to this very intensive and regular contact with new parents, German midwives are vitally important health professionals when it comes to counselling parents on health issues and the prevention of chronic diseases, especially during this vulnerable phase of transition to becoming a family.

Counselling parents before and after the birth of a child may offer a "window of opportunity" for preventing a whole range a relevant chronic allergic diseases, and midwives could play a key role in strengthening parental HL on allergy prevention [37]. It is thus important to better understand how midwives counsel on ECAP, how they translate current knowledge for parents, and how they ensure that this information can be accessed, understood, appraised, and applied by the parents in their care. To the best of our knowledge, there is, as yet, no research on how German midwives take HL into account in their daily counselling on the health topics relevant to allergy prevention, how they convey scientific evidence, and how they help parents to understand, appraise, and apply this information in their daily life. Hence, the aim of the present study is to gain insight into the experience and practices of German midwives with regard to counselling on allergy prevention and how they support parental HL.

2. Methods

An explorative study design was selected in order to capture diverse perspectives and to gain a broad insight into how midwives consider HL in their daily professional practice and how they counsel families on early childhood allergy prevention. Qualitative research allows a flexible approach to the subject, since it enables the researcher to probe interesting facets that come up spontaneously during an interview. Including the personal experiences and subjective views of midwives makes it possible to look at the topic from multiple perspectives. This approach has the potential to capture themes and topics that might not arise when working with predefined, standardized categories and assumptions [38].

We conducted 24 interviews with midwives from May 2020 to March 2021. The initial plan was to conduct face-to-face interviews, but due to the COVID-19 pandemic, which prohibited personal contact, we conducted most of the interviews via telephone. The interviews were semi-structured to enable us to maintain a focus on certain topics, while being open for aspects arising during the conversations. After some minor adaptations and changes following the first three interviews, the same interview guide was used for all interviews to ensure a certain degree of comparability. The interviewees were encouraged to speak freely and discuss their own ideas; thus, the sequence of questions did not always strictly follow the interview guide.

The interview guide (cf. Appendix A) comprised four main topics: 1, information and evidence; 2, knowledge translation and transfer; 3, promotion of health literacy; 3a, counselling of parents and health literacy; 3b, attitudes toward and experiences of health literacy/health literacy-sensitive care; and 4, health literacy concept awareness.

3. Recruitment

With qualitative research, the aim is to understand social phenomena in depth, while statistical representativeness is not a requirement [39]. In order to retrieve rich information and ensure rigor, a purposive sampling strategy was used by identifying specific groups of midwives who possessed certain characteristics relevant to the topic being studied, with a view to accessing maximum variation of perspectives (cf. Table 1) [39,40].

First, in urban areas, we expect patients' backgrounds to be more diverse in terms of socio-economic status, ethnicity, and, since the prevalence of allergic conditions is higher in urban settings, parental information needs are also expected to be different than in rural areas. Thus, the way parents are counselled might differ as well. Bearing this in mind, we intended to recruit from both types of catchment areas. Second, in Germany, there has been a recent shift with regard to the professional education of midwives. Until January 2020, vocational training of three or five years was sufficient to become a midwife. Since then, a bachelor's degree has become a mandatory requirement. Thus, the education of midwives varies widely, and we assume this might have an impact on counselling and knowledge of health literacy as a concept as well. Our aim was therefore to recruit midwives with different educational backgrounds. Third, we assumed that the length of professional experience would have an effect on how midwives counsel parents and that, in this regard, there might be a significant difference between older midwives with a lot of professional experience and younger, less experienced midwives. Thus, we aimed to include both groups into the sample.

We excluded midwives working solely in clinical settings as the time provided to counsel parents on ECAP in the hospital setting is considered too short. We also excluded midwives with less than two years of professional experience.

Table 1. Inclusion criteria of midwives participating in this study.

Inclusion Criteria	Description
Catchment area	Rural vs. urban
Education	Professional training vs. bachelor's/master's
Professional experience	15 years + vs. less than 15 years

To recruit suitable interviewees, contact was established with the Associations of Midwifery in Bavaria, Lower Saxony, and North Rhine-Westphalia. With the support of the associations, a call for participation was sent to the midwives who belonged to these associations and put on the websites. Midwives who contacted us were asked about their education and professional experience, as well as the catchment area of their professional activities and were then, if their answers were appropriate, included in our study. Thus, we had an initial sample of midwives, which was completed by subsequent snowballing and personal contacts. Further cold calling was performed in order to recruit midwives working in rural areas as these were underrepresented in the sample (for further details cf. Figure 1).

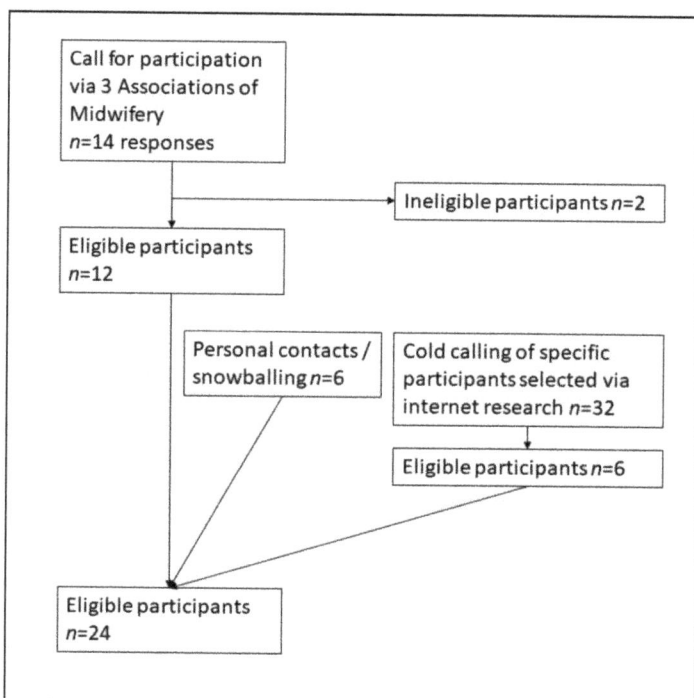

Figure 1. Flowchart of recruiting process.

After conducting 15 interviews, the research team (JvS, EMG, JC) began to discuss the topics and themes in the data to establish whether data saturation had been reached. The researchers agreed after 20 interviews that no more new topics or themes had emerged. Four additional interviews were conducted to ensure data saturation was reached [41].

4. Sample

All of the midwives are female, between 26 and 63 years old, and live in Bavaria (n = 17), North Rhine-Westphalia (n = 1), or Lower Saxony (n = 6). Their professional experience ranges from three to 23 years. Seven midwives in our sample hold a university degree, four have completed special training regarding allergy (prevention), mostly with a focus on breastfeeding. Concerning the catchment areas, 14 interviewees work in villages/small towns (<20,000 inhabitants), ten work in a medium-sized to large town (>20,000 inhabitants) (cf. Table 2).

Table 2. Midwives included in our study.

	Midwives (n = 24)
Catchment area	
Village/small town (<20,000 inhabitants (IN))	14
Medium-sized/large town (>20,000 IN)	10
Education	
Vocational training	17
bachelor's/master's	7
Professional experience	
<10 years	12
>10 years	12

5. Analysis

The duration of the interviews was between 32 and 68 min. A total of 23 interviews were conducted via telephone, and one was conducted face to face. All interviews were audio recorded and transcribed verbatim. Initially, three interviews were jointly discussed and coded by three researchers (JvS, EMG, JC) using ATLAS.ti (v8). Codes were developed deductively, based on the interview guide, and inductively derived from emerging themes in the interview data. After this initial joint coding phase, the rest of the interviews were coded independently by the researcher using the jointly developed codes. Each interview was coded by two researchers. Codes were compared and differences discussed until consensus was reached. This was followed by a thorough and detailed content analysis conducted by the three researchers [42–44]. Themes and overarching topics were identified and enriched with the most pertinent quotes [45]. The study follows the COREQ standard for collecting, preparing, and reporting qualitative research results [46].

6. Informed Consent and Confidentiality, Ethics Approval

The study has received ethical approval from the Ethics Committee of the University of Regensburg (18-1205-101). All information from the study and informed consent documents issued to study participants were approved by the Ethics Committee of the University of Regensburg. Participation in the study was only possible after providing informed consent to the audio recording and scientific use of the interviews.

7. Results

Only five of the midwives interviewed, all of whom held a university degree, were aware of HL as a concept and what it entails. However, although the theoretical concept or the term "health literacy" was not known by many of our interviewees, most of the participating midwives possessed the implicit knowledge and skills needed to identify the HL level and varying information needs of parents.

7.1. Assessment of Parental HL and Knowledge on ECAP

In order to explore how and to what extent midwives assess the ECAP-related HL of parents, we asked them to describe how they assess parental HL and how they take differences into account when counselling families on ECAP. Almost all of the midwives reported that it was important for them to somehow assess the pre-existing knowledge of parents regarding the care of their children. Moreover, they took the parents' ability to absorb new information into account, enabling them to adapt their counselling to the specific needs. The midwives put emphasis on "meeting parents where they are", which they described as a core skill of midwifery.

> *Some want things explained in simple terms, and to others you have to explain or prove everything down to the last comma. I try to convey information in a way that is understandable to them. In other words, I meet them where they are. I don't need to come up with any scientific explanations for someone who is rather "simple-minded". (Int 3)*

Information on parental education and employment is often collected during the anamnesis at the first meeting. Some midwives use this, along with other information, as indicators for parental HL, determining the way information is communicated during their counselling and the level of complexity conveyed.

> *Sometimes you just have to be a bit more scientific [with academics] and can give them more facts about sudden infant death syndrome and allergy prevention than with a cashier, where you say, "It's just good if your child gets breast milk". (Int 12)*

None of the midwives used formal strategies to assess parental HL. Most midwives doubt that formal screening would be helpful and are more of the opinion that it could unsettle parents as it might make them feel as though they are being "tested." The interviewees in our sample preferred to assess parental HL based on their personal "gut feeling", experience, and intuition.

> *This questionnaire stuff . . . I tend to have the feeling that it would take me away from the women. It would become so scientific. They don't want that. It's such a vulnerable time [. . .]. They want to talk a lot. And if you allow that, it's very easy to understand these women and work with them. You know exactly what you have to say and how you can take good care of them. (Int 2)*

All interviewees reported that close personal contact with the mothers and families is the most important prerequisite to assess parental HL and information needs regarding ECAP. During conversations and close interaction with parents, the midwives feel confident in their ability to form an accurate impression of parental HL and information needs on ECAP.

> *So, you quickly realize in a personal conversation, how much information you can give at once. Whether you can do it en bloc or whether you have to convey it in portions. That is individual, always different. Every person is different. And then you always have to see how it is received. Is it understood? How is it implemented? And then you just have to look at it step by step, how is it working? And that's how it's passed on. (Int 16)*

Besides personal contact, visual impressions can also serve to assess parental information needs and HL. Most midwives perform home visits; thus, the midwives receive a visual impression of the family's living environment which helps them estimate parental HL and knowledge on ECAP. Specifically, factors such as cleanliness, the child's sleeping arrangements, visible food and drinks (fruits vs. sweets on the table), accessibility of ashtrays, toys (plastic vs. wood), and pets are considered in the context of assessing ECAP.

> *Of course, there is a pattern. First, when I enter, I observe: Is it clean? Is it tidy or chaotic? What kind of furniture does the person have? How is the person dressed? What*

kind of food, what kind of creams are standing around? These are all things that are subconsciously absorbed. If the baby only wears cotton clothes, then [. . .] you can start on a different level [. . .]. And if, to put it bluntly, you only see plastic toys with a thousand lights and noises and only potato chips and coke, then you have to start off differently. (Int 21)

7.2. Counselling on ECAP: Evidence-Based Knowledge and Support of Parental HL

Most midwives were aware of having a window of opportunity in early childhood to influence the occurrence of allergies by fostering preventive behavior in parents. Some interviewees were convinced that the timing of counselling on ECAP is crucial for effectively reaching parents. They felt it was most helpful to address new parents as early as possible during the first pregnancy, during antenatal counselling, for example, to provide them with more complex evidence-based (ECAP) information, since parents have more resources to absorb and appraise information before the child is born.

It is very, very important that I have these conversations [on ECAP] with them during pregnancy, when the woman is full of anticipation and wants to do everything right anyway. Once the child is born and crying and the mother is going completely crazy, it doesn't really help anymore. It's very important to find a good time during pregnancy when the woman is eager to learn and the partner is hopefully also there. Then you can reach them really well. (Int 15)

I think you actually only have a chance to really reach a first-time mother. A second or third-time mother feeds as she sees fit anyway. (Int 21)

Concerning the midwives' roles as professional health counsellors, the interviewees saw themselves as providers of scientifically sound information on ECAP and other health-related subjects and as such encouraged the parents to trust their advice.

I always say, "I explain everything. If there's anything you don't understand, please ask." I also always tell parents, "Better to ask me before you Google anything on the Internet. I'm the expert. I can answer that for you and I'll try to answer it in a way that you understand". (Int 10)

The midwives in our sample were generally aware that allergies are a chronic disease that can potentially have a significant negative impact on someone's quality of life. There are differences in perceptions of what actually constitutes an allergy though. Some midwives did not consider hay fever an allergy, which became clear when they were asked if they themselves had allergies.

Apart from this, almost all midwives seemed to be aware of current recommendations regarding allergy prevention and knew about the shift in evidence regarding exposure to allergens. However, they reported rarely counselling on ECAP directly. When we asked the midwives whether and how they helped parents to access information on ECAP, most midwives reported that ECAP was not a stand-alone topic for them but was included in the counselling on health behavior in general. The most important issues in the context of allergy prevention are nutrition, especially breastfeeding or choice of formula, the (early) introduction of solid food, hygiene, use of cosmetic products (e.g., cream, detergent, wet wipes), and the avoidance of smoking.

There are a lot of allergic people. And of course, all parents want the best for their child. It [ECAP] definitely comes up in conversations, mostly when talking about breastfeeding versus bottle feeding. If formula is used, the question is what kind of formula is considered best and then it [ECAP] comes up again when solid food is introduced. (Int 22)

Allergy counselling plays a very, very minor role, mostly with people who are already allergic themselves. That's been the case since this allergy guideline changed. I think that the behavior in the case of allergy risk or higher allergy risk is actually identical to the recommendations for people with a low allergy risk, so it's not such a big issue. (Int 19)

The midwives believed that parents found ECAP-related topics easy to understand. Most midwives assumed that the fact that breastfeeding is the best nutrition for children is common knowledge and does not have to be explained scientifically. Their counselling focuses more on how to establish a comfortable breastfeeding situation for mother and child to ensure exclusive breastfeeding for at least four months, without providing any scientific information on why. Similarly, for the introduction of solid foods, the midwives focus their counselling mostly on how to start, what to begin with, and how to continue, and less on the reasons why.

> It [ECAP] automatically resonates in our work, because we advise on breastfeeding, for example. That is God-given allergy prevention. That's why it's always part of our work. And again, when we advise on weaning, it comes quite automatically that you say, okay, start feeding different solid foods in a short time while maintaining the protection of breast milk. (Int 2)

When explicit information on ECAP is provided, most midwives have to help parents appraise this information. Most midwives reported having the impression that they needed to put official guidelines and recommendations into perspective, to encourage parents to see them as a blueprint and not as a rule that needs to be strictly adhered to. For example, even if parents understand that early introduction of solid food might help prevent allergies, the child's readiness to actually eat solids may put constraints on the officially recommended blueprint.

> I try to avoid these blueprints a bit, because I find that most children simply don't eat according to a blueprint. And then the whole text on allergy prevention doesn't help if this child decides it doesn't like vegetables. (Int 9)

Thus, the key message most midwives want to give to parents regarding specific ECAP counselling is to "calm down" and rely on their parental intuition instead of trying to strictly follow evidence-based recommendations. They try to help parents appraise information and thus, make the right choices for themselves and their children.

> I think the most important thing is that they don't get carried away. Instead, they should take a more nuanced look at what information is available and what is really true. And I try to instill a bit of calmness in the parents when it comes to allergy prevention. (Int 14)

> I think it would be much more important to strengthen the women in their skills and abilities, for birth or raising children, because the women simply try too hard to follow blueprints and rules, because they read in a self-help book or because it was done like that in the past. (Int 9)

Most midwives see themselves as advisers, but they prefer to leave the final say in health-related decisions to the parents, at least as long as the decisions are not potentially life threatening for the babies.

> If a woman decides against breastfeeding, then it doesn't help if I say, the probability of allergies occurring is much higher. This doesn't help at all. You can't convert people. (Int 5)

> I emphasize the arguments again, why she should not drink coke. And then I leave it at that. I leave the responsibility to the woman. It is her life, her child, her decision. (Int 20)

Sometimes midwives seek compromises, but rather than taking an exclusively "top-down" approach to educating parents on what is evidence based, they aim at agreeing with parents on pragmatic and actionable recommendations, which take the family situation as well as individual preferences of the child and parents into account.

> And also, when women say they don't want to breastfeed, I say, "That's not a problem at all. That's your decision. But it would be great if we could put the baby to the breast at least once in the delivery room." And no mommy has turned me down yet. (Int 21)

7.3. HL-Sensitive Counselling Techniques and Materials

Health literacy-sensitive counselling techniques can help support parents in accessing, understanding, appraising, and applying information on ECAP, but also regarding health behavior in general. In the interviews it became clear that, even though most midwives are not aware of HL-sensitive counselling techniques as such, HL-supportive strategies are sometimes applied, e.g., using plain language, omission of scientific wording, etc. These interviewees also reported using these techniques not only when talking to parents with lower levels of education, but in general, since, in their experience, parents with newborn children sometimes have difficulties processing information in this challenging phase of life.

> *I really try to avoid medical terms and speak in simple language. [. . .] When I'm in an academic family, it's sometimes quicker for me to just blurt out the medical terms. But even then, if you are a parent yourself, you sometimes can't think straight. No matter what you do for a living. And then it's important that the person advising you simply takes a moment and sits down again and explains it simply, so that everyone understands it.* (Int 18)

Most midwives described the relationship with the families as being based on mutual trust. Due to the close and intimate contact, they assume that most women and families feel comfortable to ask any question they are concerned with. Hence, the midwives do not see the need for special techniques to encourage parents to ask questions.

> *I don't have the impression that parents have any inhibitions about asking me anything.* (Int 10)

Only a few midwives knew about and had tried to apply specific HL-sensitive counselling techniques, such as the teach-back method. However, they emphasized that they had done this subliminally, without the parents noticing.

> *But then I say, "We'll make a plan for breastfeeding. Now we have just discussed it, and now I would like to know how you would do it?" In other words, you don't ask directly, but you do it in a hidden way.* (Int 15)

Some midwives disliked the idea of using teach-back because it appeared too much like an exam situation to them and they feared it would be rejected by the women in their care.

> *You know whether they understood or not. I'm not testing them. I don't want to behave toward the women like a schoolteacher.* (Int 11)

Using visualizations is reported as being helpful in supporting explanations, especially with non-native speakers of German, but ECAP-specific pictograms or similar materials are difficult to obtain. Apart from demonstrating things using models or pictures, some interviewees emphasized that actually performing a task with the parents, or supervising and guiding them, has the biggest effect on parental learning.

> *Now, for example, when it comes to breastfeeding, I have various materials with me. For example, I have little balls that represent the stomach. So I always try to make it very vivid.* (Int 15)

> *A good example is always when the children are crying and I take them in my arms and speak to them in a calm voice. Then you simply practice this with the parents.* (Int 8)

Some midwives felt that written material was valuable as a way of providing parents with information, as, due to tiredness, mothers are sometimes not capable of really absorbing the information when the midwife is present. Written information material can be read in more appropriate moments and thus might be better understood.

> *I have worksheets and I leave those with the mothers, because I know, when you don't get enough sleep, all you hear is "bla bla" and you can't remember what you were told.* (Int 2)

However, most midwives doubted the benefit of handing out written information, as new mothers and families are often overwhelmed by the high amount of information they receive concerning their children.

The women get a lot of information material. I have been working in postnatal care for many years and I know that all this paper stuff is just lying around at home. During the period immediately after birth women are so preoccupied with themselves and the baby that there is very little time to look at brochures, etc. (Int 10)

In conclusion, the interviews revealed that HL-sensitive counselling techniques are applied to some extent, but not in a systematic or deliberate way.

8. Discussion

In the interviews it became clear that most midwives in our sample are not aware of HL as a concept with regard to ECAP. However, the interviewees reported that due to the comprehensive in-home care provided by midwives in Germany before, during, and after birth, their relationship with the parents is often close, thus counselling can be adapted to individual needs. Working with different types of parents was seen by the study participants as a core task of midwifery. However, assessing parental HL and counselling in an HL-sensitive and HL-supportive way is not performed systematically. Personal interaction seems to be the most important factor in establishing a basis for tailor-made counselling on ECAP, frequently supplemented by midwives' impressions of social and educational backgrounds as well as their visual impressions of the living environment.

The study also shows that midwives are aware of the possibility and importance of allergy prevention during the first months of life. They are mostly acquainted with current recommendations regarding ECAP, however, allergy prevention itself is not treated as a stand-alone topic but is mostly covered in counselling on other topics regarding infant care. Midwives consider it their duty to convey scientific information to parents and help them access, understand, appraise, and apply information, but they view their own influence on the prevention of chronic diseases as limited. They try to find compromises between official scientific recommendations and parental wishes and possibilities. Timing is seen as an important factor when it comes to providing effective advice on allergy prevention, with this preferably being done early on during the first pregnancy.

Most midwives are unfamiliar with HL-sensitive counselling techniques; however, some techniques are applied based on counselling experience and "gut feeling". Written information is perceived ambiguously.

A lack of awareness of HL as a concept among health professionals was also found in a systematic review by Rajah et al. on the perspectives of healthcare providers and patients on health literacy: The majority of the 19 studies included in the review reported inadequate knowledge and understanding of HL among health professionals. Rajah et al. also found several studies highlighting that health professionals do not regularly use formal HL assessment tools in their practice, but do use other assessments such as verbal cues, nonverbal cues, and their "gut feelings", which is similar to what was described by the midwives in our sample. The authors of the review also conclude that training of health professionals on HL and HL counselling techniques could help support patients' HL. The results of our study concerning the assessment of parental HL based on "gut feeling" and work experience are also in line with the findings of an Australian survey on how midwives assess maternal HL [47]: Out of 307 study participants, the majority (77.1%, $n = 221$) reported paying limited attention to formally assessing women's health literacy.

In our interviews it became clear that especially when it comes to topics that are assumed to be "easy" to understand, such as breastfeeding or the introduction of solid foods, HL is not something health professionals focus on. This lack of attention devoted to HL might lead to a systematic overestimation of parental HL and thus misunderstandings and, as a result, a lack of knowledge among parents, which is in line with the results of various studies on health professionals [48–51]. For example, Dickens et al. showed that, without using a validated HL screening tool, nurses tend to overestimate patients' HL.

Using the specific measurement tool "Newest Vital Sign" based on a nutrition label and six questions about it, the study showed that 63% of the patients included in the study had a high likelihood of limited HL, whereas nurses only identified 19% as such [49].

The assumption of midwives in our sample that parents are confident enough to ask any questions they have might in some cases also be misleading. Katz et al. showed in their mixed-methods study on patient-physician encounters in a hospital, that patients with a low HL level tend to ask fewer questions and thus might be less informed [52]. The relationship between midwives and families during in-home ante- and postnatal care in our study differs significantly from clinical encounters. That said, the midwives' "gut feelings" might still convey a false impression regarding parents' behavior and their ability to ask questions.

Wilmore et al. drew the same conclusions, but with regard to written material. Other than in Germany, Australian midwives seem to rely more strongly on written information material, which is distributed in the 8–12th week of gestation [53]. The Australian midwives who participated in this study were aware that this information needed to be tailored to the individual parents' needs, or at least needed to be explained according to the HL level of the parents. Similar to our study, Wilmore et al. observed that there was no specific HL screening applied and that midwives were often unaware of their patients' HL and thus not always able to provide enough support to ensure understanding [53].

The midwives in our study see themselves as responsible for supporting parents in preventing chronic health conditions in their children later in life. They also emphasize that they see the time of transition to parenthood, especially during pregnancy, as a window of opportunity for effective health counselling. In line with this, Phelan et al. describe pregnancy as a point of transition in life, which may be a "teachable moment" and as such an opportunity to positively influence health behavior [54]. During a "teachable moment" individuals can be motivated to spontaneously adopt risk-reducing behaviors. It can facilitate promoting a healthier lifestyle, e.g., healthier nutrition behavior to prevent excessive weight gain during pregnancy, but also preventive behavior, e.g., regarding allergy prevention, as women are open to learning about health-related topics during this transitional time of becoming a parent [54].

9. Practical Implications

Midwives might have the opportunity to strengthen families' HL and thus health-related behavior aimed at the prevention of chronic diseases like allergies. In order to enable them to perform HL-sensitive counselling more systematically and effectively, formal education of midwives on HL as a concept and on HL-sensitive counselling techniques would be beneficial.

It is important to convey to them the importance of systematically assessing parental HL to prevent overestimation. Thus, adequate screening instruments or strategies need to be identified and included in the formal education of midwives. Additionally, HL-sensitive counselling techniques should be explained to midwives, and they should be given the opportunity to practice these during their training in order to enable them to adequately counsel all families. Midwives with less than two years of work experience were not included in our study. However, we believe that integrating HL and HL-sensitive counselling into the curriculum of midwifery training would be especially helpful to young health professionals at the start of their careers, because these cannot draw on work experience when counselling parents with different HL levels.

Concerning ECAP, a useful approach would be to provide German midwives with tailor-made, easy-to-access evidence on ECAP and to integrate ECAP as a stand-alone topic in antenatal counselling.

All of these educational measures could strengthen the role of midwives in Germany in preventing chronic diseases by using the window of opportunity in ante- and post-natal care for effective, HL-sensitive preventive counselling.

10. Strengths and Limitations

To our knowledge, this is the first qualitative study with the aim of understanding how German midwives engage in preventive counselling, how they take HL into account, and how they apply HL counselling techniques. It is the nature of qualitative research to draw on a small sample of participants. Therefore, our results cannot be generalized for all German midwives. However, qualitative studies do not claim to produce representative data but are meant to provide an in-depth insight into a specific topic. Our interviews, lasting up to one hour, were very much in depth and enabled us to gain a thorough understanding of the daily working life of midwives. Additionally, we were able to recruit a broad sample of midwives regarding age and experience and could thus capture a wide variety of different perspectives. Moreover, we were able to recruit midwives from different regions of Germany. However, it is not representative for all midwives. We supplemented our initial recruiting via the German Associations of Midwifery in a specific manner, by contacting midwives individually via cold-calling and personal contacts, while considering the criteria for inclusion.

Due to the COVID-19 pandemic, we had to conduct telephone interviews, during which some information might have been lost (e.g., context of interview situation, etc.). However, interviews could be scheduled more flexibly in terms of location and time, which might have facilitated the arrangement and implementation of interviews for the midwives.

We cannot rule out that participants with a special interest in ECAP and HL might have been more willing to participate in such a time-consuming interview study. Therefore, the interviewees were possibly better informed on ECAP or more aware of HL than the average German midwife and might have focused more on HL-sensitive counselling than others. Another limitation also concerns the sample: the educational level of the participants was fairly high, with 7 out of 24 midwives holding a university degree in subjects which go beyond "classic" midwifery, e.g., nursing science. This may indicate a strong interest in topics which lie beyond their daily work as midwives.

11. Conclusions

Midwives are health professionals who support families at a vulnerable and transitional time. As they are close to families, they may have an impact on the prevention of chronic diseases, like allergies, and preventive health behavior in general. They have the opportunity to enhance parents' HL and thus to empower them to make informed choices on preventive behavior for their children. The midwives included in the sample of our qualitative study were mostly unaware of the concept of HL, formal screening strategies for parental HL, and HL-sensitive counselling techniques. This would suggest that further research on HL-sensitive counselling on ECAP on a larger scale is needed, in order to assess midwives' awareness of the relevance of HL and their routine application of HL-sensitive counselling techniques in a broader, representative sample. Results of such future research could provide the basis for an intervention aimed at strengthening the HL-sensitive counselling capabilities of midwives in the prevention of allergies and other chronic diseases.

Author Contributions: J.C. developed the concept and design of the study. J.v.S., E.-M.G. and J.C. developed the interview guide, J.v.S. and E.-M.G. conducted the interviews, J.v.S., E.-M.G. and J.C. analyzed and interpreted the data. J.v.S. drafted and finalized the manuscript. J.C. contributed to and supported the writing of the manuscript. All authors have read and agreed to the published version of the manuscript.

Funding: This research study is funded by the German Research Foundation (DFG, grant number: FOR 2959 CU 438/1-1) and is a sub-project of the HELICAP Research Group on ECAP-related HL (www.helicap.org, accessed on 1 March 2022).

Institutional Review Board Statement: The Ethics Committee of the Medical Faculty of the University of Regensburg approved this study (18-1205-101).

Informed Consent Statement: Written consent was obtained from all study participants in accordance with the ethics approval. Participation was voluntary. Financial incentives for participation were offered.

Data Availability Statement: The data presented in this study are available on request from the corresponding author. The data are not publicly available due to the need to preserve the anonymity of the interview partners.

Acknowledgments: We would like to thank all of our interview partners for sharing their insights and experiences with us.

Conflicts of Interest: The authors declare that they have no competing interests.

Appendix A. Interview Guide

Interview guide for midwives on ECAP and health literacy
Topics/questions:
Introduction

1. How is early childhood allergy prevention relevant in your routine counselling?
    a. When and with whom do you address this topic?
    b. What is the most important message you want to convey to parents concerning allergy prevention? Do you make a difference between low- and high-risk groups?
    c. Which topics also matter in your counselling on early childhood allergy prevention (prompts: e.g., nutrition, living environment, early exposure to allergens)?

Information and evidence

1. What are your main sources to keep yourself informed about health topics (especially allergy prevention)?
2. Are you satisfied with the available information?
    a. Do you feel well informed? Why? Why not?
    b. Is there anything that would help to keep up to date?
3. How do you handle inconsistent and changing information? (e.g., avoidance of allergens vs. early confrontation with allergens)
    a. How did/do you feel about a key message of your consultation changing due to new research findings?

Knowledge Translation and implementation

1. We have just talked about how you keep yourself up to date on health-related recommendations: What are you doing with this knowledge (in your head) to make it applicable/use it for your practice?
2. How do you incorporate this knowledge into your daily work?
    a. Do you pass on specific scientific information to your patients (on ECAP)?
        i. If yes, could you give an example of how you pass on this information to your patients?
        ii. What helps you to pass on your knowledge to parents?
3. Is there anything that could be improved to facilitate health-related counselling of parents?

Promotion of health literacy

A. *Counselling of parents and health literacy*
    1. How do you deal with different patients (e.g., level of knowledge, education, migration background) in counselling and transfer of knowledge? Do you differentiate? Could you give an example?
    2. How do you assess the level of knowledge and information demand of parents?

a. How do you notice that you have to explain a lot/in a way that is easy to understand?
b. Do you consciously use strategies to assess what kind of information and support needs parents have? If yes, which ones do you use?
3. Do you think parents are well informed regarding allergy prevention? How do you recognize that?
4. What previous knowledge or lay conceptions do parents bring up in counselling?
5. What opportunities do you see to support parents regarding the access to information and appraising it? Could you give some examples from your everyday practice?
6. Do you provide your patients with information sources so they can inform themselves about health topics (e.g., allergy prevention)? Which sources do you consider (not) helpful?
7. Do you use certain strategies during counselling to make sure the parents understand everything? (e.g., simple language, avoidance of special language, drawing pictures, teach-back etc.) Do you encourage parents to ask questions? How?
8. How do you ensure that parents apply your health behavior recommendations?

B. *Attitudes towards and experiences with health literacy/health literacy-sensitive care.*
1. How well do you feel educated/trained to counsel your patients according to their (information) needs?
2. Do you personally see a need of further information/training on the issues we have talked about? If yes, what would be important topics to you?
3. How should academic results/recommendations be prepared and made available so that you can use them efficiently in consultations?

HL concept awareness
1. Have you heard of the term "health literacy" in the context of your work or in advanced training courses?

References

1. Sørensen, K.; van den Broucke, S.; Fullam, J.; Doyle, G.; Pelikan, J.; Slonska, Z.; Brand, H. Health literacy and public health: A systematic review and integration of definitions and models. *BMC Public Health* **2012**, *12*, 80. [CrossRef] [PubMed]
2. Bitzer, E.M.; Sørensen, K. Gesundheitskompetenz—Health Literacy. *Gesundheitswesen* **2018**, *80*, 754–766. [CrossRef] [PubMed]
3. Berkman, N.D.; Sheridan, S.L.; Donahue, K.E.; Halpern, D.J.; Crotty, K. Low health literacy and health outcomes: An updated systematic review. *Ann. Intern. Med.* **2011**, *155*, 97–107. [CrossRef] [PubMed]
4. Kickbusch, I.; Pelikan, J.M.; Apfel, F.; Tsouros, A.D. *Health Literacy: The Solid Facts*; World Health Organization: Copenhagen, Denmark, 2013.
5. Fernandez, D.M.; Larson, J.L.; Zikmund-Fisher, B.J. Associations between health literacy and preventive health behaviors among older adults: Findings from the health and retirement study. *BMC Public Health* **2016**, *16*, 596. [CrossRef]
6. Shaker, M.S.; Schwartz, J.; Ferguson, M. An update on the impact of food allergy on anxiety and quality of life. *Curr. Opin. Pediatr.* **2017**, *29*, 497–502. [CrossRef]
7. Blaiss, M.S.; Hammerby, E.; Robinson, S.; Kennedy-Martin, T.; Buchs, S. The burden of allergic rhinitis and allergic rhinoconjunctivitis on adolescents: A literature review. *Ann. Allergy Asthma Immunol.* **2018**, *121*, 43–52.e3. [CrossRef]
8. Peters, R.L.; Koplin, J.J.; Gurrin, L.C.; Dharmage, S.C.; Wake, M.; Ponsonby, A.-L.; Tang, M.L.K.; Lowe, A.J.; Matheson, M.C.; Dwyer, T.; et al. The prevalence of food allergy and other allergic diseases in early childhood in a population-based study: HealthNuts age 4-year follow-up. *J. Allergy Clin. Immunol.* **2017**, *140*, 145–153.e8. [CrossRef]
9. Asher, M.I.; Montefort, S.; Björkstén, B.; Lai, C.K.W.; Strachan, D.P.; Weiland, S.K.; Williams, H.; ISAAC Phase Three Study Group. Worldwide time trends in the prevalence of symptoms of asthma, allergic rhinoconjunctivitis, and eczema in childhood: ISAAC Phases One and Three repeat multicountry cross-sectional surveys. *Lancet* **2006**, *368*, 733–743. [CrossRef]
10. Jarosz, M.; Syed, S.; Błachut, M.; Badura Brzoza, K. Emotional distress and quality of life in allergic diseases. *Wiad Lek* **2020**, *73*, 370–373. [CrossRef]
11. Caffarelli, C.; Di Mauro, D.; Mastrorilli, C.; Bottau, P.; Cipriani, F.; Ricci, G. Solid Food Introduction and the Development of Food Allergies. *Nutrients* **2018**, *10*, 1790. [CrossRef]
12. Schäfer, T.; Bauer, C.-P.; Beyer, K.; Bufe, A.; Friedrichs, F.; Gieler, U.; Gronke, G.; Hamelmann, E.; Hellermann, M.; Kleinheinz, A.; et al. S3-Guideline on allergy prevention: 2014 update: Guideline of the German Society for Allergology and

Clinical Immunology (DGAKI) and the German Society for Pediatric and Adolescent Medicine (DGKJ). *Allergo J. Int.* **2014**, *23*, 186–199. [CrossRef]
13. Waggoner, M.R. Parsing the peanut panic: The social life of a contested food allergy epidemic. *Soc. Sci. Med.* **2013**, *90*, 49–55. [CrossRef]
14. Colver, A. Are the dangers of childhood food allergy exaggerated? *BMJ* **2006**, *333*, 494–496. [CrossRef]
15. Shenker, N.S. The resurgent influence of big formula. *BMJ* **2018**, *362*, k3577. [CrossRef]
16. Gharachourlo, M.; Mahmoodi, Z.; Akbari Kamrani, M.; Tehranizadeh, M.; Kabir, K. The effect of a health literacy approach to counselling on the lifestyle of women with gestational diabetes: A clinical trial. *F1000Research* **2018**, *7*, 282. [CrossRef]
17. Nawabi, F.; Krebs, F.; Vennedey, V.; Shukri, A.; Lorenz, L.; Stock, S. Health Literacy in Pregnant Women: A Systematic Review. *Int. J. Environ. Res. Public Health* **2021**, *18*, 3847. [CrossRef]
18. Dennis, S.; Williams, A.; Taggart, J.; Newall, A.; Denney-Wilson, E.; Zwar, N.; Shortus, T.; Harris, M.F. Which providers can bridge the health literacy gap in lifestyle risk factor modification education: A systematic review and narrative synthesis. *BMC Fam. Pract.* **2012**, *13*, 44. [CrossRef]
19. Berni Canani, R.; Leone, L.; D'Auria, E.; Riva, E.; Nocerino, R.; Ruotolo, S.; Terrin, G.; Cosenza, L.; Di Costanzo, M.; Passariello, A.; et al. The effects of dietary counseling on children with food allergy: A prospective, multicenter intervention study. *J. Acad. Nutr. Diet* **2014**, *114*, 1432–1439. [CrossRef]
20. Gagliardi, A.R.; Abdallah, F.; Faulkner, G.; Ciliska, D.; Hicks, A. Factors contributing to the effectiveness of physical activity counselling in primary care: A realist systematic review. *Patient Educ. Couns.* **2015**, *98*, 412–419. [CrossRef]
21. Jenssen, B.P.; Bryant-Stephens, T.; Leone, F.T.; Grundmeier, R.W.; Fiks, A.G. Clinical Decision Support Tool for Parental Tobacco Treatment in Primary Care. *Pediatrics* **2016**, *137*, e20154185. [CrossRef]
22. Stevens, Z.; Barlow, C.; Kendrick, D.; Masud, T.; Skelton, D.A.; Dinan-Young, S.; Iliffe, S. Effectiveness of general practice-based physical activity promotion for older adults: Systematic review. *Prim. Health Care Res. Dev.* **2014**, *15*, 190–201. [CrossRef]
23. Farmanova, E.; Bonneville, L.; Bouchard, L. Organizational Health Literacy: Review of Theories, Frameworks, Guides, and Implementation Issues. *Inquiry* **2018**, *55*, 46958018757848. [CrossRef]
24. Brach, C.; Keller, D.; Hernandez, L.; Baur, C.; Parker, R.; Dreyer, B.; Schyve, P.; Lemerise, A.J.; Schillinger, D. Ten Attributes of Health Literate Health Care Organizations. *NAM Perspect.* **2012**, *2*, 1–27. [CrossRef]
25. Allenbaugh, J.; Spagnoletti, C.L.; Rack, L.; Rubio, D.; Corbelli, J. Health Literacy and Clear Bedside Communication: A Curricular Intervention for Internal Medicine Physicians and Medicine Nurses. *MedEdPORTAL* **2019**, *15*, 10795. [CrossRef]
26. Badaczewski, A.; Bauman, L.J.; Blank, A.E.; Dreyer, B.; Abrams, M.A.; Stein, R.E.K.; Roter, D.L.; Hossain, J.; Byck, H.; Sharif, I. Relationship between Teach-back and patient-centered communication in primary care pediatric encounters. *Patient Educ. Couns.* **2017**, *100*, 1345–1352. [CrossRef]
27. Coleman, C.; Hudson, S.; Pederson, B. Prioritized Health Literacy and Clear Communication Practices For Health Care Professionals. *Health Lit. Res. Pract.* **2017**, *1*, e91–e99. [CrossRef]
28. Vamos, C.A.; Thompson, E.L.; Griner, S.B.; Liggett, L.G.; Daley, E.M. Applying Organizational Health Literacy to Maternal and Child Health. *Matern. Child Health J.* **2019**, *23*, 597–602. [CrossRef]
29. De Walt, D.A.; Hink, A. Health literacy and child health outcomes: A systematic review of the literature. *Pediatrics* **2009**, *124* (Suppl. 3), S265–S274. [CrossRef]
30. DeWalt, D.A.; Dilling, M.H.; Rosenthal, M.S.; Pignone, M.P. Low parental literacy is associated with worse asthma care measures in children. *Ambul. Pediatr.* **2007**, *7*, 25–31. [CrossRef]
31. Stafford, J.D.; Goggins, E.R.; Lathrop, E.; Haddad, L.B. Health Literacy and Associated Outcomes in the Postpartum Period at Grady Memorial Hospital. *Matern. Child Health J.* **2021**, *25*, 599–605. [CrossRef]
32. Gagnon, A.J.; Sandall, J. Individual or group antenatal education for childbirth or parenthood, or both. *Cochrane Database Syst. Rev.* **2007**, *3*, CD002869. [CrossRef] [PubMed]
33. Venter, C.; Clayton, B.; Dean, T. Infant nutrition part 2: The midwife's role in allergy prevention. *Br. J. Midwifery* **2008**, *16*, 791–803. [CrossRef]
34. BZgA. Hebammenbetreuung—Ihr Gutes Recht | kindergesundheit-Info.de. 2021. Available online: https://www.kindergesundheit-info.de/themen/ernaehrung/0-12-monate/hebammenbetreuung/ (accessed on 1 October 2021).
35. Sander, M.; Albrecht, M.; Loos, S.; Stengel, V. Studie zur Hebammenversorgung im Freistaat Bayern. 2018. Available online: https://www.stmgp.bayern.de/meine-themen/fuer-hebammen-und-entbindungspfleger/ (accessed on 1 March 2022).
36. Wilhelmova, R.; Hruba, D.; Vesela, L. Key Determinants Influencing the Health Literacy of Pregnant Women in the Czech Republic. *Zdr. Varst.* **2015**, *54*, 27–36. [CrossRef] [PubMed]
37. Royal, C.; Gray, C. Allergy Prevention: An Overview of Current Evidence. *Yale J. Biol. Med.* **2020**, *93*, 689–698. [PubMed]
38. Ritchie, J. (Ed.) *Qualitative Research Practice: A Guide for Social Science Students and Researchers*; SAGE: Los Angeles, CA, USA, 2011.
39. Mays, N.; Pope, C. Rigour and qualitative research. *BMJ* **1995**, *311*, 109–112. [CrossRef]
40. Palinkas, L.A.; Horwitz, S.M.; Green, C.A.; Wisdom, J.P.; Duan, N.; Hoagwood, K. Purposeful Sampling for Qualitative Data Collection and Analysis in Mixed Method Implementation Research. *Adm. Policy Ment. Health* **2015**, *42*, 533–544. [CrossRef]
41. Saunders, B.; Sim, J.; Kingstone, T.; Baker, S.; Waterfield, J.; Bartlam, B.; Burroughs, H.; Jinks, C. Saturation in qualitative research: Exploring its conceptualization and operationalization. *Qual. Quant.* **2018**, *52*, 1893–1907. [CrossRef]

42. Mayring, P. Qualitative Content Analysis: Theoretical Foundation, Basic Procedures and Software Solution. 2014. Available online: https://nbn-resolving.org/urn:nbn:de:0168-ssoar-395173 (accessed on 31 January 2022).
43. Schreier, M. *Qualitative Content Analysis in Practice*; SAGE: London, UK, 2012.
44. Kuckartz, U. *Qualitative Inhaltsanalyse. Methoden, Praxis, Computerunterstützung*, 4th ed.; Beltz Juventa: Weinheim, Germany; Basel, Switzerland, 2018.
45. Patton, M.Q. *Qualitative Research & Evaluation Methods*, 3rd ed.; SAGE: Thousand Oaks, CA, USA, 2009.
46. Tong, A.; Sainsbury, P.; Craig, J. Consolidated criteria for reporting qualitative research (COREQ): A 32-item checklist for interviews and focus groups. *Int. J. Qual. Health Care* **2007**, *19*, 349–357. [CrossRef]
47. Creedy, D.K.; Gamble, J.; Boorman, R.; Allen, J. Midwives' self-reported knowledge and skills to assess and promote maternal health literacy: A national cross-sectional survey. *Women Birth* **2020**, *34*, e188–e195. [CrossRef]
48. Bass, P.F.; Wilson, J.F.; Griffith, C.H.; Barnett, D.R. Residents' ability to identify patients with poor literacy skills. *Acad. Med.* **2002**, *77*, 1039–1041. [CrossRef]
49. Dickens, C.; Lambert, B.L.; Cromwell, T.; Piano, M.R. Nurse overestimation of patients' health literacy. *J. Health Commun.* **2013**, *18* (Suppl. 1), 62–69. [CrossRef]
50. Safeer, R.S.; Keenan, J. Health Literacy: The Gap between Physicians and Patients. *AFP* **2005**, *72*, 463–468. Available online: https://www.aafp.org/afp/2005/0801/p463.html (accessed on 1 March 2022).
51. Rogers, E.S.; Wallace, L.S.; Weiss, B.D. Misperceptions of medical understanding in low-literacy patients: Implications for cancer prevention. *Cancer Control* **2006**, *13*, 225–229. [CrossRef]
52. Katz, M.G.; Jacobson, T.A.; Veledar, E.; Kripalani, S. Patient literacy and question-asking behavior during the medical encounter: A mixed-methods analysis. *J. Gen. Intern. Med.* **2007**, *22*, 782–786. [CrossRef]
53. Wilmore, M.; Rodger, D.; Humphreys, S.; Clifton, V.L.; Dalton, J.; Flabouris, M.; Skuse, A. How midwives tailor health information used in antenatal care. *Midwifery* **2015**, *31*, 74–79. [CrossRef]
54. Phelan, S. Pregnancy: A "teachable moment" for weight control and obesity prevention. *Am. J. Obstet. Gynecol.* **2010**, *202*, 135.e1–135.e8. [CrossRef]

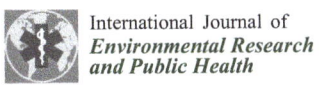

Article

Organizational Health Literacy in a Hospital—Insights on the Patients' Perspective

Johanna Sophie Lubasch [1,*], Mona Voigt-Barbarowicz [1], Nicole Ernstmann [2], Christoph Kowalski [3], Anna Levke Brütt [1] and Lena Ansmann [1]

1 Department of Health Services Research, University of Oldenburg, 26129 Oldenburg, Germany; mona.voigt-barbarowicz@uol.de (M.V.-B.); anna.levke.bruett@uol.de (A.L.B.); lena.ansmann@uol.de (L.A.)
2 Center for Health Communication and Health Services Research (CHSR), Department of Psychosomatic Medicine and Psychotherapy, University Hospital Bonn, 53127 Bonn, Germany; nicole.ernstmann@ukbonn.de
3 German Cancer Society (DKG), 14057 Berlin, Germany; kowalski@krebsgesellschaft.de
* Correspondence: johanna.lubasch@uol.de; Tel.: +49-441-798-4606

Abstract: Health literacy-sensitive communication has been found to be an important dimension of organizational health literacy measured from the patients' perspective. Little is known about the role of health literacy-sensitive communication in complex care structures. Therefore, our aim was to assess which hospital characteristics (in terms of process organization) and patient characteristics (e.g., age, chronic illness, etc.) contribute to better perceptions of health literacy-sensitive communication, as well as whether better health literacy-sensitive communication is associated with better patient reported experiences. Data were derived from a patient survey conducted in 2020 in four clinical departments of a university hospital in Germany. Health literacy-sensitive communication was measured with the HL-COM scale. Data from 209 patients (response rate 24.2%) were analyzed with a structural equation model (SEM). Results revealed that no patient characteristics were associated with HL-COM scores. Better process organization as perceived by patients was associated with significantly better HL-COM scores, and, in turn, better HL-COM scores were associated with more patient-reported social support provided by physicians and nurses as well as fewer unmet information needs. Investing into good process organization might improve health literacy-sensitive communication, which in turn has the potential to foster the patient–provider relationship as well as to reduce unmet information needs of patients.

Keywords: health literacy-sensitive communication; patient–professional relationship; HL-COM; information needs; patient survey

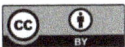

1. Introduction

The multidimensional concept of health literacy was originally developed in the 1970s [1]. It has gained increased attention ever since the U.S. Department of Education released a report in 1993 showing that a high percentage of the country's adult population may have insufficient literacy skills to understand written information needed to engage in health-related activity [2]. Congruent with this finding, the European Health Literacy Survey (HLS-EU) involving eight EU member states revealed that a high percentage of the population did not have adequate health literacy [3]. It defined individual health literacy as "[. . .] people's knowledge, motivation and competences to access, understand, appraise, and apply health information in order to make judgments and take decisions in everyday life concerning healthcare, disease prevention and health promotion to maintain or improve quality of life during the life course" [4]. In Germany, several initiatives aiming to strengthen health literacy in the population stress the importance of individual skills and abilities in searching, understanding, evaluating, and applying health-relevant information [5,6].

In recent decades, an increase of studies concerning individual health literacy can be observed; these studies have investigated the associations between health literacy and health outcomes [7], health literacy of patients with different diseases [8–10], health literacy of different patient groups [11,12], health literacy interventions [13,14] and health literacy assessment tools [15]. Studies revealed that low health literacy was associated with higher hospitalization rates, greater use of emergency care, lower preventive health care use (e.g., cancer screening or vaccination) as well as an unhealthy lifestyle (e.g., physical activity), and poorer health behavior (e.g., medication adherence and self-management skills) [7,16–20]. Low socioeconomic status (SES), migration background, and older age were found to be associated with lower health literacy levels [21–26]. Moreover, considering that chronic conditions require a high degree of self-management [27,28] and that the ability for self-management may be impaired when health literacy is low [16,17,20], improving health literacy clearly has the potential to prevent the development of chronic diseases, or at least the occurrence of comorbidities [17,29], and to reduce the associated burdens. In line with this idea, previous results show that fostering health literacy could contribute to lower healthcare costs [30].

1.1. Concept of Organizational Health Literacy

Beyond the individual-based definition—of finding, understanding, evaluating, and applying health information [4]—health literacy is now understood to be a much more complex construct. Attention has shifted to the specific context in which health care is delivered, since health literacy involves the interaction with health services and other societal institutions [22]. Thus, patients' ability to understand medical information and navigate the care process is associated with the demands placed on them by the health care system [31–33]. In this process, the specific organizational context in which care is delivered can help to compensate for patients' limited health literacy [31]. Health literacy is therefore currently considered to be the product of the interaction between individuals' capabilities and the health literacy demands and complexities of the health care system [34]. To characterize and assess organizational conditions and efforts to help patients navigate the system, the concept of health literate health care organizations—also known as organizational health literacy—has emerged [35]. Brach et al. [35] defined the following ten attributes of health literate healthcare organizations:

1. Has leadership that makes health literacy integral to its mission, structure, and operations.
2. Integrates health literacy into planning, evaluation measures, patient safety, and quality improvement.
3. Prepares the workforce to be health literate and monitors progress.
4. Includes populations served in the design, implementation, and evaluation of health information and services.
5. Meets the needs of populations with a range of health literacy skills while avoiding stigmatization.
6. Uses health literacy strategies in interpersonal communications and confirms understanding at all points of contact.
7. Provides easy access to health information and services and navigation assistance.
8. Designs and distributes print, audiovisual, and social media content that is easy to understand and act on.
9. Addresses health literacy in high-risk situations, including care transitions and communications about medicines.
10. Communicates clearly what health plans cover and what individuals will have to pay for services.

1.2. Organizational Health Literacy in Hospitals

The results of previous publications indicate that the ten attributes defined by Brach et al. [35] are implemented by hospitals with varying degrees of success [36–38].

Moreover, previous results show that organizational health literacy scores vary by hospital ownership [37,38]. However, the results remain inconclusive as to whether scores are highest in private [37,39] or university hospitals [38]. The results of the validation study of the health literate health care organization ten item questionnaire (HLHO-10) from Kowalski et al. [40] revealed that organizational health literacy is associated with the patients' perception of having received adequate information during their hospital stay. In other studies, associations were found between HLHO-10 scores and patient satisfaction [39] as well as the healthcare professionals' (HCP) perception of the quality of care [37]. All things considered, research on basic correlations with organizational health literacy in hospitals is limited, whereas many studies focus on interventions to foster organizational health literacy in hospitals.

1.3. Interventions, Barriers, and Facilitators of Organizational Health Literacy in Hospitals

Studies on interventions for fostering organizational health literacy predominantly focus on interventions supporting patients, e.g., through materials (e.g., informative flyers or brochures) or through digital support (e.g., apps) improving patient education or access to health information [41]. Other studies evaluated the effect of interventions targeting hospital staff, such as communication training, and further studies examined the effect of interventions supporting hospital governance (e.g., development and use of organizational health literacy tools) [41]. The successful implementation of organizational health literacy was found to be associated with organizational and institutional culture and leadership (e.g., priority of and commitment to health literacy), the design of the intervention (e.g., having change champions or procedures, policies, and protocols supporting health-literate practice), and available resources (e.g., time and money) [42–44]. Moreover, organizational health literacy was found to be fostered by high staff awareness, by knowledge and skills concerning organizational health literacy, and by the sharing of responsibilities for measures concerning organizational health literacy and practices across multiple people in the organization (e.g., using frameworks or guides) [42,45]. What has also proven to be beneficial is to tailor the intervention specifically to the needs of the organization, and to use appropriate tools for baseline assessments of current practice to inform gaps in organizational health literacy as well as for monitoring processes during implementation [45–47].

Tools assessing organizational health literacy are predominantly designed to be assessed by HCPs or key informants of hospitals [40,48,49]. To also allow taking the patient perspective into account, Ernstmann et al. [50] developed a scale for measuring aspects of organizational health literacy from the patients' perspective, namely the HL-COM scale. The development phase of the scale entailed theoretical work, during which an item pool based on the ten attributes of organizational health literacy by Brach et al. [35] was generated. However, the subsequent item prioritization by cancer patients and psychometric testing resulted in a reduced item pool measuring health literacy-sensitive communication (HL-COM) as a subdimension of organizational health literacy that can be assessed by and seems to be relevant for patients [50]. Through the items, patients assess factors, such as whether they were asked if they understood information or documents, whether they were encouraged to ask questions, or whether it was ensured that they understood consent forms they signed. The HL-COM thereby measures an important aspect of organizational health literacy from the patients' perspective. In the validation study, the instrument was found to be associated with patient enablement [50].

1.4. Research Question

Organizational health literacy can help to compensate for patients' limited individual health literacy. For patients, health literacy-sensitive communication was found to be the most salient dimension of organizational health literacy that can be assessed by them [50]. Therefore, fostering health literacy-sensitive communication could potentially help to improve organizational as well as individual health literacy. However, to our knowledge, little is known about the factors influencing health literacy-sensitive communication in hospitals or about the effect of good health literacy-sensitive communication on other outputs of healthcare in hospitals. Therefore, the aim of our study was to assess which factors might contribute to better perceptions of health literacy-sensitive communication, as well as whether better health literacy-sensitive communication is associated with better patient reported experiences.

The factors that our analysis model (see Figure 1) assumed to have an impact on health literacy-sensitive communication were selected based on the communication framework of Feldman-Stewart et al. [51]. This framework emphasizes that patient–professional communication is influenced by individual characteristics of the interacting persons as well as by the environment in which it takes place. The individual characteristics were chosen according to the characteristics that have been found to be associated to individual health literacy, namely education, migration background, age, and number of chronic diseases [17,21–26,29] (see Figure 1). Moreover, we assumed that individual health literacy itself might have an impact on health literacy-sensitive communication. As an environmental factor, process organization (e.g., coordination between wards as well as professions or waiting times) was assessed since it has already been found to be associated with patient–professional interaction in hospitals [52,53]. Previous studies assumed that professionals working in hospitals with worse process organization have fewer resources available for adequate interaction with their patients [53]. Our research questions were the following:

1. Are individual patient characteristics, in terms of education, migration background, age, number of chronic diseases, and individual health literacy associated with the patients' perception of health literacy-sensitive communication?
2. Is the hospital's process organization as perceived by patients associated with health literacy-sensitive communication?

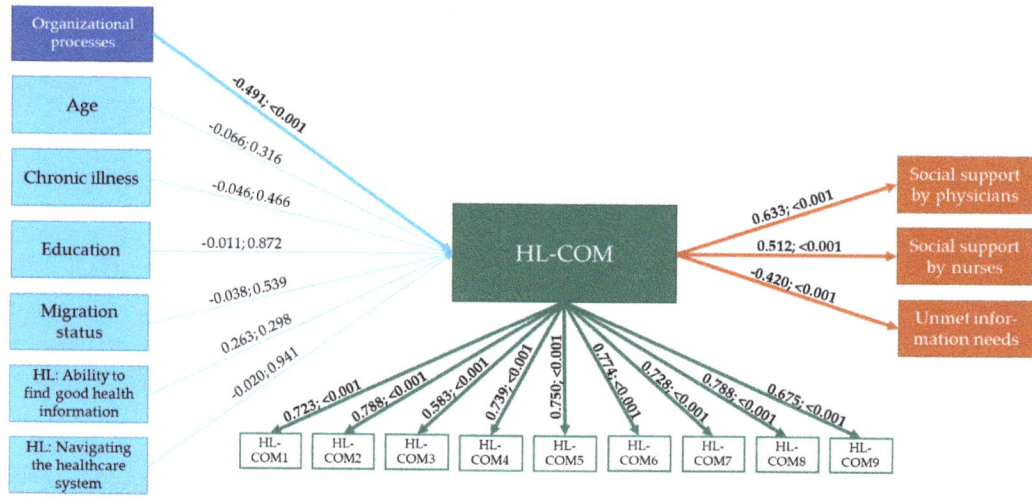

Figure 1. Results of the structural equation model with standardized model estimates and p-values.

The factors that our analysis model (see Figure 1) assumed to be influenced by health literacy-sensitive communication were selected based on the results of previous publications. On the one hand, the literature revealed that good patient–professional communication was key for the patient–professional-relationship [54], and that providing the patient with information fosters a supportive patient–professional relationship [55]. In our model, we therefore assumed that the provision of social support—as part of the patient–professional relationship—might be associated with health literacy-sensitive communication. On the other hand, previous publications revealed that organizational health literacy was associated with the adequacy of information patients received during their hospital stay [40]. We therefore assumed that health literacy-sensitive communication might improve the provision of health information. This resulted in the following research questions:

3. Is health literacy-sensitive communication associated with social support provided by physicians and nurses?
4. Is health literacy-sensitive communication associated with unmet information needs of patients?

2. Materials and Methods

Data were collected within the PIKoG study 'As made for us—Improving professional health literacy in hospitals' [56]. The study aims at co-designing, implementing, and evaluating a communication concept for clinical departments of a hospital. The communication concept was developed to improve health literacy at the levels of the healthcare organization, healthcare professionals, and patients. For our analysis, we used data from a patient survey conducted in 2020 prior to the implementation of the communication concept.

2.1. Study Site

The study was conducted in acute inpatient care at a university hospital. This non-profit general hospital in north-western Germany offers approximately 400 beds. Four out of eleven clinical departments of this hospital (oncology, gynecology, orthopedics, and visceral surgery) participated in the study.

2.2. Sample

Patients were eligible for inclusion in the study if they were: (1) older than 18 years of age, (2) hospitalized for at least two nights in one of the four participating clinical departments, and (3) able to fill in the questionnaires in one of the available languages (i.e., German, English, Russian, Turkish, or Polish), either alone or with the support of a friend or relative. Moreover, the study team offered help with filling in the questionnaire to facilitate the participation of illiterate or semi-literate patients. Of 2049 eligible patients, 897 patients were asked to participate in the defined period, 473 consented to participate in the study, and 217 returned T0 and T1 questionnaires (response rate: 24.2%). Thereof, 209 completed all items relevant for the present analysis.

2.3. Recruitment

On their day of admission, patients treated as inpatients in the clinical departments in September through December 2020 were asked to participate in the study. Patients who had given verbal consent were provided with written study information, a consent form, and the questionnaire. Participants were asked to return the completed consent form with the address sheet and the questionnaire in sealable envelopes to mailboxes in the hospital. All patients were surveyed twice: at hospital admission (T0) and at hospital discharge (T1). Sociodemographic data as well as individual health literacy scores were assessed at T0. Data on health literacy-sensitive communication were assessed at T1. The T1 questionnaire was sent to the participants' home address after their discharge or—if possible—handed to them in the hospital on the day of discharge. Participants were reminded to return the questionnaire twice, according to Dillman's method [57].

2.4. Measures

Patient data were collected with questionnaires. Quality assurance during study execution was safeguarded by the standards of questionnaire development [58,59], pretesting [60], and data processing with the Teleform® software (Version 16.5.1, Electric Paper Informationssysteme GmbH, Lueneburg, Germany).

Health literacy-sensitive communication was assessed using the validated questionnaire HL-COM [50]. The HL-COM consists of 9 items rated on a four-point Likert scale ranging from 1 ('I disagree') to 4 ('I fully agree') (Cronbachs' alpha = 0.911) [50] (for all items, see Table 1). The scale was calculated if at least 70% of items (6 items) were answered by summing up all item scores and dividing them by the number of answered items. Higher values on the HL-COM scale indicate better health literacy-sensitive communication.

Table 1. Items of HL-COM and frequency of response options.

Item	Content		Response Options [1]				Mean Score
			1	2	3	4	
HL-COM1	I was made to feel that it is important for me to understand the information about my disease and treatment.	n [a] %	9 4.3	31 14.8	113 54.1	53 25.4	3.03
HL-COM2	I was asked if I understood all information or documents.	n [a] %	12 5.7	47 22.5	85 40.7	64 31.6	2.96
HL-COM3	Verbal information about my disease and treatment was additionally provided in writing.	n [a] %	25 12.0	47 22.5	67 32.1	68 32.5	2.86
HL-COM4	Terms and abbreviations were explained to me.	n [a] %	18 8.6	50 23.9	99 47.4	41 19.6	2.78
HL-COM5	People spoke slowly and clearly to me.	n [a] %	5 2.4	27 12.9	94 45.0	82 39.2	3.21
HL-COM6	I was encouraged to ask questions if I didn't understand something.	n [a] %	10 4.8	53 25.4	78 37.3	67 32.1	2.97
HL-COM7	Written materials were additionally explained to me.	n [a] %	15 7.2	54 25.8	94 45.0	43 20.6	2.81
HL-COM8	When signing consent forms, efforts were made to ensure that I understood everything.	n [a] %	6 2.9	40 19.1	92 44.0	68 32.5	3.08
HL-COM9	My results were explained comprehensively to me.	n [a] %	6 2.9	37 17.7	96 45.9	68 32.5	3.09

[1] 1: I disagree, 2: I somewhat disagree, 3: I somewhat agree, 4: I fully agree. [a] Summation of the number of respondents for each item might not equal to 209 since some patients had missing values on single items. The scale was calculated if at least 70% of items (6 items) were answered.

The following sociodemographic and disease-related patient characteristics were collected: sex, age group, education, employment situation, type of health insurance, migration background, chronic diseases, diagnosis, and length of hospital stay. The clinical department in which the patient was treated was derived from the patient's medical record.

The general health literacy of patients was measured using the German version of the Health Literacy Questionnaire (HLQ) [61,62]. It consists of 44 items (sample item 'I make plans for what I need to do to be healthy') in 9 subscales: feeling understood and supported by healthcare providers (4 items, Cronbachs' alpha = 0.805); having sufficient information to manage my health (4 items, Cronbachs' alpha = 0.781); actively managing my health (5 items, Cronbachs' alpha = 0.829); social support for health (5 items, Cronbachs' alpha = 0.713); appraisal of health information (5 items, Cronbachs' alpha = 0.796); ability to actively engage with healthcare providers (5 items, Cronbachs' alpha = 0.871); navigating the healthcare system (6 items, Cronbachs' alpha = 0.833); ability to find good health information (5 items, Cronbachs' alpha = 0.823); and understand health information well enough to know what to do (5 items, Cronbachs' alpha = 0.711) [61]. Subscales 1 through 5 are rated on a four-point Likert scale ranging from 1 ('Strongly disagree') to 4 ('Strongly agree'), and subscales 6 through 9 are rated on a five-point Likert scale ranging from 1 ("Cannot do or Always difficult") to 5 ('Always easy') [61], with higher values indicating higher levels of individual health literacy. The scales were calculated according to the HLQ handbook.

Process organization during the hospital stay was measured with six items (Cronbachs' alpha = 0.842), which were developed within the Cologne Patient Questionnaire [63,64] (sample item: 'Here at the hospital, the right hand sometimes didn't know what the left hand was doing.'). The items had to be rated using four response options, ranging from 'strongly disagree' to 'strongly agree', with higher values indicating more problems with process organization. The scale was calculated if at least 70% of items (4 items) were answered by summing up all item scores and dividing them by the number of answered items.

The scales measuring the patients' perceptions of social support from physicians as well as nurses were also developed within the Cologne Patient Questionnaire [63,64]. Both scales have already been validated (physicians: Cronbachs' alpha = 0.924) [65] (nurses: Cronbachs' alpha = 0.928), and each consists of three items (sample items: 'The physicians supported me in a way that made it easier for me to deal with my illness.'; 'I could rely on the nurses when I had problems with my illness.'). The items had to be rated using four response options, ranging from 'strongly disagree' to 'strongly agree', with higher values indicating more support. Each scale was calculated if at least 70% of items (2 items) were answered by summing up all item scores and dividing them by the number of answered items.

To assess the information needs of patients, they answered 'yes' or 'no' to the question of whether they would have wished to have more information concerning the following aspects: (1) 'healthy lifestyle (diet, alcohol, smoking etc.)'; (2) 'physical burden in everyday life'; (3) 'mental burden in everyday life'; (4) 'self-help groups'; (5) 'books and brochures about their disease'; (6) 'health promoting measures'; and (7) 'help and care at home'. The number of times a patient stated 'yes' was then summed and served as a measure of unmet information needs (with higher values indicating more unmet needs).

2.5. Data Analysis

The associations between health literacy-sensitive communication and patient characteristics, process organization, and patient–provider relationships were analyzed within a comprehensive structural equation model (SEM) (see Figure 1). According to the HLQ handbook, missing data for the HLQ items were imputed using the expectation maximization (EM) algorithm. No further imputations were conducted since missing data for each variable were below 5%. Of the 217 patients who completed T0 and T1, 209 patients had no missing data on the variables of interest, which formed the basis for the present analysis. According to Kline et al. [66], an ideal sample size-to-parameters ratio would be 20:1. Consequently, 200 patients are sufficient to estimate a model with 10 parameters. Therefore, only two of the nine subscales of the HLQ were included, namely 'Navigating the healthcare system' and 'Ability to find good health information'. The subscales were selected by conducting a prior SEM containing only HL-COM and the nine subscales of the HLQ (results not displayed). Only the HLQ subscales which showed significant associations in this prior SEM were included in the final SEM. To develop and test the SEM, the maximum likelihood estimation procedure [66] of Mplus Version 8.2 (Muthen & Muthen, Los Angeles, CA, USA) was used. The recommended thresholds were used to determine a good model fit of the SEM: root mean square error of approximation (RMSEA) 0.08–0.5, standardized root mean square residual (SRMR) < 0.5, and incremental fit indexes (comparative fit index (CFI) and Tucker–Lewis index (TLI) close to 0.90 and 0.95) [67]. IBM® SPSS® 26.0 (IBM Corporation, Armonk, NY, USA) was used for descriptive analysis. A significance level of α = 0.05 was chosen.

2.6. Ethical Considerations and Trial Registration

The study was conducted in accordance with the Declaration of Helsinki in its current version (World Medical Association (WMA), 2013). A study protocol was approved by the Ethics Committee of the Medical Faculty of Oldenburg (number: 2019-148) before the study started. All study participants were asked to provide written informed consent based on current data protection regulations. All study participants were informed that participation in the study is voluntary. All personal identifiers were pseudonymized. Data security has been approved by all institutions involved in data collection. The identifying data are stored separately from the research data.

The study has been registered in the German Clinical Trials Register (DRKS) (trial registration number: DRKS00019830).

3. Results

The majority of participants in the sample were female (63.2%) and older than 50 years (62.7%) (see Table 2). Three quarters of participants reported having at least one chronic condition (76.1%), whereof 30.1% and 26.3% indicated having one or two chronic conditions, respectively (see Table 3). The most common chronic conditions were high blood pressure (30.1%), overweight/obesity (23.0%), and cancer (21.5%). Most patients were treated in the departments of orthopedics (38.8%) and gynecology (34.4%). Mean scores of the two HLQ subccales were 3.63 for 'navigating the healthcare system' and 3.67 for 'ability to find good health information' (range 1–5) (see Table 4).

Table 2. Sociodemographic characteristics of the sample (n = 209).

		n [a]	%
Sex	Female	132	63.2
	Male	75	35.9
	Diverse	1	0.5
	Missing	1	0.5
Age	18–29 years	18	8.6
	30–39 years	19	9.1
	40–49 years	41	19.6
	50–59 years	57	27.3
	60 years or older	74	35.4
Education	Lower secondary school education or less	41	19.6
	Intermediate secondary school education	81	38.8
	University entrance qualification	87	41.6
Migration status	Without	190	90.9
	With	19	9.1
Health insurance status	Public	164	78.5
	Public with additional private insurance	15	7.2
	Private	29	13.9
	Other	1	0.5

[a] Due to rounding, percentages might not add up to exactly 100%.

The mean scale score of HL-COM was 2.98 (range 1–4) (see Table 4), with scores for item 5 ('People spoke slowly and clearly to me') being the highest (see Table 1). Mean scale scores of process organization, social support by physicians, and social support by nurses were 1.76, 3.16, and 3.51, respectively (range 1–4) (see Table 4). On average, patients reported unmet needs concerning one or two of the seven aspects.

The model fit indices indicated good model fit (see Table 5). The model results revealed no statistically significant associations between patient characteristics and HL-COM scores. All other constructs of the model showed significant associations with HL-COM scores. Worse process organization was associated with lower HL-COM scores (-0.491, p-value < 0.001) (see Figure 1). Moreover, higher HL-COM scores were associated with higher perceived levels of social support provided by physicians (0.633, p-value < 0.001) and nurses (0.512, p-value < 0.001). Furthermore, higher HL-COM scores were associated with fewer unmet information needs of patients (0.420, p-value < 0.001).

Table 3. Disease and diagnosis related characteristics of the sample (n = 209).

		n [a]	%
Number of chronic diseases	0	50	23.9
	1	63	30.1
	2	55	26.3
	3	17	8.1
	4	17	8.1
	>4	7	3.4
Chronic diseases (multiple answers possible)	High blood pressure	63	30.1
	Overweight/obesity	48	23.0
	Cancer	45	21.5
	Mental illness	32	15.3
	Cardiovascular disease	24	11.5
	Lung disease (chronic bronchitis/COPD/asthma)	18	8.6
	Arthritis or rheumatism	16	7.7
	Diabetes	13	6.2
	Kidney disease	7	3.3
	Stroke	4	1.9
	Other diseases	61	29.2
	No chronic disease	52	23.9
Clinical division in which the patient was treated	Oncology	2	1.0
	Visceral surgery	54	25.8
	Gynecology	72	34.4
	Orthopedics	81	38.8
Number of nights spent in hospital	≤3	71	33.9
	4–6	75	35.9
	7–9	39	18.7
	>9	20	8.8
	Missing	4	1.9

[a] Due to rounding, percentages might not add up to exactly 100%.

Table 4. Descriptive statistics of the latent constructs and unmet information needs.

	Possible Range	Mean	SD [1]	Observed Range	Min	Max	Cronbachs' α
Health literacy-sensitive communication	1–4	2.98	0.65	3.00	1.00	4.00	0.911
Process organization	1–4	1.76	0.65	3.00	1.00	4.00	0.842
Social support provided by physicians	1–4	3.16	0.70	3.00	1.00	4.00	0.924
Social support provided by nurses	1–4	3.51	0.64	2.67	1.33	4.00	0.928
Unmet information needs	0–7	1.59	1.92	7.00	0.00	7.00	-
Health literacy: Navigating the healthcare system	1–5	3.63	0.57	3.17	1.67	4.83	0.833
Health literacy: Ability to find good health information	1–5	3.67	0.58	3.20	1.60	4.80	0.823

[1] SD = standard deviation.

Table 5. Fit indices of the structural equation model.

	X^2	Df	Cronbachs' α	RMSEA	SRMR	TLI	CFI
Threshold			≥0.7	≤0.08	≤0.08	≥0.90	≥0.90
SEM	832	521	0.911	0.048	0.070	0.920	0.926

X^2: chi square; Df: degrees of freedom; RMSEA: root mean square error of approximation; SRMR: standardized root mean square residual; CFI: comparative fit index; TLI: Tucker–Lewis index.

4. Discussion

Health literacy-sensitive communication measures are an important aspect of organizational health literacy that is relevant for patients. To our knowledge, this is the first study to investigate the role of health literacy-sensitive communication in a hospital setting from the patient view. The results of the SEM revealed that better processes organization was associated with significantly better health literacy-sensitive communication. Moreover, patients who gave higher ratings for health literacy-sensitive communication felt more supported by physicians and nurses and had fewer unmet information needs.

4.1. Interpretation within the Context of the Wider Literature

Concerning the association between organizational processes and health literacy-sensitive communication, we can confirm the assumptions of previous literature that problems with process organization negatively affects the patient–professional interaction [52,53]. Hence, our results are in line with the communication framework developed by Feldman-Stewart et al. [51], which suggests patient–professional interactions to be influenced by the context in which they take place. A possible explanation for this might be that physicians and nurses working in hospitals with worse process organization might have fewer ressources to interact with their patients because they are preoccupied with managing these processes [53,68]. Hence, deficits in process organization might reflect as stress and high workload among physicians and nurses [53].

Moreover, our results revealed that better health literacy-sensitive communication is associated with more perceived social support provided by physicians and nurses. Hence, our results confirm previous research findings that identified patient–provider communication as a key determinant for good patient–provider relationships [54], and defined the provision of information as an element contributing to a supportive patient–provider relationship [55]. Furthermore, the results of our study revealed that whenever health literacy-sensitive communication was rated better, patients' unmet information needs were significantly lower. We thereby confirm the results from Kowalski et al. [40], who found significant associations between organizational health literacy and the adequacy of information provided by hospitals as perceived by patients. Our results imply that health literacy-sensitive communication plays an important role in patients' information seeking process.

Our data did not confirm our assumption that individual patient characteristics that were previously found to be associated with individual health literacy are also associated with the perception of health literacy-sensitive communication. In our sample, age, education, migration status, and chronic illness were not found to be associated with health literacy-sensitive communication. While these characteristics have been found to be associated with individual health literacy [17,21–26,29], our results are partly in line with previous findings on associations between patient characteristics and patients' reports of communication with healthcare providers. Previous results concerning the association between age, educational level, ethnicity, native language, and comorbidities and patient–provider communication or interaction are inconsistent, and partially do not show any significant associations [52,53,68–70]. However, neither our data nor previous data deliver any explanation for the findings. It remains unclear how to interpret these results. Possible explanations are: (1) communication does not vary according to patient characteristics; (2) the perception of communication does not vary according to patient characteristics; (3) vulnerable patient groups are underrepresented; (4) the different patient groups in the sample did not have differing communication needs; (5) different communication needs of the patient groups were already met; or (6) a combination of these or other reasons led to the results.

4.2. Strengths and Limitations

A strength of our study is the comprehensive examination of different factors influencing health literacy-sensitive communication within one SEM. SEM has emerged as the method of choice when considering complex patterns of relationships or differences between a multitude of variables [66]. However, like any cross-sectional study, this study is not suitable for examining causality. Moreover, we conducted the study in only one hospital. Since patients were treated in four different clinical departments of the hospital, we believe that the heterogeneous group of patients participating in our study reflects the patient diversity found in hospitals. However, assessing associations between organizational health literacy and environmental factors would require analyzing several hospitals to allow comparisons between them. Furthermore, we are aware that a response rate of only one quarter is relatively low. One reason for this might be the COVID-19 pandemic, which has created uncertainty among hospital patients and reduced their willingness to participate in studies. In anticipation of this effect, we chose a recruitment period that was less impacted by the pandemic. Unfortunately, we were unable to perform a non-responder analysis. Moreover, our study is at risk of common method bias since the predictor variables and the outcome measure were both reported in the same patient survey.

4.3. Implications for Practice and Research

The findings of our study suggest that better health literacy-sensitive communication contributes to fewer unmet information needs of patients. To foster health literacy-sensitive communication, communication training for healthcare professionals might be implemented, which has already been found to be a suitable measure for this purpose [41]. Special care should be taken to explain terms and abbreviations, and to combine verbal and written information (handing out verbal information in written form and verbally explaining written information), since these were the items that were rated lowest by the patients in our sample as well as in the validation sample [50].

Additionally, improving patient health literacy requires wider changes within healthcare organizations, as emphasized by the concept of health-literate healthcare organizations [35]. Such changes range from generating information flyers or brochures for improving patient education or access to health information, to supporting hospital governance by evaluating and managing efforts to become a health-literate healthcare organization [41]. The need for changes on the organizational level is supported by the findings of our study. The results revealed that investing in better organized processes may foster health literacy-sensitive communication. Therefore, health policy and hospital management should strive to create conditions to optimize processes in hospitals in a patient-centered way. This might be achieved by restructuring workplaces or implementing standardized work processes to foster well-organized and effective work processes as previously suggested in the context of hospital discharge [71].

To address the limitations of our study, future studies should be conducted in more than one hospital to allow consideration of between-hospital differences in health literacy-sensitive communication. Furthermore, the role of patient characteristics should be clarified in future studies in order to be able to address possible individual communication needs (e.g., due to chronic illness or education level) in interventions improving health literacy-sensitive communication. Moreover, efforts should be made to determine the professionals' perspective on organizational health literacy and to compare it with the patients' perspective to be able to assess whether patients and professionals share the same concept of health literate healthcare organizations.

5. Conclusions

This study provides preliminary evidence on the important role played by health literacy-sensitive communication—as a key dimension of organizational health literacy—in the healthcare of patients in hospitals. Promoting health literacy-sensitive communication may be an important measure for reducing patients' unmet information needs. Besides communication training, improving the hospitals' process organization might contribute to better health literacy-sensitive communication and improved relevant outputs. Furthermore, health literacy-sensitive communication is not only an important dimension of organizational health literacy but might have the potential to improve the patient–professional relationship—as demonstrated here in terms of the provision of social support.

Author Contributions: Conceptualization, J.S.L., M.V.-B., A.L.B. and L.A.; methodology, J.S.L., N.E., C.K. and L.A.; software, J.S.L., M.V.-B. and L.A.; validation, L.A.; formal analysis, J.S.L. and M.V.-B.; investigation, J.S.L. and M.V.-B.; resources, L.A.; data curation, J.S.L. and M.V.-B.; writing—original draft preparation, J.S.L.; writing—review and editing, M.V.-B., N.E., C.K., A.L.B. and L.A.; visualization, J.S.L.; supervision, L.A.; project administration, L.A. and A.L.B.; funding acquisition, L.A. and A.L.B. All authors have read and agreed to the published version of the manuscript.

Funding: This research was funded by the Federal Ministry of Health on the basis of a resolution of the German Bundestag, grant number 2519FSB519.

Institutional Review Board Statement: The study was conducted according to the guidelines of the Declaration of Helsinki and approved by the Ethics Committee of the Medical Faculty of Oldenburg (number: 2019-148; date of approval: 23 January 2019).

Informed Consent Statement: Informed consent was obtained from all subjects involved in the study.

Data Availability Statement: The data presented in this study are available on request from the corresponding author.

Acknowledgments: We would like to thank the participating clinical departments, all employees as well as all patients for participating in the surveys. Moreover, we would like to thank Giulia Hollje and Hannah Nordmann for their active support in the recruitment of patients.

Conflicts of Interest: The authors declare no conflict of interest. The funders had no role in the design of the study; in the collection, analyses, or interpretation of data; in the writing of the manuscript; or in the decision to publish the results.

References

1. Simonds, S.K. Health Education as Social Policy. *Health Educ. Monogr.* **1974**, *2*, 1–10. [CrossRef]
2. U.S. Department of Education. *Adult Literacy in America: A First Look at the Findings of the National Adult Literacy Survey*; NCES 93275; U.S. Department of Education: Washington, DC, USA, 1993.
3. HLS-EU Consortium. Comparative Report of Health Literacy in Eight EU Member States, The European Health Literacy Survey HLS-EU. 2012. Available online: http://cpme.dyndns.org:591/adopted/2015/Comparative_report_on_health_literacy_in_eight_EU_member_states.pdf (accessed on 25 September 2021).
4. Sørensen, K.; Van den Broucke, S.; Fullam, J.; Doyle, G.; Pelikan, J.; Slonska, Z.; Brand, H. Health literacy and public health: A systematic review and integration of definitions and models. *BMC Public Health* **2012**, *12*, 80. [CrossRef]
5. Nationaler Aktionsplan Gesundheitskompetenz. Available online: https://www.nap-gesundheitskompetenz.de/ (accessed on 7 June 2021).
6. Ernstmann, N.; Bauer, U.; Berens, E.-M.; Bitzer, E.M.; Bollweg, T.M.; Danner, M.; Dehn-Hindenberg, A.; Dierks, M.L.; Farin, E.; Grobosch, S.; et al. DNVF Memorandum Gesundheitskompetenz (Teil 1)—Hintergrund, Relevanz, Gegenstand und Fragestellungen in der Versorgungsforschung. *Gesundheitswesen* **2020**, *82*, e77–e93. [CrossRef] [PubMed]
7. Berkman, N.D.; Sheridan, S.L.; Donahue, K.E.; Halpern, D.J.; Crotty, K. Low Health Literacy and Health Outcomes: An Updated Systematic Review. *Ann. Intern. Med.* **2011**, *155*, 97–107. [CrossRef]
8. Kilfoyle, K.A.; Vitko, M.; O'Conor, R.; Bailey, S.C. Health Literacy and Women's Reproductive Health: A Systematic Review. *J. Women's Health* **2016**, *25*, 1237–1255. [CrossRef]
9. Al Sayah, F.; Majumdar, S.R.; Williams, B.; Robertson, S.; Johnson, J.A. Health Literacy and Health Outcomes in Diabetes: A Systematic Review. *J. Gen. Intern. Med.* **2013**, *28*, 444–452. [CrossRef]
10. Cajita, M.I.; Cajita, T.R.; Han, H.-R. Health Literacy and Heart Failure: A Systematic Review. *J. Cardiovasc. Nurs.* **2016**, *31*, 121–130. [CrossRef]
11. Fleary, S.A.; Joseph, P.; Pappagianopoulos, J.E. Adolescent health literacy and health behaviors: A systematic review. *J. Adolesc.* **2018**, *62*, 116–127. [CrossRef] [PubMed]
12. Bröder, J.; Okan, O.; Bauer, U.; Bruland, D.; Schlupp, S.; Bollweg, T.M.; Saboga-Nunes, L.; Bond, E.; Sørensen, K.; Bitzer, E.-M.; et al. Health literacy in childhood and youth: A systematic review of definitions and models. *BMC Public Health* **2017**, *17*, 361. [CrossRef]
13. Fernández-Gutiérrez, M.; Bas-Sarmiento, P.; Albar-Marín, M.J.; Paloma-Castro, O.; Romero-Sánchez, J.M. Health literacy interventions for immigrant populations: A systematic review. *Int. Nurs. Rev.* **2018**, *65*, 54–64. [CrossRef]
14. Berkman, N.D.; Sheridan, S.L.; Donahue, K.E.; Halpern, D.J.; Viera, A.; Crotty, K.; Holland, A.; Brasure, M.; Lohr, K.N.; Harden, E.; et al. Health literacy interventions and outcomes: An updated systematic review. *Evid. Rep. Technol. Assess.* **2011**, *199*, 1–941.
15. Liu, H.; Zeng, H.; Shen, Y.; Zhang, F.; Sharma, M.; Lai, W.; Zhao, Y.; Tao, G.; Yuan, J.; Zhao, Y. Assessment Tools for Health Literacy among the General Population: A Systematic Review. *Int. J. Environ. Res. Public Health* **2018**, *15*, 1711. [CrossRef] [PubMed]
16. Med, J.K.P.; Hasan, S.M.; Barnsley, J.; Berta, W.; Fazelzad, R.; Papadakos, C.J.; Giuliani, M.E.; Howell, D. Health literacy and cancer self-management behaviors: A scoping review. *Cancer* **2018**, *124*, 4202–4210. [CrossRef]
17. Buja, A.; Rabensteiner, A.; Sperotto, M.; Grotto, G.; Bertoncello, C.; Cocchio, S.; Baldovin, T.; Contu, P.; Lorini, C.; Baldo, V. Health Literacy and Physical Activity: A Systematic Review. *J. Phys. Act. Health* **2020**, *17*, 1259–1274. [CrossRef] [PubMed]
18. Oldach, B.R.; Katz, M.L. Health literacy and cancer screening: A systematic review. *Patient Educ. Couns.* **2014**, *94*, 149–157. [CrossRef]
19. Geboers, B.; Brainard, J.S.; Loke, Y.K.; Jansen, C.J.M.; Salter, C.; Reijneveld, S.A.; De Winter, A.F. The association of health literacy with adherence in older adults, and its role in interventions: A systematic meta-review. *BMC Public Health* **2015**, *15*, 903. [CrossRef]

20. Mackey, L.M.; Doody, C.; Werner, E.L.; Fullen, B. Self-Management Skills in Chronic Disease Management: What Role Does Health Literacy Have? *Med. Decis. Mak.* **2016**, *36*, 741–759. [CrossRef]
21. Van Der Heide, I.; Rademakers, J.; Schipper, M.; Droomers, M.; Sørensen, K.; Uiters, E. Health literacy of Dutch adults: A cross sectional survey. *BMC Public Health* **2013**, *13*, 179. [CrossRef] [PubMed]
22. Sørensen, K.; Pelikan, J.M.; Röthlin, F.; Ganahl, K.; Slonska, Z.; Doyle, G.; Fullam, J.; Kondilis, B.; Agrafiotis, D.; Uiters, E.; et al. Health literacy in Europe: Comparative results of the European health literacy survey (HLS-EU). *Eur. J. Public Health* **2015**, *25*, 1053–1058. [CrossRef]
23. Schaeffer, D.; Berens, E.-M.; Vogt, D. Health Literacy in the German Population. *Dtsch. Aerzteblatt Int.* **2017**, *114*, 53–60. [CrossRef]
24. Naus, T. Health literacy in EU immigrants: A systematic review and integration of interventions for a comprehensive health literacy strategy. *Eur. J. Public Health* **2016**, *26*, 26. [CrossRef]
25. Berens, E.-M.; Vogt, D.; Messer, M.; Hurrelmann, K.; Schaeffer, D. Health literacy among different age groups in Germany: Results of a cross-sectional survey. *BMC Public Health* **2016**, *16*, 1151. [CrossRef]
26. Kobayashi, L.C.; Wardle, J.; Wolf, M.S.; Von Wagner, C. Aging and Functional Health Literacy: A Systematic Review and Meta Analysis. *J. Gerontol. Ser. B* **2016**, *71*, 445–457. [CrossRef] [PubMed]
27. Allegrante, J.P.; Wells, M.T.; Peterson, J.C. Interventions to Support Behavioral Self-Management of Chronic Diseases. *Annu. Rev. Public Health* **2019**, *40*, 127–146. [CrossRef]
28. Grady, P.A.; Gough, L.L. Self-Management: A Comprehensive Approach to Management of Chronic Conditions. *Am. J. Public Health* **2014**, *104*, e25–e31. [CrossRef]
29. Liu, L.; Qian, X.; Chen, Z.; He, T. Health literacy and its effect on chronic disease prevention: Evidence from China's data. *BMC Public Health* **2020**, *20*, 690. [CrossRef]
30. Palumbo, R. Examining the impacts of health literacy on healthcare costs. An evidence synthesis. *Health Serv. Manag. Res.* **2017**, *30*, 197–212. [CrossRef] [PubMed]
31. Rudd, R.E.; Renzulli, D.; Pereira, A.; Daltory, L. Literacy demands in health care settings: The patient perspective. In *Understanding Health Literacy: Implications for Medicine and Public Health*; Schwartzberg, J.G., VanGeest, J., Wang, C., Eds.; American Medical Association: Chicago, IL, USA, 2005; ISBN 1579476309.
32. Nutbeam, D. The evolving concept of health literacy. *Soc. Sci. Med.* **2008**, *67*, 2072–2078. [CrossRef]
33. Baker, D.W. The meaning and the measure of health literacy. *J. Gen. Intern. Med.* **2006**, *21*, 878–883. [CrossRef] [PubMed]
34. Institute of Medicine. *Organizational Change to Improve Health Literacy: Workshop Summary*; National Academies Press: Washington, DC, USA, 2013.
35. Brach, C.; Keller, D.; Hernandez, L.; Baur, C.; Parker, R.; Dreyer, B.; Schyve, P.; Lemerise, A.J.; Schillinger, D. *Ten Attributes of Health Literate Health Care Organizations*; NAM Perspectives: Washington, DC, USA, 2012; Volume 2. [CrossRef]
36. Howe, C.J.; Adame, T.; Lewis, B.; Wagner, T. Original Research: Assessing Organizational Focus on Health Literacy in North Texas Hospitals. *AJN, Am. J. Nurs.* **2020**, *120*, 24–33. [CrossRef]
37. Bonaccorsi, G.; Romiti, A.; Ierardi, F.; Innocenti, M.; Del Riccio, M.; Frandi, S.; Bachini, L.; Zanobini, P.; Gemmi, F.; Lorini, C. Health-Literate Healthcare Organizations and Quality of Care in Hospitals: A Cross-Sectional Study Conducted in Tuscany. *Int. J. Environ. Res. Public Health* **2020**, *17*, 2508. [CrossRef] [PubMed]
38. Hayran, O.; Ataç, Ö.; Orhan, Ö. Assessment of Organizational Health Literacy in a Group of Public, Private and University Hospitals in Istanbul. *J. Health Syst. Policies (JHESP)* **2019**, *1*, 47–59.
39. Hayran, O.; Özer, O. Organizational health literacy as a determinant of patient satisfaction. *Public Health* **2018**, *163*, 20–26. [CrossRef]
40. Kowalski, C.; Lee, S.-Y.D.; Schmidt, A.; Wesselmann, S.; Wirtz, M.A.; Pfaff, H.; Ernstmann, N. The health literate health care organization 10 item questionnaire (HLHO-10): Development and validation. *BMC Health Serv. Res.* **2015**, *15*, 47. [CrossRef]
41. Zanobini, P.; Lorini, C.; Baldasseroni, A.; Dellisanti, C.; Bonaccorsi, G. A Scoping Review on How to Make Hospitals Health Literate Healthcare Organizations. *Int. J. Environ. Res. Public Health* **2020**, *17*, 1036. [CrossRef] [PubMed]
42. Farmanova, E.; Bonneville, L.; Bouchard, L. Organizational Health Literacy: Review of Theories, Frameworks, Guides, and Implementation Issues. *Inq. J. Health Care Organ. Provis. Financ.* **2018**, *55*, 46958018757848. [CrossRef]
43. Kaper, M.; Sixsmith, J.; Meijering, L.; Vervoordeldonk, J.; Doyle, P.; Barry, M.M.; De Winter, A.F.; Reijneveld, S.A. Implementation and Long-Term Outcomes of Organisational Health Literacy Interventions in Ireland and The Netherlands: A Longitudinal Mixed-Methods Study. *Int. J. Environ. Res. Public Health* **2019**, *16*, 4812. [CrossRef]
44. Palumbo, R. Leveraging Organizational Health Literacy to Enhance Health Promotion and Risk Prevention: A Narrative and Interpretive Literature Review. *Yale J. Biol. Med.* **2021**, *94*, 115–128. [PubMed]
45. Meggetto, E.; Kent, F.; Ward, B.; Keleher, H. Factors influencing implementation of organizational health literacy: A realist review. *J. Health Organ. Manag.* **2020**, *34*, 385–407. [CrossRef]
46. Weaver, N.L.; Wray, R.J.; Zellin, S.; Gautam, K.; Jupka, K. Advancing Organizational Health Literacy in Health Care Organizations Serving High-Needs Populations: A Case Study. *J. Health Commun.* **2012**, *17*, 55–66. [CrossRef] [PubMed]
47. Jessup, R.L.; Osborne, R.H.; Buchbinder, R.; Beauchamp, A. Using co-design to develop interventions to address health literacy needs in a hospitalised population. *BMC Health Serv. Res.* **2018**, *18*, 989. [CrossRef]
48. Dietscher, C.; Lorenc, J.; Pelikan, J.M. *Piloting of the "Self-Assessment Tool to Investigate the Organizational Health Literacy of Hospitals" following the Vienna Concept of a Health Literate Health Care Organization*; Ludwig Boltzmann Institute: Vienna, Austria, 2015.

49. Trezona, A.; Dodson, S.; Osborne, R.H. Development of the Organisational Health Literacy Responsiveness (Org-HLR) self-assessment tool and process. *BMC Health Serv. Res.* **2018**, *18*, 694. [CrossRef]
50. Ernstmann, N.; Halbach, S.; Kowalski, C.; Pfaff, H.; Ansmann, L. Measuring attributes of health literate health care organizations from the patients' perspective: Development and validation of a questionnaire to assess health literacy-sensitive communication (HL-COM). *Z. Evidenz Fortbild. Qual. Gesundh.* **2017**, *121*, 58–63. [CrossRef]
51. Feldman-Stewart, D.; Brundage, M.; Tishelman, C. A conceptual framework for patient-professional communication: An application to the cancer context. *Psycho-Oncology* **2005**, *14*, 801–809. [CrossRef]
52. Ansmann, L.; Wirtz, M.A.; Kowalski, C.; Pfaff, H.; Visser, A.; Ernstmann, N. The impact of the hospital work environment on social support from physicians in breast cancer care. *Patient Educ. Couns.* **2014**, *96*, 352–360. [CrossRef] [PubMed]
53. Lubasch, J.; Lee, S.; Kowalski, C.; Beckmann, M.; Pfaff, H.; Ansmann, L. Hospital Processes and the Nurse-Patient Interaction in Breast Cancer Care. Findings from a Cross-Sectional Study. *Int. J. Environ. Res. Public Health* **2021**, *18*, 8224. [CrossRef]
54. Honavar, S.G. Patient–physician relationship—Communication is the key. *Indian J. Ophthalmol.* **2018**, *66*, 1527–1528. [CrossRef] [PubMed]
55. Caplan, G. *Support Systems and Community Mental Health, Lectures on Concept Development*; Behavioral Publications: Pasadena, CA, USA, 1974.
56. Lubasch, J.S.; Voigt-Barbarowicz, M.; Lippke, S.; De Wilde, R.L.; Griesinger, F.; Lazovic, D.; Villegas, P.C.O.; Roeper, J.; Salzmann, D.; Seeber, G.H.; et al. Improving professional health literacy in hospitals: Study protocol of a participatory codesign and implementation study. *BMJ Open* **2021**, *11*, e045835. [CrossRef]
57. Dillman, D.A. *Mail and Telephone Surveys: The Total Design Method*; John Wiley & Sons: New York, NY, USA, 1978; ISBN 0471215554.
58. Bradburn, N.M.; Sudman, S.; Wansink, B. *Asking questions: The Definitive Guide to Questionnaire Design for Market Research, Political Polls, and Social and Health Questionnaires*; John Wiley & Sons: New York, NY, USA, 2004; ISBN 978-0-7879-7088-8.
59. Groves, R.M.; Fowler, F.J.; Couper, M.P.; Lepkowski, J.M.; Singer, E.; Tourangeau, R. *Survey Methodology*, 2nd ed.; John Wiley & Sons: Hoboken, NJ, USA, 2011; ISBN 9780470465462.
60. Prüfer, P.; Rexroth, M. Two-phase pretesting. In *Querschnitt: Festschrift für Max Kaase*; Mohler, P.P., Ed.; ZUMA: Mannheim, Germany, 2000; ISBN 3924220204.
61. Osborne, R.H.; Batterham, R.W.; Elsworth, G.R.; Hawkins, M.; Buchbinder, R. The grounded psychometric development and initial validation of the Health Literacy Questionnaire (HLQ). *BMC Public Health* **2013**, *13*, 658. [CrossRef] [PubMed]
62. Nolte, S.; Osborne, R.H.; Dwinger, S.; Elsworth, G.R.; Conrad, M.L.; Rose, M.; Härter, M.; Dirmaier, J.; Zill, J.M. German translation, cultural adaptation, and validation of the Health Literacy Questionnaire (HLQ). *PLoS ONE* **2017**, *12*, e0172340. [CrossRef]
63. Ansmann, L.; Kowalski, C.; Pfaff, H. Ten Years of Patient Surveys in Accredited Breast Centers in North Rhine-Westphalia. *Geburtshilfe Frauenheilkd.* **2016**, *76*, 37–45. [CrossRef] [PubMed]
64. Pfaff, H. (Ed.) *The Cologne Patient Questionnaire (CPQ): Development and Validation of a Questionnaire to Assess Patient Involvement as a Therapist*; Asgard-Verlag: Sankt Augustin, Germany, 2003; ISBN 3537743718.
65. Ommen, O.; Wirtz, M.A.; Janssen, C.; Neumann, M.; Ernstmann, N.; Pfaff, H. Validation of a theory-based instrument measuring patient-reported psychosocial care by physicians using a multiple indicators and multiple causes model. *Patient Educ. Couns.* **2010**, *80*, 100–106. [CrossRef]
66. Kline, R.B. *Principles and Practice of Structural Equation Modeling*, 4th ed.; Guilford Press: New York, NY, USA, 2016; 534p.
67. Schumacker, R.E.; Lomax, R.G. *A Beginner's Guide to Structural Equation Modeling*, 4th ed.; Routledge Taylor & Francis Group: New York, NY, USA; London, UK, 2016; ISBN 9781138811904.
68. Ansmann, L.; Kowalski, C.; Ernstmann, N.; Ommen, O.; Pfaff, H. Patients' perceived support from physicians and the role of hospital characteristics. *Int. J. Qual. Health Care* **2012**, *24*, 501–508. [CrossRef] [PubMed]
69. Dad, T.; Tighiouart, H.; Lacson, E., Jr.; Meyer, K.B.; Weiner, D.E.; Richardson, M.M. Hemodialysis patient characteristics associated with better experience as measured by the In-center Hemodialysis Consumer Assessment of Healthcare Providers and Systems (ICH CAHPS) survey. *BMC Nephrol.* **2018**, *19*, 340. [CrossRef]
70. Van Der Veer, S.N.; Arah, O.A.; Visserman, E.; Bart, H.A.J.; De Keizer, N.F.; Abu-Hanna, A.; Heuveling, L.M.; Stronks, K.; Jager, K.J. Exploring the relationships between patient characteristics and their dialysis care experience. *Nephrol. Dial. Transplant.* **2012**, *27*, 4188–4196. [CrossRef] [PubMed]
71. Nowak, M.; Swora, M.; Karbach, U.; Pfaff, H.; Ansmann, L. Associations between hospital structures, processes and patient experiences of preparation for discharge in breast cancer centers: A multilevel analysis. *Health Care Manag. Rev.* **2021**, *46*, 98–110. [CrossRef]

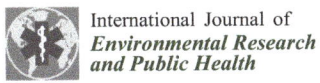

Study Protocol

The Health Literacy in Pregnancy (HeLP) Program Study Protocol: Development of an Antenatal Care Intervention Using the Ophelia Process

Maiken Meldgaard [1,*], Rikke Damkjær Maimburg [2,3,4], Maiken Fabricius Damm [2], Anna Aaby [1], Anna Peeters [5] and Helle Terkildsen Maindal [1]

1. Department of Public Health, Aarhus University, 8000 Aarhus, Denmark; aaby@ph.au.dk (A.A.); htm@ph.au.dk (H.T.M.)
2. Department of Obstetrics and Gynecology, Aarhus University Hospital, 8000 Aarhus, Denmark; rmai@clin.au.dk (R.D.M.); maikda@rm.dk (M.F.D.)
3. Department of Clinical Medicine, Aarhus University, 8000 Aarhus, Denmark
4. School of Nursing and Midwifery, Western Sydney University, Locked Bag 1797, Penrith, NSW 2751, Australia
5. Institute for Health Transformation, Deakin University, Geelong, VIC 3220, Australia; anna.peeters@deakin.edu.au
* Correspondence: mme@ph.au.dk; Tel.: +45-2364-1410

Abstract: A pregnant woman needs adequate knowledge, motivation, and skills to access, understand, appraise, and apply health information to make decisions related to the health of herself and her unborn baby. These skills are defined as health literacy: an important factor in relation to the woman's ability to engage and navigate antenatal care services. Evidence shows variation in levels of health literacy among pregnant women, but more knowledge is needed about how to respond to different health literacy profiles in antenatal care. This paper describes the development protocol for the HeLP program, which aims to investigate pregnant women's health literacy and co-create health literacy interventions through a broad collaboration between pregnant women, partners, healthcare providers, professionals, and other stakeholders using the Ophelia (Optimising Health Literacy and Access) process. The HeLP program will be provided at two hospitals, which provide maternity care including antenatal care: a tertiary referral hospital (Aarhus University Hospital) and a secondary hospital (the Regional Hospital in Viborg). The Ophelia process includes three process phases with separate objectives, steps, and activities leading to the identification of local strengths, needs and issues, co-design of interventions, and implementation, evaluation, and ongoing improvement. No health literacy intervention using the Ophelia process has yet been developed for antenatal care.

Keywords: health literacy; inequality; intervention development; health literacy responsiveness; organizational health literacy; co-design; pregnancy; health promotion

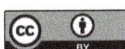

1. Introduction

Globally, social inequality is documented in the use and outcomes of antenatal care [1,2], even in social welfare states such as Denmark [3,4]. Socio-economic factors including low educational level, low income, and ethnicity are associated with a higher risk of obstetric complications and poor health outcomes for the mother and her child, including gestational diabetes mellitus, maternal stress and depression, low birth weight, preterm birth, stillbirth, and congenital malformations [2–8].

Health literacy is also associated with socio-economic factors [9,10] and seems to follow a social gradient; a phenomenon whereby people who are less advantaged in terms of socioeconomic position have poorer health compared to those who are more advantaged [11,12]. Several studies have investigated health literacy among pregnant women and show that health literacy levels in this group depend on e.g., employment status, ethnicity, and education [13,14]. Low health literacy might be associated with less antenatal care attendance and engagement [15–17], less knowledge about medication use in pregnancy [18,19], lower self-efficacy [17,20], depression [21], and smoking [22,23] among pregnant women. Existing evidence is inconsistent, and further knowledge about associations between health literacy, socio-economic factors, and pregnancy outcomes is needed.

Health literacy is a multi-dimensional concept, which can be defined as a person's knowledge, motivation, and skills to access, understand, appraise, and apply health information to make decisions in everyday life concerning one's own health [13,24]. Closely related to health literacy is organizational health literacy, which can be defined as "the way in which services, organizations, and systems make health information and resources available and accessible according to health literacy strengths and limitations" [25]. The World Health Organization (WHO) recommends a health literacy focus and responsiveness in preventive services to respond to inequality [26–28].

The Ophelia (Optimising Health Literacy and Access) process is used to guide co-design—a method to involve and engage relevant stakeholders in the process—of interventions to improve health literacy and equity in healthcare services [29]. The Ophelia process was developed and tested by Professor Richard Osborne and team in nine different primary health care settings [30]. They found it suitable as a framework to guide the generation of intervention ideas and respond to inequity in health care services. The Ophelia process has further been used as a methodological foundation for quite a few intervention projects [31–33], and findings show that the co-creative nature of the process can improve understanding of the needs and vulnerabilities of specific population groups in relation to health literacy [32]. A recent publication describes seven flagship European National Health Literacy Demonstration Projects (NHLDPs) conducted in different healthcare settings that focus on different non-communicable diseases but are similar in their use of the Ophelia methodological process [33].

Health literacy interventions in antenatal care could potentially improve knowledge, behavior, and ultimately reproductive outcomes. Only a few health literacy interventions have been developed specifically for pregnant women in antenatal care [34], and to the best of our knowledge, the Ophelia process has not previously been tested in antenatal care. Further research is warranted to investigate the role of pregnant woman's health literacy-specific needs in relation to the development of effective initiatives.

The HeLP program aims to investigate pregnant women's health literacy and co-create health literacy interventions based on local knowledge. Interventions will be developed through a broad collaboration between pregnant women, partners, healthcare providers, professionals, and other stakeholders using the Ophelia (Optimising Health Literacy and Access) process. This paper describes the development protocol for the HeLP program.

2. Materials and Methods

2.1. Setting and Study Population

The HeLP program will be conducted at two primary intervention sites, the tertiary referral hospital, Aarhus University Hospital, and the secondary hospital, Regional Hospital in Viborg. The annual number of births is approximately 5000 and 2200 at each site, respectively. The two sites handle the midwifery consultations during antenatal care. The two intervention sites differ in size, location, and organization. The inclusion of both sites is an attempt to increase the representativeness of the study population. During the development of interventions, external collaborators and other sites will potentially be identified, e.g., general practice. The study population in the HeLP program includes pregnant women referred to antenatal care at Aarhus University Hospital, Denmark, or the Regional Hospital Viborg, Denmark.

All pregnant women in Denmark have free-of-charge access to maternity care including antenatal, intrapartum, and post-partum care. The basic antenatal program is described in Figure 1 and includes three consultations in general practice and five consultations with a midwife (study sites). The first antenatal visit is normally in general practice where the pregnancy is confirmed. After the first consultation, the general practitioner forwards information after consent to the midwifery clinic affiliated with the hospital obstetric department through the woman's electronic patient journal (EPJ). Medical, obstetric, or psychosocial factors detected in relation to the woman or the home, which entails specific attention, are normally specified in the women's record. A specific care level classification of the pregnant woman is based on a risk assessment concerned with the woman's history, socio-economic determinants including life circumstances, age, and obstetric, social, and mental risk factors, and is a professional judgment that may be changed during the pregnancy. The woman's health literacy level is not systematically evaluated.

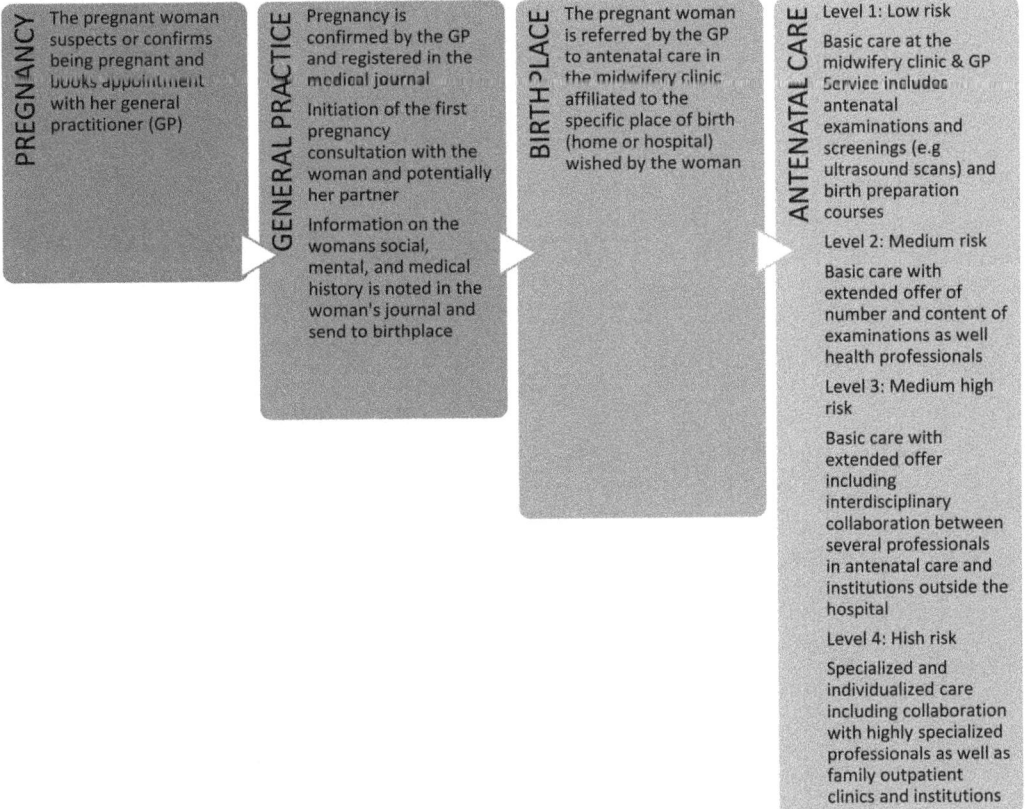

Figure 1. Organization of Danish antenatal care.

The Danish Health Authority recommends a four-level division of maternity care to secure the necessary support in relation to obstetric, social, and mental risk challenges [35]. The recommended four-level division is elaborated in Figure 1.

2.2. The Ophelia Process

The methodological foundation for the HeLP program is the Ophelia process, which was inspired by methodologies such as intervention mapping, quality improvement collaborative, and realist synthesis [36–39].

The Ophelia process provides a practical and systematic method to identify local strengths, barriers, needs and issues, and co-design of an intervention based on this local knowledge. The process is divided into three phases with separate steps and associated activities:

- Phase one: Identification of local strengths, needs, and issues includes Step 1. Project set-up Step 2. Data collection and/or extraction Step 3. Consultation to identify new ideas
- Phase two: co-design of interventions Step 4. Intervention design Step 5. Intervention planning Step 6. Intervention development and refinement
- Phase three: implementation, evaluation, and ongoing improvement Step 7. Implementation and evaluation Step 8. Development of an ongoing improvement strategy

The Ophelia process in the HeLP program, including planned activities for the different phases and steps, is elaborated in Figure 2.

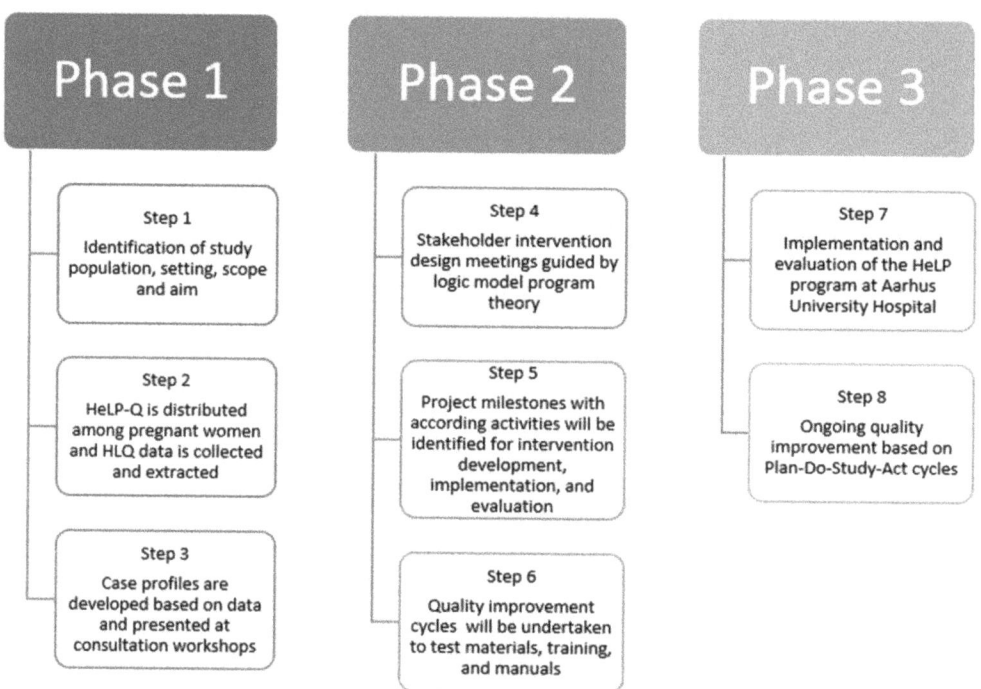

Figure 2. The Ophelia process—three phases and according steps in the HeLP program.

2.3. Phase One: Identification of Local Strengths, Needs, and Issues

Step 1. Project set-up

Step 1. *Focuses on identifying project focus, scope and aim of the HeLP program. The HeLP collaboration, organization, and according roles and responsibilities will be established.*

The HeLP program will be a broad collaboration between a large Danish research institution, Aarhus University, and two Danish hospitals, Aarhus University Hospital, and the Regional Hospital in Viborg. The program will be organized with a steering committee, a management team, and a working team. Representatives from each collaborating organ will be represented at each level. This study protocol and the above description of setting, study population, focus, scope, and aim were established and developed in close collaboration between the HeLP steering committee, the HeLP management team, and the HeLP working team.

Step 2. Data collection and extraction

Step 2. *Focuses on establishment of a data collection plan, data collection and extraction of data. Required ethical approvals will be obtained. Moreover, materials for the consultation workshops will be prepared.*

To identify local needs, a mapping of health literacy strengths and challenges through a comprehensive health survey, the HeLP-Questionnaire (HeLP-Q), will be carried out among the study population. The HeLP-Q will be developed specifically for the HeLP program and will include general health questions, items about socio-economic factors, and questions from already validated surveys (Cambridge Worry Scale (CWS) [40], the Edinburgh Postnatal Depression Score (EPDS) [41], Three-Item Loneliness Scale (TILS) [42], and the Health Care Climate Questionnaire (HCCQ) [43]). To measure health literacy, we will include the validated Health Literacy Questionnaire (HLQ) of 44 questions in total [44,45]. The HLQ consists of nine scales that will be analyzed separately: (1) feeling understood and supported by healthcare providers, (2) having sufficient information to manage my health, (3) actively managing my health, (4) social support for health, (5) appraisal of health information, (6) ability to actively engage with healthcare providers, (7) navigating the healthcare system, (8) ability to find good health information, and (9) understand health information well enough to know what to do. To further map digital health literacy competencies, we will include two domains from the eHealth Literacy Questionnaire (eHLQ) [46,47]. It will take approximately 20 min to fill out HeLP-Q.

To enhance participation, midwives in Aarhus and Viborg will be informed about the HeLP program and instructed to hand out participation cards to pregnant women containing an access link and QR code to either a Danish or an English edition of the HeLP-Q. In addition, posters with information about the program and access links and QR codes for the questionnaire will be placed at obvious locations in the midwifery consultation waiting area in both Aarhus and Viborg. Moreover, the HeLP program will be promoted on social media sites. One-pagers with instructions will be placed in the midwives' staff room and researchers from the HeLP management team (M.M. and M.F.D.) will participate every second month in morning meetings at both study sites and inform midwives about the HeLP. We acknowledge that filling out HeLP-Q requires some level of health literacy. This may lead to differential participation according to health literacy levels and thereby a risk of selection bias. To accommodate this challenge, we plan to have research assistants present two days a week throughout the data collection period at the two study sites to assist pregnant women with expected lower health literacy to participate in the study. The assistance includes help with issues related to accessing, reading, understanding, and filling out HeLP-Q.

Data collected based on HLQ in the HeLP-Q will be analyzed to provide us with insights into the health literacy strengths and challenges of the participants. Cluster analysis (a statistical technique to group similar observations into clusters based on the observed values of several variables for each individual) will be used to identify sub-groups of pregnant women with similar patterns of HLQ scores. Then, case profiles will be developed based on the identified sub-groups. Participants are invited to consider intervention ideas, and how to respond to the pregnant women's needs, based on case profiles and identified health literacy strengths and challenges.

Step 3. Response ideas consultation workshops

Step 3. *Focuses on establishing a consultation plan as well as arrangements for the consultation workshops and carrying out the consultation workshops.*

We plan to carry out two consultation workshops with pregnant women, their partners, health professionals, and other stakeholders in antenatal care (e.g., obstetricians, general practitioners, midwives, nurses, social workers, psychologists, NGO employees). The case profiles will be presented at the first consultation workshop together with additional results from HeLP-Q. These data provide the foundation for the dialogue, discussion, and idea mapping initiating the development of health literacy interventions.

As workshops are scheduled to be held in April and June 2022, and the data collection period proceeds until August 2022, the findings we present at the workshops will be based on parts of the dataset. We expect that approximately 700 women will have filled out HeLP-Q prior to the preparation of the workshop. Participants will be asked to provide informed, written consent before attending the workshops. The consultation plan and process of the workshop are elaborated in Table 1.

Table 1. Preliminary consultation plan, HeLP.

Plan Elements	Content and Arrangements
Time Frame	Approximately Four Hours
Staff responsible	Associate Professor, PhD, and Midwife R.D.M, PhD Fellow, M.M. and Midwife, M.F.D.
Format and participants	• Approximately 25 participants for each workshop placed in 5 different discussion groups. Five participants in each group have shown to be ideal in health research focus groups [48] • Two workshops held with pregnant women, partners, family members, healthcare providers and health professionals including obstetricians, general practitioners, midwives, nurses, social workers, psychologists, NGO-employees, and other stakeholders • First workshop: results from HeLP-Q and case profiles will be presented, and participants will be instructed to make table mindmaps with intervention ideas • Second workshop: participants will be instructed to discuss and prioritize an intervention package based on the matched intervention ideas and objectives
Recruitment approach	• Pregnant women and partners will be invited to participate in workshops from the two participating sites • We plan to recruit from different settings including basic midwifery consultation and other related services which provides care for pregnant women with challenges related to physical, mental, or social health, socio-economic factors, etc. • The participating group of pregnant women and partners should preferably include a heterogeneous group • Health professionals (a broad variety of professionals working in or with antenatal care) will be invited for workshop participation from different organizational levels at the two participating sites • We plan to recruit health professionals, who work in different settings and organizational levels of antenatal care
How to capture ideas and insights	• Four research assistants and three students will be present at workshops to observe and take notes • A table manager, who are responsible for writing down during workshops will be assigned for each table • Table managers will be instructed to fill out table mindmaps summing up all ideas and thoughts • Informed consent will be sent by email and signed by participants before workshop days, and dialogues at each table will be audio recorded

2.4. Phase Two

Similar to phase two and phase three is that phase one must be completed before we are able to fully plan the content in detail for these phases. Phases two and three will be planned based on results from HeLP-Q and the consultation workshops. In alignment with the Ophelia process, we are, however, able to describe the overall activities.

Step 4. Intervention design

Step 4. *Focuses on specifying the objectives for interventions. A rapid literature review will be conducted, and we will search for existing health literacy interventions in antenatal care. Afterwards, intervention ideas from the workshop will be matched with the HeLP program intervention objectives. An intervention or a package will be selected, and a logic model will be prepared.*

Based on the results from the workshops, the HeLP management team will confirm or adjust the focus, scope, and overall aim of the HeLP program. In alignment with the Ophelia process, a rapid literature review will be conducted to identify existing interventions in this area. This will be followed by a process where the produced intervention ideas from the consultation workshops and the newly established HeLP intervention objectives are matched. Consultation workshop participants will be invited for a second consultation workshop, where the aim is to discuss and prioritize an intervention package based on the matched intervention ideas and objectives. The HeLP management team will then develop one or more first draft logic models based on the suggested intervention package using shells similar to Figure 3. Logic models will be developed based on the theory by Taylor-Powell and Henert [49], and contain inputs, outputs, and outcomes. Logic model drafts will be presented to the HeLP steering committee, and members are invited to provide feedback. Afterwards, representatives from the two participating sites will be invited for a meeting where the logic models will be discussed, and agreements will be made. The HeLP management team will refine the final logic model based on agreements from this meeting.

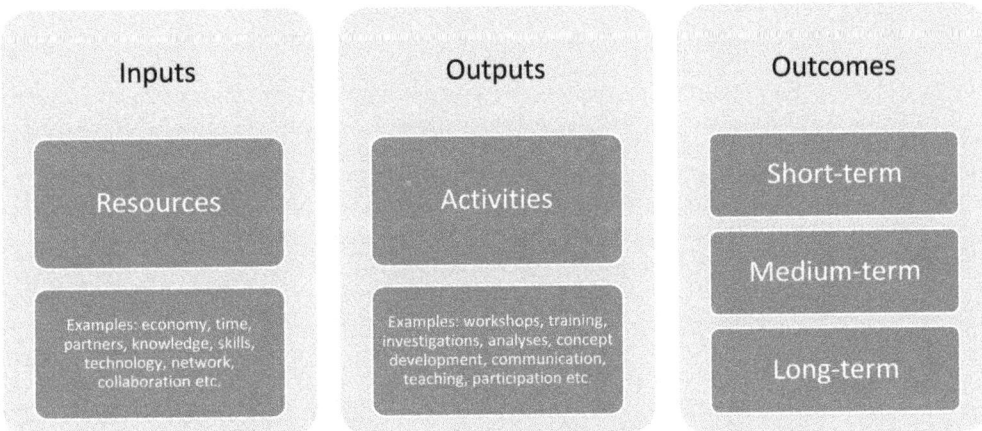

Figure 3. Outline of logic model for interventions in the HeLP program.

Step 5. Intervention planning

Step 5. *Focuses on intervention planning. Project members, timeline, and budget will be revised and confirmed. Project milestones and associated activities will be identified. Moreover, an evaluation plan will be developed and established.*

The intervention planning will proceed based on the logic model. Project milestones with according activities will be identified by the HeLP management team for intervention development, implementation, and evaluation. Materials, training, and processes will be purchased or developed in collaboration between the participating sites and the HeLP management team.

Step 6. Intervention development and refinement

Step 6. *Focuses on intervention development and refinement including performing a series of quality improvement cycles to test materials, training, manuals, and processes. Content will be refined based on findings from these cycles.*

Quality improvement cycles [50] will be undertaken by the HeLP management team to test intervention elements including materials, training, and manuals. We anticipate that quality improvement cycles will be based on the Plan-Do-Study-Act (PDSA) method [50,51].

Under 'plan', ideas for improvements related to materials, training, or manuals in HeLP will be detailed, responsibility and task assignments will be established, and expectations will be discussed and agreed upon. Moving on to 'do', where the plan is implemented and tested. Under 'study', any deviations or defects detected during the do phase will be analyzed and studied. Finally, under 'act', the learnings generated will be incorporated into the element, which was tested. Based on findings from these cycles, materials and processes will continuously be refined.

2.5. Phase Three

Step 7. Implementation and evaluation

Step 7. *Focuses on refining, implementing, and evaluating the intervention.*

In phase three, the first activity is to refine the implementation and evaluation plan. The intervention will be implemented followed by evaluation activities. Content and suitable methods used for the evaluation strategy will depend on the developed intervention and will therefore not be established before the development process is finalized. We anticipate that qualitative and mixed methods will be used to evaluate the intervention due to the potential complexity and context-bound nature [52]. The evaluation strategy will be developed with the objective to gain contextualized understandings of how the intervention works, and how it changes outcomes in practice. We expect that the evaluation strategy will contain qualitative feasibility studies [53,54]. Some of the following questions will potentially be suitable to guide the evaluation strategy in HeLP. These preliminary questions were inspired by a qualitative version of the RE-AIM (Reach, Effectiveness, Adoption, Implementation, and Maintenance) framework [55,56], a framework based on five dimensions to evaluate public health interventions.

- Reach: What factors contribute to participation/non-participation? Does the intervention reach the participants, who needs it most?
- Effectiveness: Does the intervention have a meaningful effect and benefit for participants? Are there any unanticipated outcomes of the intervention? Does the intervention work with typical pregnant women and health professionals in a real-world setting? Are the results meaningful?
- Adoption: Are interventions adopted at all organizational levels of the participating sites, by health professionals, and pregnant women? What barriers reduce intervention adoption?
- Implementation: Is the intervention delivered as intended by selected health professionals? By whom and when was the intervention implemented? What influenced implementation or lack of implementation?
- Maintenance: Is the intervention institutionalized as part of the everyday culture and norms at the participating sites?

The final outcome measures and methods used to develop an evaluation strategy in the HeLP program will be established by the HeLP management team when the intervention is developed.

Step 8. Development of an ongoing quality improvement strategy

Step 8. *Focuses on quality improvement. Intervention components will undergo continuously quality improvement in step 8 of the HeLP program.*

An ongoing quality improvement strategy [57] will be developed based on the Plan-Do-Study-Act (PDSA) method [50,51], as described under step 6.

3. Ethics

The HeLP program is approved by the Danish Data Protection Agency (2016-051-000001, 2296) and the Regional Ethics Committee. Informed consent will be collected from consultation workshop participants to audio-record table dialogue. The questionnaire will be created in the data-protected system, Research Electronic Data Capture (RedCap). Data will be cleansed, quality ensured, and anonymized by ID numbers.

4. Discussion

The HeLP program is expected to result in new knowledge of pregnant women's health literacy needs, as well as the development, implementation, and evaluation of a health literacy intervention for antenatal care, which has the potential to accommodate and respond to different levels of health literacy among pregnant women. We expect that the application of the Ophelia process will guide the co-design process successfully, entail large engagement from stakeholders and increase practical outcomes, which will benefit pregnant women, their partners, and their unborn child [30,31,33].

4.1. Strengths and Limitations

The HeLP program involves two sites: both a tertiary referral hospital and a secondary hospital. The tertiary hospital is located in Aarhus—the second largest city in Denmark (approximately 340,000 residents), while the secondary hospital is located in Viborg—a smaller Danish city (approximately 41,000 residents). The involvement of different participating sites in the HeLP program is a strength as it increases the external validity of findings. Due to the co-design process based on local knowledge, findings may not directly be reproduced in other contexts, and local adaptions may always be considered before scaling up [58].

Today, antenatal care is complex and based on a high level of patient self-management, e.g., in relation to technology use and navigation [59]. The complexity increases the risk of inequality in health and the gap between highly and less resourceful patients [60]. In the HeLP program, we seek to involve a broad variety of local stakeholders including pregnant women in vulnerable life situations. It is a strength of the HeLP program that workshop participants will be recruited from different settings and represent a heterogeneous group. Moreover, the Ophelia process has been tested in various settings and was found suitable for the successful involvement of local stakeholders including participants in vulnerable life situations [32,33]. However, we also foresee some challenges and weaknesses in the HeLP program. Engaging in a scientific project and filling out a comprehensive questionnaire requires basic health literacy skills [61]. Hence, an important group potentially eludes participation and filling out HeLP-Q. We are aware of this challenge and plan to have research assistants present at participating sites to help and support pregnant women in filling out the questionnaire.

The co-creative methodology used in the HeLP program has the potential to generate empowering processes (enable participants to gain control, develop skills, and test their knowledge) and empowering outcomes (a feeling of increased control, greater understanding, and active involvement) among participants [62]. On the other hand, some literature suggests that highly resourceful participants may dominate the co-design processes, due to their superior capital [62]. The HeLP management team needs to acknowledge and consider this challenge. For the co-design process in HeLP to succeed and produce useable and relevant practical findings, consideration of participant's motivation and professional-patient and inter-participant relationships and roles is important [62]. The HeLP management team, who is responsible for the workshops, collaboration with participants, and communication, must demonstrate an open attitude towards participants. If participants feel mistrusted by the researchers, the risk of negative attitudes towards the co-design process increases [62,63]. The researchers hold the main responsibility to set the frame, plan, structure, and organize meetings, workshops, and other collaborative activities with participants. However, they must be aware of their role and support and endorse participant empowerment [64].

The Ophelia process allows for some adaption during the process. For example, consultation workshops are scheduled to last approximately four hours each and include 25 participants. These decisions were made based on experiences from previous Ophelia processes [32] and a professional judgment. We do not know whether this timeframe and participant number are realistic and suitable in practice. If the HeLP management group experiences any challenges related to this during the first workshop, adjustments will be made before the second workshop. We will try to accommodate any challenges related to this and provide auxiliary assistance during the workshops.

Another limitation of the HeLP program is that health literacy interventions developed based on the Ophelia process need further investigation and evaluation to establish effectiveness. However, preliminary findings are promising [33].

4.2. Implementation of Findings

The development of health literacy interventions for antenatal care is important due to increasing inequality in access to antenatal care services among pregnant women [1,2,4]. A health literacy focus is needed to support and meet pregnant women's different skillset to access, understand, appraise, and apply health information and make decisions related to the health of themselves and their baby. These skills have only become more important due to the increasing complexity, and need for engagement, decision making, and use of technology in health care services [65].

In 2017, Beauchamp et al. published a paper on the systematic development and implementation of interventions to optimize health literacy and access [30]. The study showed improvements in health literacy scores, and the Ophelia process was successfully applied resulting in the development of health literacy interventions in accordance with local wisdom and organizational priorities [30]. Evidence of operationalization of the eight Ophelia principles was present at all intervention sites. Hence, (1) the operationalization was outcome focused, (2) the sites were equity driven, (3) and (5) the wisdom of local stakeholders ensured co-design, (4) and (7) intervention ideas drew on local wisdom sites focused on local health literacy needs, and (8) ideas were generated and applied across all levels of organizations. However, (6) the sustainability of the interventions needs confirmation in a long turn follow-up, as well as the improvement processes to ensure interventions remain relevant and effective [30].

In addition, Jessup et al. used the Ophelia process in hospitalized populations [66], while Anwar et al. applied the process in fishing villages in Egypt [67]. Moreover, Cheng et al. used the process with an eHealth Literacy focus [68]. Similar to these studies is that they contribute evidence supporting that the Ophelia process produces user-friendly vignettes and provides a locally driven and contextual co-design process [66–68]. However, evidence of the implementation and evaluation process in Ophelia needs further exploration as well as the sustainability of produced health literacy interventions and the ongoing process to ensure relevance and effectiveness of the interventions developed using the Ophelia process.

The HeLP program is expected to contribute new knowledge about how the Ophelia process can be used to develop health literacy interventions, which generate improvements in antenatal care and address inequity in access to services [30]. In addition, we anticipate that the HeLP program will contribute further knowledge on the effectiveness of the Ophelia process, and the operationalization of the eight Ophelia principles in antenatal intervention sites.

5. Conclusions

The HeLP program is expected to contribute new knowledge of pregnant women's health literacy needs in antenatal care and development, implementation, and evaluation of health literacy interventions. The Ophelia process will be used to co-design health literacy interventions based on local knowledge about health literacy strengths and challenges among pregnant women and improve the ability to respond to these strengths and challenges in antenatal care.

Author Contributions: Conceptualization, M.M., R.D.M., M.F.D., A.A., A.P. and H.T.M.; methodology, M.M., R.D.M., M.F.D., A.A., A.P. and H.T.M.; resources, R.D.M. and H.T.M.; writing—original draft preparation, M.M.; writing—review and editing, M.M.; visualization, M.M., R.D.M., M.F.D., A.A., A.P. and H.T.M.; supervision, R.D.M., A.A., A.P. and H.T.M.; project administration, M.M., R.D.M., M.F.D. and H.T.M.; funding acquisition, M.M., R.D.M. and H.T.M. All authors have read and agreed to the published version of the manuscript.

Funding: This study was funded by the Danish Regions and supported by Aarhus University.

Institutional Review Board Statement: The study was registered cf. General Data Protection Regulation, Aarhus University Journal number 2016-051-000001, serial number 2296.

Informed Consent Statement: Informed consent will be obtained from all subjects involved in the HeLP program.

Data Availability Statement: Not applicable.

Conflicts of Interest: The authors declare no conflict of interest.

Abbreviations

HeLP	Health Literacy in Pregnancy
Ophelia	Optimising Health Literacy and Access
WHO	World Health Organization
NHLDPs	National Health Literacy Demonstration Projects
AUH	Aarhus University Hospital
EPJ	Electronic Patient Journal
HeLP-Q	Health Literacy in Pregnancy Questionnaire
HLQ	The Health Literacy Questionnaire
eHLQ	The eHealth Literacy Questionnaire
RedCap	Research Electronic Data Capture

References

1. Adegbosin, A.E.; Zhou, H.; Wang, S.; Stantic, B.; Sun, J. Systematic review and meta-analysis of the association between dimensions of inequality and a selection of indicators of Reproductive, Maternal, Newborn and Child Health (RMNCH). *J. Glob. Health* **2019**, *9*, 010429. [CrossRef] [PubMed]
2. Yaya, S.; Ghose, B. Global Inequality in Maternal Health Care Service Utilization: Implications for Sustainable Development Goals. *Health Equity* **2019**, *3*, 145–154. [CrossRef] [PubMed]
3. Mortensen, L.H.; Helweg-Larsen, K.; Andersen, A.M. Socioeconomic differences in perinatal health and disease. *Scand. J. Public Health* **2011**, *39* (Suppl. 7), 110–114. [CrossRef] [PubMed]
4. Aabakke, A.J.M.; Mortensen, L.H.; Krebs, L. Socioeconomic inequality affects pregnancy and birth outcomes in Denmark. *Ugeskr. Laeg.* **2019**, *181*, V08180590.
5. Feleke, B.E. Determinants of gestational diabetes mellitus: A case-control study. *J. Matern Fetal Neonatal Med.* **2018**, *31*, 2584–2589. [CrossRef]
6. Ovesen, P.; Rasmussen, S.; Kesmodel, U. Effect of prepregnancy maternal overweight and obesity on pregnancy outcome. *Obstet. Gynecol.* **2011**, *118* Pt 1, 305–312. [CrossRef]
7. Nasreen, H.E.; Kabir, Z.N.; Forsell, Y.; Edhborg, M. Prevalence and associated factors of depressive and anxiety symptoms during pregnancy: A population based study in rural Bangladesh. *BMC Women's Health* **2011**, *11*, 22. [CrossRef]
8. Li, J.; Robinson, M.; Malacova, E.; Jacoby, P.; Foster, J.; van Eekelen, A. Maternal life stress events in pregnancy link to children's school achievement at age 10 years. *J. Pediatr.* **2013**, *162*, 483–489. [CrossRef]
9. Svendsen, M.T.; Bak, C.K.; Sørensen, K.; Pelikan, J.; Riddersholm, S.J.; Skals, R.K.; Mortensen, R.N.; Maindal, H.T.; Bøggild, H.; Nielsen, G.; et al. Associations of health literacy with socioeconomic position, health risk behavior, and health status: A large national population-based survey among Danish adults. *BMC Public Health* **2020**, *20*, 565. [CrossRef]
10. Pelikan, J.M.; Ganahl, K.; Roethlin, F. Health literacy as a determinant, mediator and/or moderator of health: Empirical models using the European Health Literacy Survey dataset. *Glob. Health Promot.* **2018**, *25*, 57–66. [CrossRef]
11. Bo, A.; Friis, K.; Osborne, R.H.; Maindal, H.T. National indicators of health literacy: Ability to understand health information and to engage actively with healthcare providers—A population-based survey among Danish adults. *BMC Public Health* **2014**, *14*, 1095. [CrossRef]
12. Sørensen, K.; Pelikan, J.M.; Röthlin, F.; Ganahl, K.; Slonska, Z.; Doyle, G.; Fullam, J.; Kondilis, B.; Agrafiotis, D.; Uiters, E.; et al. Health literacy in Europe: Comparative results of the European health literacy survey (HLS-EU). *Eur. J. Public Health* **2015**, *25*, 1053–1058. [CrossRef]
13. Kilfoyle, K.A.; Vitko, M.; O'Conor, R.; Bailey, S.C. Health Literacy and Women's Reproductive Health: A Systematic Review. *J. Women's Health* **2016**, *25*, 1237–1255. [CrossRef]
14. Nawabi, F.; Krebs, F.; Vennedey, V.; Shukri, A.; Lorenz, L.; Stock, S. Health Literacy in Pregnant Women: A Systematic Review. *Int. J. Environ. Res. Public Health* **2021**, *18*, 3847. [CrossRef]
15. Endres, L.K.; Sharp, L.K.; Haney, E.; Dooley, S.L. Health literacy and pregnancy preparedness in pregestational diabetes. *Diabetes Care* **2004**, *27*, 331–334. [CrossRef]

16. Poorman, E.; Gazmararian, J.; Elon, L.; Parker, R. Is health literacy related to health behaviors and cell phone usage patterns among the text4baby target population? *Arch. Public Health Arch. Belg. De Sante Publique* **2014**, *72*, 13. [CrossRef]
17. Shieh, C.; Mays, R.; McDaniel, A.; Yu, J. Health literacy and its association with the use of information sources and with barriers to information seeking in clinic-based pregnant women. *Health Care Women Int.* **2009**, *30*, 971–988. [CrossRef]
18. Lupattelli, A.; Picinardi, M.; Einarson, A.; Nordeng, H. Health literacy and its association with perception of teratogenic risks and health behavior during pregnancy. *Patient Educ. Couns.* **2014**, *96*, 171–178. [CrossRef]
19. Duggan, L.; McCarthy, S.; Curtis, L.M.; Wolf, M.S.; Noone, C.; Higgins, J.R.; O'Shea, S.; Sahm, L.J. Associations between health literacy and beliefs about medicines in an Irish obstetric population. *J. Health Commun.* **2014**, *19* (Suppl. 2), 106–114. [CrossRef]
20. Shieh, C.; McDaniel, A.; Ke, I. Information-seeking and its predictors in low-income pregnant women. *J. Midwifery Women's Health* **2009**, *54*, 364–372. [CrossRef]
21. Bennett, I.M.; Culhane, J.F.; McCollum, K.F.; Mathew, L.; Elo, I.T. Literacy and depressive symptomatology among pregnant Latinas with limited English proficiency. *Am. J. Orthopsychiatry* **2007**, *77*, 243–248. [CrossRef]
22. Arnold, C.L.; Davis, T.C.; Berkel, H.J.; Jackson, R.H.; Nandy, I.; London, S. Smoking status, reading level, and knowledge of tobacco effects among low-income pregnant women. *Prev. Med.* **2001**, *32*, 313–320. [CrossRef]
23. Smedberg, J.; Lupattelli, A.; Mårdby, A.C.; Nordeng, H. Characteristics of women who continue smoking during pregnancy: A cross-sectional study of pregnant women and new mothers in 15 European countries. *BMC Pregnancy Childbirth* **2014**, *14*, 213. [CrossRef]
24. Nutbeam, D. Health literacy as a public health goal: A challenge for contemporary health education and communication strategies into the 21st century. *Health Promot. Int.* **2000**, *15*, 259–267. [CrossRef]
25. IUHPE. Position Statement on Health Literacy: A practical vision for a health literate world. *Glob. Health Promot.* **2018**, *25*, 79–88. [CrossRef]
26. WHO. *Health Literacy—The Solid Facts*; World Health Organization: Geneva, Switzerland, 2013; Available online: www.aoos.who.int (accessed on 27 January 2022).
27. World Health Organization. Shanghai Declaration on promoting health in the 2030 Agenda for Sustainable Development. In Proceedings of the Ninth Global Conference on Health Promotion, Shanghai, China, 21–24 November 2016; Available online: www.who.int (accessed on 27 January 2022).
28. World Health Organization. *Draft WHO European Roadmap for Implementation of Health Literacy Initiatives through the Life Course*; The WHO Regional Committee for Europe: Copenhagen, Denmark, 2019.
29. Hardyman, W.; Daunt, K.L.; Kitchener, M. Value Co-Creation through Patient Engagement in Health Care: A micro-level approach and research agenda. *Public Manag. Rev.* **2015**, *17*, 90–107. [CrossRef]
30. Beauchamp, A.; Batterham, R.W.; Dodson, S.; Astbury, B.; Elsworth, G.R.; McPhee, C.; Jacobson, J.; Buchbinder, R.; Osborne, R.H. Systematic development and implementation of interventions to OPtimise Health Literacy and Access (Ophelia). *BMC Public Health* **2017**, *17*, 230. [CrossRef]
31. Batterham, R.W.; Buchbinder, R.; Beauchamp, A.; Dodson, S.; Elsworth, G.R.; Osborne, R.H. The OPtimising HEalth LIterAcy (Ophelia) process: Study protocol for using health literacy profiling and community engagement to create and implement health reform. *BMC Public Health* **2014**, *14*, 694. [CrossRef]
32. Aaby, A.; Simonsen, C.B.; Ryom, K.; Maindal, H.T. Improving Organizational Health Literacy Responsiveness in Cardiac Rehabilitation Using a Co-Design Methodology: Results from the Heart Skills Study. *Int. J. Environ. Res. Public Health* **2020**, *17*, 1015. [CrossRef] [PubMed]
33. World Health Organization; Regional Office for Europe; Bakker, M.M.; Putrik, P.; Aaby, A.; Debussche, X.; Morrissey, J. Acting together–WHO National Health Literacy Demonstration Projects (NHLDPs) address health literacy needs in the European Region. *Public Health Panor.* **2019**, *5*, 123–329.
34. Zibellini, J.; Muscat, D.M.; Kizirian, N.; Gordon, A. Effect of health literacy interventions on pregnancy outcomes: A systematic review. *Women Birth J. Aust. Coll. Midwives* **2021**, *34*, 180–186. [CrossRef] [PubMed]
35. Sundhedsstyrelsen. Anbefalinger for Svangreomsorgen. 2013. Available online: www.sst.dk (accessed on 27 January 2022).
36. Fernandez, M.E.; Ruiter, R.A.C.; Markham, C.M.; Kok, G. Intervention Mapping: Theory- and Evidence-Based Health Promotion Program Planning: Perspective and Examples. *Front. Public Health* **2019**, *7*, 209. [CrossRef] [PubMed]
37. Ovretveit, J.; Bate, P.; Cleary, P.; Cretin, S.; Gustafson, D.; McInnes, K.; McLeod, H.; Molfenter, T.; Plsek, P.; Robert, G.; et al. Quality collaboratives: Lessons from research. *Qual. Saf. Health Care* **2002**, *11*, 345–351. [CrossRef] [PubMed]
38. Nadeem, E.; Olin, S.S.; Hill, L.C.; Hoagwood, K.E.; Horwitz, S.M. Understanding the Components of Quality Improvement Collaboratives: A Systematic Literature Review. *Milbank Q.* **2013**, *91*, 354–394. [CrossRef]
39. Rycroft-Malone, J.; McCormack, B.; Hutchinson, A.M.; DeCorby, K.; Bucknall, T.K.; Kent, B.; Schultz, A.; Snelgrove-Clarke, E.; Stetler, C.B.; Titler, M.; et al. Realist synthesis: Illustrating the method for implementation research. *Implement. Sci.* **2012**, *7*, 33. [CrossRef]
40. Green, J.M.; Kafetsios, K.; Statham, H.E.; Snowdon, C.M. Factor Structure, Validity and Reliability of the Cambridge Worry Scale in a Pregnant Population. *J. Health Psychol.* **2003**, *8*, 753–764. [CrossRef]
41. Kozinszky, Z.; Dudas, R.B. Validation studies of the Edinburgh Postnatal Depression Scale for the antenatal period. *J. Affect. Disord.* **2015**, *176*, 95–105. [CrossRef]

42. Trucharte, A.; Calderón, L.; Cerezo, E.; Contreras, A.; Peinado, V.; Valiente, C. Three-item loneliness scale: Psychometric properties and normative data of the Spanish version. *Curr. Psychol.* **2021**, 1–9. [CrossRef]
43. Czajkowska, Z.; Wang, H.; Hall, N.C.; Sewitch, M.; Körner, A. Validation of the English and French versions of the Brief Health Care Climate Questionnaire. *Health Psychol. Open* **2017**, *4*, 2055102917730675. [CrossRef]
44. Maindal, H.T.; Kayser, L.; Norgaard, O.; Bo, A.; Elsworth, G.R.; Osborne, R.H. Cultural Adaptation and Validation of the Health Literacy Questionnaire (HLQ): Robust Nine-Dimension Danish Language Confirmatory Factor Model 2016 [PMC4971008]. 2016/08/19:[1232]. Available online: https://ph.au.dk/healthliteracy/projekter-og-aktiviteter (accessed on 27 January 2022).
45. Osborne, R.H.; Batterham, R.W.; Elsworth, G.R.; Hawkins, M.; Buchbinder, R. The grounded psychometric development and initial validation of the Health Literacy Questionnaire (HLQ). *BMC Public Health* **2013**, *13*, 658. [CrossRef]
46. Karnoe, A.; Furstrand, D.; Christensen, K.B.; Norgaard, O.; Kayser, L. Assessing Competencies Needed to Engage With Digital Health Services: Development of the eHealth Literacy Assessment Toolkit. *J. Med. Internet Res.* **2018**, *20*, e178. [CrossRef]
47. Kayser, L.; Karnoe, A.; Furstrand, D.; Batterham, R.; Christensen, K.B.; Elsworth, G.; Osborne, R.H. A Multidimensional Tool Based on the eHealth Literacy Framework: Development and Initial Validity Testing of the eHealth Literacy Questionnaire (eHLQ). *J. Med. Internet Res.* **2018**, *20*, e36. [CrossRef]
48. Tausch, A.P.; Menold, N. Methodological Aspects of Focus Groups in Health Research. Results of Qualitative Interviews with Focus Group Moderators. *Glob. Qual. Nurs. Res.* **2016**, *3*, 2333393616630466. [CrossRef]
49. Taylor-Powell, E.; Henert, E. *Developing a Logic Model: Teaching and Training Guide*; University of Wisconsin-Extension: Madison, WI, USA, 2008.
50. Varkey, P.; Reller, M.K.; Resar, R.K. Basics of Quality Improvement in Health Care. *Mayo Clin. Proc.* **2007**, *82*, 735–739. [CrossRef]
51. Berwick, D.M. Developing and Testing Changes in Delivery of Care. *Ann. Intern. Med.* **1998**, *128*, 651–656. [CrossRef]
52. Skivington, K.; Matthews, L.; Simpson, S.; Craig, P.; Baird, J.; Blazeby, J.; Boyd, K.; Craig, N.; French, D.; McIntosh, E.; et al. A new framework for developing and evaluating complex interventions: Update of Medical Research Council guidance. *BMJ Clin. Res. Ed.* **2021**, *374*, n2061. [CrossRef]
53. Jensen, N.H.; Aaby, A.; Ryom, K.; Maindal, H.T. A CHAT about Health Literacy—A Qualitative Feasibility Study of the Conversational Health Literacy Assessment Tool (CHAT) in a Danish Municipal Healthcare Centre. *Scand. J. Caring Sci.* **2021**, *35*, 1250–1258. [CrossRef]
54. Giangregorio, L.; Thabane, L. *Complex Interventions in Health: An Overview of Research Methods*; Routledge: London, UK, 2015.
55. Glasgow, R.E.; Vogt, T.M.; Boles, S.M. Evaluating the public health impact of health promotion interventions: The RE-AIM framework. *Am. J. Public Health* **1999**, *89*, 1322–1327. [CrossRef]
56. Holtrop, J.S.; Rabin, B.A.; Glasgow, R.E. Qualitative approaches to use of the RE-AIM framework: Rationale and methods. *BMC Health Serv. Res.* **2018**, *18*, 177. [CrossRef]
57. Brennan, S.; McKenzie, J.E.; Whitty, P.; Buchan, H.; Green, S. Continuous quality improvement: Effects on professional practice and healthcare outcomes. *Cochrane Database Syst. Rev.* **2009**, *11*, CD003319. [CrossRef]
58. Power, J.; Gilmore, B.; Vallières, F.; Toomey, E.; Mannan, H.; McAuliffe, E. Adapting health interventions for local fit when scaling-up: A realist review protocol. *BMJ Open* **2019**, *9*, e022084. [CrossRef]
59. Currell, R. The organisation of midwifery care. In *Antenatal Care: A Research-Based Approach*; Alexander, J., Levy, V., Roch, S., Eds.; Macmillan Education: London, UK, 1990; pp. 20–41.
60. Plsek, P.E.; Greenhalgh, T. The challenge of complexity in health care. *BMJ Clin. Res. Ed.* **2001**, *323*, 625–628. [CrossRef]
61. Kripalani, S.; Goggins, K.; Couey, C.; Yeh, V.M.; Donato, K.M.; Schnelle, J.F.; Wallston, K.A.; Bell, S.P.; Harrell, F.E.; Mixon, A.S.; et al. Disparities in Research Participation by Level of Health Literacy. *Mayo Clin. Proc.* **2021**, *96*, 314–321. [CrossRef]
62. Brandsen, T.; Steen, T.; Verschuere, B. (Eds.) *Co-Production and Co-Creation: Engaging Citizens in Public Services*, 1st ed.; Routledge: London, UK, 2018.
63. Ostrom, E. Crossing the great divide: Coproduction, synergy, and development. *World Dev.* **1996**, *24*, 1073–1087. [CrossRef]
64. Palumbo, R. *The Bright Side and the Dark Side of Patient Empowerment: Co-Creation and Co-Destruction of Value in the Healthcare Environment*; Springer International Publishing: Berlin/Heidelberg, Germany, 2017.
65. Clancy, C.M. Patient engagement in health care. *Health Serv. Res.* **2011**, *46*, 389–393. [CrossRef]
66. Jessup, R.L.; Osborne, R.H.; Buchbinder, R.; Beauchamp, A. Using co-design to develop interventions to address health literacy needs in a hospitalised population. *BMC Health Serv. Res.* **2018**, *18*, 989. [CrossRef]
67. Anwar, W.A.; Mostafa, N.S.; Hakim, S.A.; Sos, D.G.; Cheng, C.; Osborne, R.H. Health Literacy Co-Design in a Low Resource Setting: Harnessing Local Wisdom to Inform Interventions across Fishing Villages in Egypt to Improve Health and Equity. *Int. J. Environ. Res. Public Health* **2021**, *18*, 4518. [CrossRef]
68. Cheng, C.; Elsworth, G.R.; Osborne, R.H. Co-designing eHealth and Equity Solutions: Application of the Ophelia (Optimizing Health Literacy and Access) Process. *Front. Public Health* **2020**, *8*, 604401. [CrossRef]

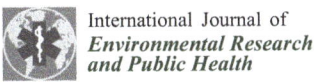

Article

Health Literacy in the Context of Implant Care—Perspectives of (Prospective) Implant Wearers on Individual and Organisational Factors

Constanze Hübner [1,*,†], Mariya Lorke [1,*,†], Annika Buchholz [2], Stefanie Frech [3], Laura Harzheim [1], Sabine Schulz [1], Saskia Jünger [4] and Christiane Woopen [5]

[1] Cologne Center for Ethics, Rights, Economics, and Social Sciences of Health (CERES), University of Cologne and University Hospital of Cologne, Universitätsstraße 91, 50931 Cologne, Germany; laura.harzheim@uni-koeln.de (L.H.); sabine.schulz@uni-koeln.de (S.S.)
[2] Department of Otolaryngology, Hannover Medical School, Carl-Neuberg-Str. 1, 30625 Hannover, Germany; buchholz.annika@mh-hannover.de
[3] Department of Ophthalmology, Rostock University Medical Center, Doberaner Str. 140, 18057 Rostock, Germany; stefanie.frech@med.uni-rostock.de
[4] Department of Community Health, University of Applied Health Sciences Bochum, Gesundheitscampus 6-8, 44801 Bochum, Germany; saskia.juenger@hs-gesundheit.de
[5] Center for Life Ethics, University of Bonn, 53113 Bonn, Germany; chwoopen@uni-bonn.de
* Correspondence: constanze.huebner@uk-koeln.de (C.H.); mariya.lorke@uni-koeln.de (M.L.)
† These authors contributed equally to this work.

Abstract: The continuous development of medical implants offers various benefits for persons with chronic conditions but also challenges an individual's, and the healthcare system's, ability to deal with technical innovation. Accessing and understanding new information, navigating healthcare, and appraising the role of the implant in body perceptions and everyday life requires health literacy (HL) of those affected as well as an HL-responsive healthcare system. The interconnectedness of these aspects to ethically relevant values such as health, dependence, responsibility and self-determination reinforces the need to address HL in implant care. Following a qualitative approach, we conducted group discussions and a diary study among wearers of a cochlear, glaucoma or cardiovascular implant (or their parents). Data were analysed using the documentary method and grounded theory. The data reveal the perceptions of implant wearers regarding the implant on (1) the ability to handle technical and ambiguous information; (2) dependence and responsibility within the healthcare system; and (3) the ethical aspects of HL. Knowing more about the experiences and values of implant wearers is highly beneficial to develop HL from an ethical perspective. Respective interventions need to initially address ethically relevant values in counselling processes and implant care.

Keywords: health literacy; decision making; values; implant care; ethical aspects; health-literacy development; cochlear implants; glaucoma implants; cardiovascular implants

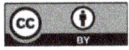

1. Introduction

The continuous development of implantable technologies offers various benefits for persons with chronic conditions, but also challenges the ability of those affected, their doctors, and the healthcare system, to deal with technical innovation. The integration of technical devices in the human body directly intermingles with individual and social values such as health, (in)dependence, responsibility and self-determination. Furthermore, implant wearers need to develop technical and health competences to keep up with a significant amount of fast-changing technical and health information. The actors involved in implant care also face the challenges of reducing barriers to information, communication and navigation for their clients. In addition, those actors may support implant wearers in their efforts to increase their quality of life *via* and *despite* constant technical upgrades and accompanying uncertainty.

Implant wearers suffer chronic conditions and often have long-term experiences with the healthcare system. Such patients may be savvy with terminology that is relevant to their conditions, but might have difficulties in other fields, such as risk communication or the appraisal of statistical information [1–3]. With respect to implant care, the knowledge about the chronic condition pairs with understanding technology- and implant-related information. Herein, two levels of health literacy (HL) become particularly relevant. On the one hand, (1) the individual level regarding competencies of handling and appraising technical and medical information as well as communication skills to engage in informed decision making has to be considered. On the other hand, (2) the organisational level with respect to the responsivity of the healthcare system to individuals' information needs with regard to their moral values and convictions is of relevance. These aspects underline the essential role of HL, referred to as the capacity of individuals to handle health- and implant-related information (individual HL) [4] and as the responsivity of the healthcare system to individuals' information needs (organisational HL) [5]. This study provides unique insights on HL in the context of implant care, since, to our knowledge, this topic has not been researched yet. Both individual and organisational HL are described in more detail in the following section.

In the individual lifeworld, wearing an implant has its medical side, where individual HL plays a significant role for organising everyday life with the implant and managing the chronic health condition. In this case, individual HL exceeds its functional dimension as the capacity to obtain, process and understand certain health-related information to be able to make appropriate health decisions [6]. It encompasses critical, communicative [7], and navigation- and technology-related HL. Critical HL relates to the critical appraisal of health information [8]; communicative HL is described as "more advanced cognitive and literacy skills, which together with social skills, can be used to actively participate in everyday activities, to extract information and derive meaning from different forms of communication and to apply new information to changing circumstances" [9] (pp. 263–264); navigation HL describes the competences of individuals to orient themselves in healthcare systems [10]; technology-related HL relates to the individual's ability to handle health-related technical information and to successfully operate technical devices. Organisational HL comprises the responsivity of the healthcare system to the information needs [6] of (prospective) implant wearers. In implant care, it therefore addresses the providers' responsibility to offer sufficient access to adequate (technical) information and enable the process of information appraisal incorporating the everyday experiences of implant wearers.

Handling medical and technology-related information is essential for decision making and living with an implant. However, as outlined above, in implant care it is also necessary to deal with the image of one's own body, adjust to the change in everyday habits and reflect on a new kind of dependence. This can be experienced and processed differently and is necessarily connected to ethically relevant values. Following a bio-psychosocial perspective, for example, *health* is not only determined by biomedical factors ("absence of disease") but also comprises mental and social components [11] which differ interpersonally. Accordingly, navigating within the healthcare system or the acceptance of implants as a treatment option can also vary, depending on the subjective understanding (in the following, prospective implant wearers (glaucoma) and children of parents with cochlear implants are also implied) of health and the individual expectations of body functionality. An implant may enable social participation [3], decelerate disease progression, or compensate for an impairment [12] but also prevents the individual from a sudden death [13]. In this context, values such as *self-determination, dependence and responsibility* play a central role, especially in terms of deciding for or against an implant (or the proxy decision that has to be made for the child) or in cases where a decision against the implant is not an actual option. This also implies that the individual is faced with a fundamentally new degree of *dependence* and *responsibility*, not only in the decision-making process [14], but also in the often lifelong management of the implant and the disease itself. The feeling of responsibility is thereby shaped by individual attitudes and competences (HL). These aspects demonstrate the relevance of social convictions on health and disease and their manifestation with regards to social participation and individual life planning.

The HL competences elaborated above can, in turn, promote ethically relevant values, emphasising the ethical relevance of HL development. This lends legitimacy to approaching HL from an ethical perspective.

Previous research has repeatedly focused on theoretical and conceptual dimensions of HL and its operationalisation [15], as well as different types of HL and empirical data assessing the HL of different populations [16]. There is also research on the ethical dimensions of HL more generally [3,17,18], whereas Watson (2019) [3] offers recommendations for HL development in the context of implant care. Two further studies address empowerment and communicative responsibility [19,20]. Nonetheless, these are not directly related to HL in the context of implant care and ethics, but rather provide an area of analogy for the better contextualisation of this article. The ethical approach to HL and HL development in the field of implant care is new in the existing research landscape. This study adds a further perspective on HL in relation to implantable technology.

Given the complexity and entanglement of implant care, HL, and ethics, it is essential to learn more about the perspectives and values of implant wearers and incorporate their experiences into the research process. This may help identify gaps in the published research and provide information and perspectives on the ethical and social values related to health technologies [21–23]. Exploring lived experiences of implant wearers can help to understand how ethical values are reflected in implant care and offer references for ethically meaningful HL development. This study presumes that individual values and social convictions affect individual and organisational HL in implant care. At the same time, HL promotes various ethical values. HL development in the field of implant care is therefore strongly influenced by ethically relevant values and an ethical responsibility itself.

As part of a joint project, this study aims to offer insights into the individual processes of navigating medical and technical information of cochlear-, glaucoma- or cardiovascular-implant wearers as well as decision making in implant care, which is characterised by constant innovations and technical upgrades. Against this background, we sought to shed light on the connection of HL and ethics in implant care and investigate possibilities for HL development. The leading research questions are: (1) What fosters HL development in the context of implant care from an ethical and patient-centred perspective? (2) How can HL initiatives in implant care be enhanced by the insights of implant wearers?

2. Materials and Methods

Following a qualitative approach, group discussions as well as diaries constitute appropriate methods to explore individual perspectives and opinions on implant care, shared understandings or controversies, which evolve through a dynamic discussion with others [24], and to capture contextual experiences in a direct and longitudinal manner [25]. This approach is well-suited to identifying different aspects of decision making, experiences in navigating the healthcare system and quality of life, as well as to obtain insights into the everyday lives of implant wearers and the associated aspects of dealing with implants in a wide range of situations (doctor's visits, check ups, medication, everyday errands, social relationships, everyday activities). Therefore, remunerated group discussions (GDs) (N = 6) and a diary study (DS) (n = 13) with individuals wearing cochlear, glaucoma or cardiovascular implants, and parents of children with a cochlear implant, were conducted. Since the data-collection period coincided with the COVID-19 pandemic, both methods had to be adjusted to an online setting. Ethics approval was obtained in November 2020 (Nr: 20-1176_1) by the Medical Faculty of the University of Cologne. According to the research plan, the study had to be conducted in the period between November 2020 and October 2021. The decision for the time span of the study was based on two main factors: (1) based on previous experience, the researchers anticipated a difficult recruiting process in the field of glaucoma and cardiovascular implants and (2) data collection and analysis were performed in an iterative process.

The data were analysed following the documentary method [1] and the principles of grounded theory [26]. For data validation and methodologically well-founded ways of gaining knowledge from different perspectives [27], a triangulation of methods [28] and of researchers [29] was performed.

2.1. Recruitment

Participants were recruited in cooperation with the clinical project partners (patient registries of hospitals) or online by contacting organisers of support groups and relevant forums. Participants were selected via purposive sampling based on the eligibility criteria shown in Table 1.

Table 1. Eligibility criteria for group discussions and diary study.

	Inclusion	Exclusion
Cochlear	Group 1: Post-lingual deafness and implantation; middle age Group 2a: Pre-lingual deafness and implantation in childhood Group 2b: Parents of participants from group 2a Minimum time after CI [A] implantation: 12 months Minimum age: 18 years	Age < 18 years
Glaucoma	Group 1: Drug therapy (drops) only Group 2: Micro-stent ± drug therapy (drops) Adults ($\geq$50 years) with open-angle glaucoma [B] Minimum time after implantation: 6 months Minimum time of diagnosis and start of drug therapy: 12 months Visual acuity in the better eye $\geq$ 30%.	Age < 50 years
Cardiovascular	Cardiovascular implants Minimum time after implantation: 6 months Minimum age: 18 years	Age < 18 years
General in- and exclusion	Written informed consent of the patients Language skills: German language skills that allow participation in the study	Cognitive or physical limitations that do not allow study participation

[A] CI = cochlear implant. [B] Due to recruitment difficulties of implant wearers with glaucoma, inclusion criteria were adjusted to normal pressure glaucoma and a minimum age of 18 years. The adjustment of the criteria applies to 2 individuals from the DS.

A great number of cochlear-implant wearers (post-lingual) were interested in study participation. In collaboration with the Hannover Medical School, purposive sampling focused on the following participant characteristics to cover the diversity of implant wearers: sex, age, experience with the implant, complications after surgery, and communication skills. The number of (prospective) glaucoma and cardiovascular-implant wearers was manageable, so that all interested persons could participate in the study after having provided written consent.

2.2. Group Discussions

The GDs were conducted via *GoToMeeting* in compliance with data protection regulations. In advance, the participants received detailed instructions on using the platform. Technical support via telephone or e-mail was provided before and during the discussion. A team of three researchers was responsible for conducting the GDs: one moderator, technical support and a substitute moderator in case of technical difficulties.

Between December 2020 and April 2021, a total of six GDs with (prospective) implant wearers (or with parents of children wearing a cochlear implant) of cochlear (N = 3), glaucoma (N = 2) and cardiovascular (N = 1) implants were conducted. The number of participants varied within the groups between 2–9 persons. Across all areas, 26 individuals participated in GDs (Table 2).

Table 2. Group discussions.

Implant	Group Discussion	n = 26 [1]	Date of Realisation	Participants	Length
Cochlear	GD1CI	n = 9	8 December 2020	Post-lingually deafened	2 h
	GD2aCI	n = 2	8 December 2020	Pre-lingually deafened	2 h
	GD2bCI	n = 4	9 December 2020	Parent of a child with CI	2 h
Glaucoma	GD1Gl	n = 6	22 March 2021	Glaucoma	2 h
	GD2Gl	n = 2	24 March 2021	Glaucoma with stent surgery	2 h
Cardiovascular	GD1C	n = 3	29 April 2021	Cardiovascular implants (passive)	2 h
	Two individual interviews (Interview I2aC, Interview I2bC)		7 May 2021	The interviews were conducted with two persons who had technical difficulties and therefore could not participate in the group discussion.	1 h each

[1] Plus two interviews.

All GDs were recorded using *GoToMeeting* and audio recording (as a back-up). For method evaluation purposes, participants were provided with an internet link for a brief online questionnaire.

The course of each GD was supported by a power-point presentation, which included introductory slides containing researchers' affiliations, several communication rules and information about data-protection requirements. In the beginning, participants were asked to freely associate to a list of keywords related to implant ethics and previously identified through literature research (e.g., "quality of life", "decision making", "care") (see, Appendix A, Table A1). The presentation continued with guiding questions regarding disease- or implant-related decision making, handling of information and future prospects. Subsequently, the participants were given the opportunity to comment or address further aspects. The moderators let the conversations run as freely as possible and only intervened when necessary (e.g., for time-management purposes). The aim was to support the natural flow of the conversation and to ensure active participation by everyone [22].

2.3. Diary Study

For this study, the DS complemented the data generated via GDs and interviews. The design of the method was developed referring to the checklist by Janssens et al. [21]. The participant information and the supporting materials developed for the DS were based on the preliminary analysis of the GDs (see Appendix B, Table A2). The aim was to shed light on certain aspects, illuminate them in greater depth, and to reveal aspects that had not yet been discussed in the GDs. To increase compliance, participants were offered personalised feedback reports based on their recordings [21]. A total of $n = 13$ individuals were recruited for the DS: seven wearing cochlear, four glaucoma and two cardiovascular implants (see Table 3.). Apart from the written study information, the participants were also introduced (either via video conference or by telephone) to the exact procedure, the contents, as well as data-protection issues by a research assistant. Study participants kept their diaries for 4 weeks and could contact the researchers at any time. The duration of the diary study was chosen in order to minimise participant burden, on the one hand, and to obtain a representative picture of the daily life of persons with implants on the other hand. This included both during-the-week and weekend records, which covered the time span of 4 weeks. This approach aligns with existing research (see, e.g., Ref. [21]).

Table 3. Diaries.

Participants	Time Period [1]	Indication
DCI1	21 June–18 July	Post-lingually deafened
DCI2	21 June–18 July	Post-lingually deafened
DCI3	21 June–18 July	Pre-lingually deafened
DCI4	21 June–18 July	Pre-lingually deafened
DCI5	21 June–18 July	Pre-lingually deafened
DCI6	21 June–18 July	Parent of a child with CI
DCI7	21 June–18 July	Parent of a child with CI
DGl1	26 June–22 August	Glaucoma with stent surgery
DGl2	2 August–29 August	Glaucoma with stent surgery
DGl3	9 August–5 September	Glaucoma with stent surgery
DGl4	2 August–29 August	Glaucoma
DC1 [2]	5 July–1 August	Cardiovascular implant (passive)
DC2	12 July–8 August	Cardiovascular implant (passive)

[1] Data collection took place between June and September in 2021. [2] Participant DC1 also participated in an individual interview which was analysed along with the GD.

Participants submitted their records on a weekly basis and could keep handwritten or digital diaries. In the handwritten format, each participant received blank templates and pre-stamped envelopes to return the completed diaries each week. Participants who chose to keep a digital diary received the exact same template in *Microsoft Word* format and could complete their entries using a computer. The individual diary parts were reviewed by the researchers upon reception, followed by a weekly feedback conversation. The final conversation served to review the entire recording period in order to evaluate the method, similarly to the GDs. Additional data generated by these conversations were documented by the researchers and included in the analysis.

2.4. Analysis

Data from the GDs and the DS (incl. the corresponding notes taken by the researchers during the feedback discussions) were analysed based on Bohnsack's documentary content analysis [23] and grounded theory [24], whereby the grounded theory was the superordinate research style. Since the grounded theory implies a non-linear and iterative research process, data collection and data analysis were conducted in a circular process; the development of the diary study was based on a preliminary analysis of the data from the GDs. Once complete, the data from the GDs and DS were then analysed in a process combining the documentary analysis and the grounded theory. The aim of this approach was not only to methodically triangulate the data, but also to provide an *in-width* and *in-depth* analysis [25]. Inductive thematic saturation and sufficient depth of understanding was achieved in the analytical process of the data from the GDs and the DS. This process was performed in the following three consecutive phases.

Phase 1: Reconstruction of the thematic outline by means of formulating interpretation (documentary analysis) and memos (grounded theory)

The recordings of the GDs were transcribed, and the diary entries were put into a standard digital format. The handwritten diaries were typed so that a homogeneous diary collection of all participants was created. The three researchers (C.H., M.L and S.S.) independently reviewed the material line by line and reconstructed the central thematic lines. Thereby, two different levels of statements were differentiated—descriptive (what was discussed, e.g., situations, experiences, diagnoses, etc and analytical (why does this matter, e.g., attitudes, values, beliefs, etc.) [23]—and memos were recorded. The three researchers compared and discussed their work and collaboratively selected the themes and text sections that were to be included in the next analytical step.

Phase 2: Exploration of the collective orientation patterns (documentary analysis) and open coding (grounded theory)

In the second phase, the selected text sections were further analysed by means of the documentary analysis using reflective interpretation and collective orientation patterns were elaborated. Furthermore, the memos (recorded in the first step) were analysed and related to the founded patterns so that an additive interpretation took place. This step was again independently performed by each of the three researchers. The systems of collective orientation patterns were then compared, discussed and merged, so that an integrative system was finally created for each type of implant. Parallel to the reflective and additive interpretation, data were coded by means of open coding using the principles of grounded theory [24], so that the orientation frameworks could be further substantiated by different specifications of the pattern. Coding was divided among the research team, with each coded transcript being cross-checked by a different researcher. Any conflicts were resolved in discussions among the three researchers.

Phase 3: Type formation (documentary analysis) and abductive reasoning (grounded theory)

In the third phase, the authors searched for thematic cross-connections between the collective orientation patterns from the three different implant fields; at the same time, the different cases along the orientation patterns within each implant field were also compared, informing the type formation (documentary analysis). In this stage, the theoretical memos were also included in the analysis. In order to relate the data and the type formation to theoretical reasoning (already noted in the memos), explanatory hypotheses [26] (which were heuristic in character) were formulated (grounded theory). Each hypothesis disclosed specific collective orientation patterns which emerged in the second phase of the analysis (e.g., training on technology use) and was then related to known concepts of health literacy and ethical values (e.g., technology handling as part of the functional health literacy and perceptions on technology as a factor for self-determination). The resulting hypotheses on health literacy in implant care were then cross-verified along the transcripts. This step allowed for elaborating on the different types of health-literate behaviour following the principles of the documentary analysis [23].

2.5. Participants

Twenty-eight participants took part in the GDs and thirteen in the DS (total $n = 41$). One participant with cochlear implant and one participant with a cardiovascular implant participated in both methods. In total, 15 participants with cochlear implant or parents of children wearing cochlear implants took part in three GDs ($n = 2$ pre-lingual, $n = 9$ post-lingual and $n = 4$ parents of children wearing cochlear implants); 8 individuals suffering from glaucoma took part in two GDs ($n = 6$ no implant and $n = 2$ with implant); 3 wearers of cardiovascular implants took part in one GD ($n = 3$); two further participants with cardiovascular implants could not actively participate in the GD due to technical difficulties or bad internet connection and were additionally interviewed via telephone ($n = 2$) along the same question script used during the GDs.

Regarding the DS, 7 participants wearing a cochlear implant or having a child with cochlear implant submitted their diary notes. Moreover, 4 individuals suffering from glaucoma and 2 participants with cardiovascular implants participated in the study. The sample characteristics are described in Table 4.

Table 4. Sample characteristics.

		Cochlear [1]		Glaucoma		Cardiovascular [1]	
		GD	DS	GD	DS	GD [3]	DS
Total		15	7	8	4	5	2
Gender	Female	11	5	5	2	4	1
	Male	4	2	3	2	1	1

Table 4. Cont.

		Cochlear [1]		Glaucoma		Cardiovascular [1]	
		GD	DS	GD	DS	GD [3]	DS
Age	18–30	2	4	-	-	-	-
	31–40	3	1	-	-	-	-
	41–50	4	1	-	1	-	-
	51–60	2	-	2	-	2	1
	61–70	3	1	4	2	-	-
	≥71	1	-	2	1	3	1
Living conditions	Alone	-	-	2	2	2	1
	With partner	6	4	6	2	3	1
	With relative	3	1	-	-	-	-
	With partner and relatives	6	2	-	-	-	-
Education	Abitur (graduated high school)	10	6	6	4	1	-
	Advanced technical college certificate	2	-	1	-	2	1
	Intermediate school diploma	2	1	1	-	1	1
	Secondary school diploma	1	-	-	-	1	-
Implant status	Implant wearer	11	5	6	4	5	2
	No implant [2]	4	2	2	-	-	-
Marital Status	Single	3	4	1	1	1	1
	Married	10	3	4	2	3	-
	Widowed	-	-	-	1	1	-
	Divorced	-	-	1	-	-	-
	In separation	1	-	-	-	-	1
	n.s.	1	-	2	-	-	-
Cultural background	German	15	5	7	3	5	1
	Bi-cultural	-	2	1	1	-	-
Native language	German	14	6	7	4	5	2
	Other	-	1	1	-	-	-
	n.s.	1	-	-	-	-	-
Religion	Non-denominational	7	2	5	1	2	2
	Denomination	8	5	2	3	3	-
	n.s.	-	-	1	-	-	-
Occupation (multiple answers possible)	Healthcare	3	3	1	-	1	-
	Social services	2	-	-	-	-	1
	Science	-	-	3	-	1	-
	Economics	2	2	1	1	1	1
	Administration	3	-	-	-	-	-
	Commerce	-	-	1	-	-	-
	Industry	1	-	-	2	1	1
	IT	3	1	-	1	-	-
	Craft	-	-	-	1	-	-
	Art/Culture/Design	-	1	1	-	-	-
	Service	-	1	-	-	-	-
	other	1	1	1	1	1	-
	n.s.	-	-	-	1	-	-
Employment status	Employed full-time	4	2	2	-	-	-
	Employed part-time	4	2	1	-	-	-
	In education/study	2	2	-	-	-	-
	Retired	5	1	5	3	4	1
	Job-seeking	-	-	-	1	1	1

[1] One participant in the group of cochlear and one participant in the cardiovascular implants participated in both methods. [2] In the case of cochlear implants, this accounts for parents of children with CI and in the field of glaucoma, this accounts for glaucoma patients without implants. [3] Incl. two interviews. n.s.—not specified, GD—group discussion, DS—diary study.

3. Main Findings

The major collective orientation patterns for all three clinical fields refer to (1) information and individual perceptions; (2) appraisal, dependence and responsibility; and (3) implant-related values. The further specifications of the patterns vary for each type of implant, according to the specifics of the implant, the therapy or the disease, as well as the two qualitative methods. The collective orientation patterns and their specifications can be found in Appendix C, Table A3.

3.1. Information and Perceptions Regarding the Implant, Technology and Disease

Data analysis revealed the perceptions of the implant as well as one's own attitudes towards medical technology as collective orientation patterns, in the context of perceptions regarding the implant, damage prevention, control over one's implant and health in everyday life, and finding and dealing with information, especially with regard to decision making. This not only refers to the knowledge and information about the implant, its handling and user experience, but also to the perception on the implant in relation to the body.

3.1.1. Perceptions on the Implant as a Physical Object

In the case of **cochlear** implants, the implant was perceived as part of the body and wearing it evoked a sense of normalcy blending in with everyday life. Participants described their perceptions on the implant as follows:

> "[. . .] to the extent that you experience that the technology becomes part of you, that is also fascinating [. . .]." (GD1CIA9)

> "You can simply take part in life in a normal way [. . .], is like a pair of glasses, that you simply put on and then go through your everyday life in a normal way, with no restrictions, but having a technical device with you without really noticing it". (GD2aCIB2)

A mother of a child wearing a cochlear implant described the CI as "a piece of jewellery" also demonstrating her positive attitude and presumably also the positive attitude of her child towards the implant device.

Similarly, to implant wearers with a CI, implant wearers with a **cardiovascular** implant described:

> "The implant/band is part of oneself, completely normal, it is like wearing glasses." (DC2)

For implants that are physically less visible, such as **glaucoma** stents, the data demonstrate that the implant itself was hardly noticeable. A participant described this in the GD as follows:

> "I do not perceive the stent as a foreign body or in any other special way." (DGl1)

Nevertheless, the following explanation of a GD participant demonstrates that, even if the implant itself is not perceived physically, it could be indirectly noticeable through certain accompanying symptoms:

> "I have to say that these XEN stents have created filtering blebs in the eyes, [. . .] not formed intentionally, and they are also on the surface of the eye [. . .], so that when you blink, the eyelid rubs over them, which is a mechanical irritation every time. That is what I experience as a direct consequence of these implants." (GD2GlB1)

3.1.2. Perceptions on Implant's Functioning and Damage Prevention

Besides perceiving the implant as a physical object within the body, the perceptions on the implant's functioning, combined with the relevant information and knowledge, play an important role in everyday life and well-being. In the case of **cardiovascular** implants, this became especially apparent with the implant and its technological functioning being perceived as one of two extremes: supporting and enabling versus thought-consuming and inhibiting. On the one hand, the perception of the implant as reliably functioning and failure-free can elicit a certain level of trust and feeling of security in one's own physical body and establish a sense of normality. This was described by a participant as follows:

"After the successful tape-laying my optimism returned and today I definitely have the feeling (wrongly?!), that at least I will not die of this one day. I have a feeling of invulnerability in this area, as stupid as that may sound! Despite all existing physical limitations, also because of my age. But it is a good feeling !!!" (DC2)

On the other hand, worrying about a possible implant failure can become very consuming in everyday life. The concern about possible damage to the implant due to stress was particularly relevant; in the same vein, the implant itself was also perceived as a source of stress or anxiety and therefore, in a way, also harmful for its own functioning:

"I am afraid that this permanent stress (caused by the implant) will damage the implant. Actually, this thinking determines the day. This question comes up all the time." (DC1)

Being aware of the implant and the perception of its functioning is a prerequisite for another aspect of implant care which was also mentioned in this quotation: damage prevention.

For persons with **glaucoma**, damage prevention mainly refers to preventing the progression of the disease in order to avoid blindness. In this regard, a possible measure is controlling the intraocular pressure either with an implant or with drop therapy, which may be necessary in addition to the implant. Participants regularly wrote about drop therapy in their diaries, describing the administration of eye drops as a kind of ritual (1) and depicting its integration in everyday life (2):

"The evening ritual. Left Trisopt right Xalacom dropped." (DGl4)

"Eye drops are always in the bag and a reminder is set in the phone so I drip every three hours." (DGl1)

Since intraocular pressure cannot be perceived physically, there is no direct way for implant wearers to know if the pressure is regulated effectively. In the context of damage prevention, this gave rise to feelings of uncertainty as well as the desire to gain more control over the measurement of intraocular pressure and thus over the disease. An increased interest in technical innovations was communicated during the discussion, paired with scepticism towards the state-of-the-art glaucoma treatments in medicine:

"[. . .] aren't there ways to measure intraocular pressure constantly over a longer period of time [...]? That would primarily be a question of a reliable and self-applicable technique. Are the researchers from the university perhaps better informed? I haven't heard anything about it yet, but such technology would perhaps be also a way of guiding patients towards [...] being able to control themselves better with this data, instead of blindly relying on [...] data collected in one single point of time (during the medical check by the doctor)." (GD1GlB2)

Similar to the case of glaucoma implants, self-monitoring and self-knowledge were important assets among participants wearing **cardiovascular** implants when it comes to controlling disease progression and maintaining implant functioning:

"I also measure myself, my coagulation value every week. I know exactly where there are risks, where there are no risks and what is just as important [. . .]." (GD1CB2)

"I've been keeping detailed records since I was discharged from rehab after the heart attack: weight, diuretic dose, blood pressure, exercise profile. So that I can recognise a connection in case of possible strong changes." (DC2)

With regards to **cochlear** implants, damage prevention mainly refers to the prevention of material damage to implant parts such as the speech processor and batteries (not waterproof). The concept of damage, here, was more on a technological level related to external influences in everyday life:

"X (diarist's child) is missing her processor of the second CI for a third day in a row. We had quests on the weekend and there was a water battle [. . .]. X got so wet, so that one of the battery cases got also a load of water. Since Friday evening, X is only unilaterally supported by the CI." (DCI7)

3.1.3. Information and Knowledge Related to the Implant and the Disease

With regards to cochlear implants, individual's general interest in innovation and positive attitude towards technology may incite efforts to improve the quality of hearing with the implant, as well as the wish for a more precise technology adjustment. One participant (pre-lingually deafened) described this as follows:

"I'm [. . .] interested in innovations, I also look at something newer from time to time, but what would be even more interesting for me would be if you can make more [. . .] progress in the [...]. technical settings. That you can make even finer adjustments to the sound quality, [...] that would be even easier for us." (GD2aCIB1)

The capability to avert implant failure, or ensure or optimise (in the case of CI) functioning presupposes sufficient information and knowledge about the implant, technology and disease and empowers patients to handle the implant and disease in everyday life.

Overall, information seems to be mainly obtained through internet research, exchanges in a private context (self-help groups, family, friends, random encounters, etc.) or consultations with health professionals. Participants with **glaucoma** refer to the internet as an important source of up-to-date information that was also considered reliable (1); participants also reported positive developments (especially in recent times) in finding adequate information online (2):

"[. . .] I have informed myself mainly via the internet, the glaucoma forum was essential. You can find really good information there. Then also on the university pages. And I tried to read some of the publications." (GD2GlB2)

"[...] it has somehow become clear to me that medical knowledge changes significantly over the years and the assessments of it, so that it is good if you try to keep up to date as intensively as possible, and of course that is better today than it used to be via the internet [...]." (GD1GlB1)

A participant in the **cochlear** group discussion also referred to the internet as a source of information in interaction with healthcare professionals and described:

"I'm on the internet a lot and find out about things on the internet or through other contacts, if I've picked up something new somewhere, I look it up more on the internet and when I'm stuck, I ask experts who might already know more about it and ask where I can look up something else." (GD2aCIB1)

In light of the fact that, e.g., negative side effects of the implant are not always communicated transparently in the care system (see Section 3.2.), the exchange in the peer group was also considered important. One participant wearing a CI (post-lingually deafened) explained:

"I find that increasingly important, I mean I know my family, [...] we have a lot of experience that we can exchange, but for example the neck tension, which I have only just learned here that it also affects others, I just don't know that and from the XY [healthcare institution], [...] so far I have been rather dismissed that it doesn't come from the CI. I think it would be nice if there was [...] a closed platform where you can exchange [...]." (GD1CIA6)

The notion was similar in the **glaucoma** group discussion; information from the peer group was also considered crucial in general, where the self-help groups were seen as a space for information exchange, networking and discussing (1) and were also perceived as empowering for participants in terms of decision-making processes (2):

"[. . .] for me, the self-help group is clearly a tool to inform myself [...] the self-help groups are an organisation that already exists and where you can definitely network, where you can query, where you can discuss." (GD1GlB4)

"I (have) talked to many patients [...] who just had an operation [...]. Then I had the feeling: "Okay, I can assess a little bit what people experience" and then I also talked to the doctors-they also wanted to do a seepage cushion operation on me. [...] So 15, 16 years ago, there were at least half of the seepage cushion surgeries that didn't work. And since it was absolutely necessary for me, I had the feeling: "Well, now I'm smart enough and I can assess it for myself" and then I said: "No, I don't want to", because my pressure values were really good. [...] I got information from my fellow patients and then I did a lot of research on the internet and through the self-help group [. . .]." (GD1GlB3)

Similarly, the Heart Foundation was perceived as an important source of *information* for participants with **cardiovascular** implants. It offered an opportunity to exchange information and to gain technology- or disease-related knowledge through peers:

"That's why I went to the Heart Foundation, there's a lot of information there [...]. Of course, I know that there are people who see the whole thing more casually, according to the motto the doctor has to make me healthy, but after my valve operation I had a rehab that was especially for people with heart valve diseases and you could see that most people had already dealt with it [...] that there are possibilities and I like to take the information from the rehab to avoid further damage, [. . .], to keep myself fit and to get the best out of the situation." (GDCB3)

Attitudes towards implant technology (see Section 3.2) interact with the medical and technical information on the implant and were considered essential for decision-making. As a result, participants felt the necessity to inform themselves as extensively as possible. A parent of a child with CI described the feeling of being left alone with the decision and explained:

"[. . .] it was an incredibly difficult decision. I also obtained information where it was available, but as a parent you are relatively alone, and it's a decision that you don't make for yourself, but for your child, and there are also certain risks, and not just the health risks." (GD2bCIB2)

The complexity of this information environment is also characterised by the high speed of technological progress in the **cochlear** implant area. This puts implant wearers in the position of informing their doctors on technical features and functioning. A participant wearing a CI said:

"There are different implants, they are always developing and that is of course important, because I always feel as if I have to inform the doctors about what works and what doesn't work or which direction it goes in or what it does to you." (GD1CIA1)

In the context of a perceived lack of knowledge of doctors, however, a diarist with **glaucoma** reflected on uncertainty in the research context in one of the feedback interviews; in their opinion, receiving uncertain or lacking information results from low levels of existing knowledge about the disease and its causes in general, so that doctors cannot make any well-founded statements. A study author took field notes during the telephone call with participant DGl1 after the first week of diary keeping and made the following note:

"Uncertainty among patients (and doctors) is caused by a lack of research into the causes of glaucoma. Since the causes are not known, it is difficult to assess the chances of success for the treatment as a whole. Control of symptoms works to some extent, but it is difficult to assess how and with what prospects a progression of the destruction of the optic nerve can be prevented. The patient sees the reason not so much in the lack of information by doctors, but in the fact that doctors themselves cannot make precise statements and recommendations because there is a lack of knowledge and research in this area." (study author Sa.S)

Against this background, participants wished for a more holistic approach regarding glaucoma, as one participant in the GD stated:

"[. . .] that you also perceive the eye as a component of the brain and the whole body, and that you have to make sure that it is also properly cared for. [...] That not only the purely mechanical treatment in the eye, but also this peripheral view should be expanded" (GD1GlB4)

In light of a perceived lack of knowledge about the disease, participants felt the desire to contribute to the research processes by providing information on their individual disease peculiarities. A participant in the GD explained:

"What would really be close to my heart is to find more cooperation, with researchers on the subject of glaucoma, because there are so many glaucoma patients who have now also decided to get informed and to observe themselves with their peculiarities in relation to glaucoma, so I think we could really contribute a lot to this, because the doctors don't have glaucoma themselves and we know a lot of what they don't know." (GD1GlB3)

In the group of **cardiovascular**-implant wearers, gathering information about surgery conditions and techniques was very important for participants, since it enabled them to assess their own needs and wishes concerning the therapy. The process of decision making in view of the prevailing medical assessment versus individual fears and uncertainties was described by one group discussion participant as follows:

"When the heart valve doesn't work as it used to, then you get weaker, [...] it's a long process over many years and then my doctor said, "well, you know, you have to deal with it, in your case it can be done quite well today, the heart valve can be replaced quite well". [...] then you get to know what that means, you are cut open from the neck to the navel, then the whole chest is opened up, [...] and (as I) was already afraid of this thing, [...] (the information about this minimally invasive operation method) came naturally just at the right time, then I enquired, they told me "you are too young", "what does too young mean?" I said, "I'm 77 now", "yes, we don't actually do that until you're over 80", and so I looked into it and [...], the Heart Foundation offers all kinds of information, not just the material on the website or the brochures they have, you can also talk to cardiologists there, and so it was clear to me from the start that if it's an option for me, I want to have it." (GD1CB3)

Feeling well informed about the implant and the disease empowered patients and reinforced their efforts to seek, find and communicate health information. Evaluating such information adequately and applying the gained knowledge and experiences in the care context were considered essential for the successful management of the health condition. This process also raises issues of (critical) appraisal and one's awareness of (in-)dependence and responsibility, which are presented in the next section.

3.2. Appraisal, Dependence and Responsibility

The comprehensive appraisal and application of gained knowledge and experiences are considered essential for coping within the healthcare setting. Participants repeatedly described their experiences of insufficient counselling, trust in patient–doctor communication and a lack of transparency regarding the differences in quality of care. In particular, taking an active patient role was described as an important skill.

3.2.1. Appraisal of Information and Disease

A particularly important issue for participants with **glaucoma** was glaucoma care itself; it was perceived as illness-centred, determined by an isolated view on the eye leaving scarcely any room for a holistic approach. Such an illness-centred approach was perceived as unsatisfactory by the participants and evoked frustration towards the treatment environment. This resulted in a feeling of being solely individually responsible for one's own health (1) and negative experiences within the doctor–patient relationship expressing a perceived lack of sensitivity and belittlement as follows (2):

> "You shouldn't leave everything to the doctor [...] ... I can only say from my experience that I would already be dead if I had always followed the doctor's advice, and you also have to listen to your own gut feeling about the story very carefully, because the doctors don't know you that well. So, you have to deal with the subject yourself and not leave everything to the doctors." (GD1GlB5)

> "Yes, well I noticed at our glaucoma meetings that many ophthalmologists simply dismiss it, do not answer questions and simply downplay the whole topic." (GDGl1B5)

Participants in this group not only felt responsible for informing others about glaucoma but also for appraising relevant information in an opaque information environment with many different sources. In a diary feedback conversation, one participant (DGl1) with glaucoma also emphasised the struggle of critically appraising information and making up their own mind against many different opinions. Against this background, exchanging information within the peer group, or with friends, acquaintances and doctors present important means of appraising information.

Among participants with **cardiovascular** implants, the process of appraisal was weighted differently depending on their medical history: participants who had a sudden cardiac condition and concomitant emergency surgery were engaged in appraising their health in line with cardiac-disease prevention and healthy living only after the implantation (1); participants who were aware of their heart problems were also concerned about a healthy lifestyle but had had additional time to appraise recommendations and risks on surgery options in more detail and actively partook in their care provision (2):

> "I mean, for a year now I've been thinking about almost nothing but health and about [...] doing everything to live healthily in order to grow old and have a good quality of life, and health is something I can perhaps influence myself by trying to live healthily and yes, it's actually about that every day." (GD1CB1)

> "I wanted to keep my heart valve at all costs, I wanted it to be repaired, then after a long search, [...] I found a hospital [...] where the head doctor reconstructed the heart valve. He told me at the time that the chance was about 50%, but I did it anyway and it went wrong, [...] Well, after five and a half years I had to go back to the operating table and then I got the mechanical heart valve [...]. Since then, things have gone uphill, and then I decided to pass on my knowledge so that other people don't have to search like that, and I applied to the Heart Foundation and started working there straight away, and the heart valve I have now, I can live with it, I can cope with it, I know what's going on, [...]." (GD1CB2)

The last quotation also suggests that the patient's role in the process of knowledge appraisal (active demanding versus passive receiving) may determine both the perceived quality of care and the patient–doctor relationship.

3.2.2. The Role of the Active Patient

The participants in the **cardiovascular** GD described how they perceive their role in the process of knowledge appraisal and explained how they prepare themselves for medical consultations in order to be able to critically question a doctor's advice and recommendation:

> "[...] you have to [...] educate yourself, you have to inform yourself, you always have to learn and that's what I do every time, now I have another routine cardiology appointment on Monday and I've already written down some questions and you just have to and that's what I've learned, that it makes sense if you present yourself as an educated, informed patient and not like an idiot who listens to everything they say, how great it all is. [...]." (GD1CB1)

Similarly, in the **cochlear** GDs, the importance of assuming an active patient role–being proactive in care management, claiming certain services and taking responsibility in the context of provision of care—was accentuated. This was perceived as a prerequisite for imparting empowerment:

> "I lodged an objection and explained to them on two pages my facts as I see it [...] and that I don't think it's okay that the health insurance company thinks otherwise and that it wouldn't be vital for us (decision for or against financing the aqua-case), and I explained my thoughts to them and got it accepted [...]." (GD2aCIB1)

The importance of individual assertiveness and communication skills regarding the equity in quality of care was also described by participants suffering from **glaucoma**. For effective dealing of the disease, it was considered essential to be able to claim adequate care, initiate diagnostics and treatment, as well as to obtain sufficient counselling:

> "[...] there are also people in our group who can't articulate themselves so well verbally or who are rather quiet and reserved and they won't get what others can enforce because they [who are more articulate] can deal better with the doctors." (GD1GlB3)

> "[...] if you can't open your mouth or you don't know what question to ask the ophthalmologist, then you're in trouble." (GD1GlB6)

A related topic discussed among participants was the doctor's reaction to such an active and assertive patient role. In the case of participants suffering from glaucoma, the varying quality of care, the low transparency with regard to the experience of the clinics with MIGS and a lack of empathy hampered the coordination of treatment. One participant explained:

> "[doctors] react in an offended way [...] when you have already been somewhere else, and perhaps also in another clinic [...]. I have experienced several times that the doctors react very insulted: "Oh, you have already been somewhere else, so we won't do anything more for you, because then you should go to where you have already been". (GD1GlB1)

In the case of **cardiovascular** implants, the coordination of therapy and aftercare was considered as a decisive component for successfully dealing with the disease. One participant evaluated his experiences in retrospect:

> "Yes, there's a world of difference between having it (the implant), wanting it and getting it (laughs), it was a long process. I applied and then they told me, "[...], pay attention, so this is a relatively new procedure", [...]. I got it, it went well and [...], even if I were to fall over now, I've lived with it for two years [...] I'm glad that I have it and hope that it's a [...] biological part in there, but I didn't even ask whether it's from pigs or cattle, I know that it's been adapted with my blood and set up, so that's how I got it." (GD1CB3)

3.2.3. Dependence on the Healthcare System and the Implants

Considering patient's dependence on good care quality, experiences with insufficient consultation were perceived as frustrating. The need for assertiveness seemed to arise from a feeling of *dependence* on the healthcare system and the implants themselves. With regards to **cochlear** implants, the feeling of dependence directly relates to the production of manufacturers (functionality, technical state and range of functions of the respective implant-make) and indirectly to the access to alternative care services (after implantation). Participants of the cochlear GD described this as follows:

> "I got the first (implant) in 2012 and now the second in 2020, even though (my hearing) was actually already very bad, I waited so long because I always had [...] in the back of my mind that I was making myself dependent on the technology [...]." (GD1CIA6)

> "We are not unhappy, but it is still the case that we would not have the chance to say that we are no longer happy, so we'll just change. [...] we are dependent on the implant manufacturer making the same technical progress as the others, so that we don't always

look enviously at the others and see what they have just developed, but that they [...] catch up." (GD2bCIB3)

A similar feeling of dependence on technology and manufacturers, but particularly with a focus on participation in certain activities of everyday life, was described in a diary entry by a cochlear implant wearer:

"Artone 3 Max headphones that connect to CI seem to be broken. I've noticed that I'm really lost without headphones; I hope that the problem can be solved quickly. I do a lot with headphones: I have a university seminar coming up I'm totally surprised by how much this thing with the headphones is bothering me, but technology is also pretty important at the moment & if one thing is missing that I urgently need, then the whole situation is pretty annoying." (DCI4)

In the context of **glaucoma**, the issue of dependence manifested itself in drop therapy. Although applying drops was seen as an integral part of everyday life by most study participants, it was also referred to as burdensome with regards to the side effects of the medication or the necessity of continuous use. One participant of the GD described this dependence as follows:

"I hope that there will be even better eye drops in the future, [. . .] that you don't have to apply so often and that this feeling of constantly having to think about it and this 'the day is timed according to eye drops' will simply decrease a little. [. . .] ... You always have the feeling that you are never completely free of it, that there are only four or five hours in between the drops, [. . .]." (GD2GIB1)

A dependence on the implant and accompanying medicinal care was also evident in patients with **cardiovascular** implants. Since there is an increased risk of mortality and physical limitations in the case of unsuccessful or non-treatment, "no treatment" or a decision against an implant is not a real alternative. This is especially the case when the implant is inserted due to an emergency. One participant described this feeling of dependence as follows:

"[. . .] if I had stayed at home, I would be dead now [...] and in the meantime I'm learning more and more, I'm questioning my medication, because I also notice that some things just don't really work [...], because I know that if I don't take certain things, then I'll feel bad at some point [...]." (GD1CB1)

3.2.4. Attitudes, Coping and Responsibility

Acceptance was considered as a way of handling such feeling of dependence among both participants with cardiovascular and cochlear implants, although the mortality aspect was relevant only in the context of **cardiovascular** implants:

"[...] I accept that I have heart disease and I'm grateful above all that I'm doing so well and accept this stent, so if I ... there I also thought about, that in principle I would probably accept everything that prolongs my life, or that helps me." (GD1CB1)

In the case of **cochlear** implants not only acceptance but also a self-confident attitude towards the implant in interactions with others seemed to play a significant role as a way of coping:

"Some people, if they don't know me and my CIs very well, seem irritated and stop talking, even though I can still hear. If it happens that I have to change the battery, I say something like 'I have to change my battery for a moment, I can still hear you with the other side, keep talking'." (DCI5)

"I usually also explain what I have on my head, because the devices stand out and people don't dare ask questions. So, I explain it proactively, which always goes down well with the counterpart and also has a likeable effect." (DCI3)

Another way of handling the feeling of dependence was gaining control over the knowledge on medical issues and participants' own body. Participants with **glaucoma**, e.g., were well-versed in the technical language regarding the glaucoma disease and saw this as a part of self-responsible disease management. One participant self-monitored their vision to prepare and inform future medical appointments and to be aware of variations in their visual acuity. The results were meticulously (self-)analysed (comparing both eyes, controlling the vision during different activities and times of day) and described in the diary as follows:

> "Distance visual acuity left as good as after standing up (=very good), right noticeably less than after standing up. Visual acuity at medium distance (approx. 3 m) good on the left, surprisingly worse on the right, ditto even for short reading distance (50 cm), where the left visual acuity was good, the right at best sufficient. Reading on the computer clearly better on the left than on the right." (DGl3)

In the case of **cardiovascular** implants, being well-informed in terms of individual responsibility was manifested regarding individual risk–opportunity assessments of one's own physical capacity, life planning, healthy-living choices and experience-based acquisition of medical knowledge:

> "I used to do a lot of sports, [. . .] but in that respect you do think about it, whether you go a bit further away for skiing or whatever, it doesn't really have much of an effect on my normal life, it's just that you've become more cautious when it comes to taking risks or going further away, which is what you used to do." (GDCB3)

> "I have also given some cardiologists further training, that is, when I go on holiday to other countries, for example warmer countries, [...], different diet, that my coagulation value changes again, just from the temperature, I should know that, if I get diarrhea what do I do there, but if you measure yourself, you are always on the better side and then you can help yourself. [...]." (GDCB2)

Effective interaction within the implant care setting requires an adequate and well-balanced appraisal of information. Firstly, being well-informed (Section 3.1), secondly, being able to critically appraise and apply information and ultimately, to be assertive within the care environment are factors that lead to a certain degree of independence and support patients to act responsibly in their own care management (Section 3.2). All these aspects influence and are influenced by ethically relevant (individual) values. These interactions are described in the next section.

3.3. Implant-Related Values

The data of this study illuminate the role of some value-laden issues in implant care related to the impact of implants on self-determination, irreversibility of the treatment, perception of emotional and physical burden in everyday life, identity and vicarious decision making, equity, participation, and discrimination experiences. These were differently weighted and represented among the three different groups of participants according to the disease and type of implant.

3.3.1. Self-Determination in the Context of Treatment Irreversibility and Perceptions of Good Life

In the case of **cochlear implants**, the fast pace of technological development paired with the irreversibility of the implantation impeded the process of decision making. Thereby, the execution of patient autonomy in the sense of self-determination can be strongly influenced by this circumstance. Participants described challenges in adequately assessing the consequences of living with an implant in general as well as in regard to a specific implant brand. A participant wearing a CI described this as follows:

> "[. . .] the brands of course have very different options, and when I got my first implant in 2012, I was [...] informed a bit about what options there are and what was recommended for me [...] and I also understood everything and the technology, but nevertheless it wasn't clear to me at that moment what I was choosing [. . .] and also not what the

consequences were. [...] That's fixed and because it's in your head you can't change it. You can't just say 'I'm going to go out and buy something new', because that doesn't work with the implant, but you have to live with the choice you've made, maybe by chance. Self-determination was not possible at that moment. Of course, it's not possible to look into the future, you don't know which manufacturer will be the forerunner at some point [...], I know that too, but this self-determination is actually lost at some point, where no one can do anything about it, but I find that considerable and also very unjust in part." (GD1CIA6)

This quotation also suggests some ethically relevant issues that challenge individuals in the process of *deciding for* and *living with* an implant: the feeling of injustice due to the perceived randomness of the technological up-to-datedness of implant delivery and probable inequity in implant care.

In the case of **glaucoma**, value-laden issues were mainly discussed with regards to subjective perceptions of a good life and the fear of blindness in the context of decision making on therapy and health management. The data show that dealing with the uncertainties around the glaucoma, especially in terms of its causes, influencing factors and prognosis, were perceived as limiting, both on an emotional and physical level. In particular, participants felt driven in their own care management by the impending loss of sight. Two participants suffering from glaucoma (without implant) described:

"[...] I think the quality of life is limited [...] So you are afraid of losing your eyesight completely on the one hand and that can sometimes lead to you sleeping very badly over a certain period. And the other thing is that if you really can't see well anymore, then you can't do everything. [...] for example, photography [...], that's also one of my hobbies, you can't do it as well as with two functioning eyes. And in this respect, the quality of life is limited overall in a certain way." (GD1GlB4)

"I would have rather run to the ophthalmologist every day because I simply didn't know what the pressure was like and it was very, very erratic and I couldn't really live with it because it ... well, it pulled me down psychologically even more than I already was [...]. So, what do you do when the drops are no longer enough? Usually surgery, but if the surgery doesn't work either-what do you do? So, you are faced with a very big dilemma [...]". (GD1GlB5)

Other participants did not perceive any impairments (in the sense of a subjectively lower quality of life) directly caused by the implant (1). Participants reported that they did not have any thoughts about the implant in everyday life, except when, for example, irregularities or uncertainties in the functioning were detected during a doctor's check-up (2):

"As the stent is not noticeable to me, it has no impact on my quality of life." (DGl1)

"When Dr. XY measured the eye pressure [...], it was 19 in both eyes, which he thought was a little too high. It could be a small blockage in the implant. [...] If it was a blockage, it should be removed in about 6–9 months by a small operation [...] This situation moved me emotionally, because it would be an operation on my still better eye, and the fear that something could worsen my vision. It is strange that you have an implant in your eye and you think that's it forever without any problems and then you find out that there might be a blockage without noticing anything like that." (DGl2)

The findings regarding **cardiovascular** implants differed from the other two types of implants. This was primarily due to the fact that implant wearers were confronted with the possibility of dying due to their cardiovascular disease in the case of implant failure. The data predominantly provided insights in the role of anxiety, the psychological burden of participants' encounter with their own mortality, trust in the technology and cohesion within the community. The fear of dying vis-à-vis the gratitude of being alive influences individual's values and quality of life. One participant expressed his experience of gratitude as follows:

"[. . .] I was totally grateful that I survived that, that I was so lucky, [. . .], if I had stayed at home, I would be dead now and this gratitude then also subsided at some point [. . .] at the end of the day, I have a high quality of life because I'm just grateful that I'm still here [. . .]." (GD1CB1)

The data show that the medical history (emergency situation vs. already-known cardiac problems) determined which issues are relevant for the individual in the context of implant care. Furthermore, they emphasised psychological components that play a significant role in the everyday experience with the implant. Among the participants who were implanted as a result of a medical emergency, aspects of uncertainty (1), and disenchantment (2) were particularly significant, whereas participants with a known cardiac problem were able to reflect on and prepare for the implantation resulting in an increased sense of security and resilience (3):

"[. . .] since the cardiac arrest, I was dead for about two minutes and my whole life revolves around safety, [...] and in principle I am constantly questioning whether I have to go to the emergency room again and [...] I don't really feel safe." (GD1CB1)

"Since the operation, everything has been constantly going downhill. Only problems, [. . .] that can't be good." (DC1)

"I don't have that (fear), although of course you think about it, especially when you get arrhythmias again, but I'm not afraid in that sense. But I also suspect that it's because I was able to prepare for it for a long time and wanted to have it and also got it [...] it still works, [...] I'm glad." (GD1CB3)

3.3.2. Identity and Participation

The data of this study show that concerns in terms of identity issues and participation also play a role in the process of decision making and handling life with an implant. In the case of **cochlear** implants, the general attitudes toward hearing impairment in society (especially when negative) may cause or reinforce tension and uncertainty. In the case of parents who need to make the decision on implantation for their child, some complemental factors directly or indirectly related to the implant and the hearing disability of the child come into play. These include, e.g., access to education and inclusion as well as language and identity in the context of the Deaf culture. A mother of a child wearing CI explained in one of the GDs:

"[. . .], that we had to decide whether or not to go ahead with the implantation. That was also a big aspect for us, how does she deal with it, does she want it at all, because she was just at an age where she could not yet decide with us and we had to decide completely for our child and we have always said that was the most difficult decision of our lives, because everything else can be revised somewhere, but such an implantation sets somewhere a final point and the child must then organise its life with it. [. . .]." (GD2bCIB2)

A mother of a child with CI described such emotional tensions as follows:

"[. . .] as parents, we already had a stomach ache because we took this decision away from him, so I also documented it [...] in a letter [...] so that we could show him why we made this decision. [...] But of course we did it on the advice of the doctors, so that he would benefit as much as possible and later [...] be able to live a more self-determined life, because he would have better hearing. [. . .]." (GD2bCIB3)

From a health-related perspective, belonging to a certain group of individuals who share similar experiences plays a significant role among implant wearers regarding their identity. Being part of a self-help group, e.g., meets the need for commitment and agency.

In the case of **cochlear** implants, such belonging is strongly connected to the Deaf culture or the ability to communicate in a way that allows participation. Especially among pre-lingually deafened individuals or parents of children who obtained an implant at an early age, such belonging is related to communication (communicating equally in both the hearing and non-hearing world):

"[...] it is very important for her education that she learns sign language. At the same time, she also learns a little bit to deal with other children outside of the school environment in the normal sphere or normal life [...]." (GD2bCIB2)

In the case of participants with cardiovascular implants, it became apparent that a heart disease and the accompanying confrontation with one's own mortality increased participants' need for exchange with other affected persons and promoted one's own commitment. The participants with **cardiovascular** implants explained that shared experiences with cardiovascular diseases contributed to the development of a (partially life-changing) collective identity of those affected. It was perceived that this factor reinforces cohesion and self-conception within the group:

"I'm also a member of the Heart Foundation and I've noticed that all the people who are somehow involved with heart problems are very special kind of persons who are incredibly helpful and simply loving [...] ... I can call them all and they help each other and also the professor I'm in contact with there, they're all really nice people and that's why I say heart is something special." (GD1CB1)

These quotations disclose one further significant ethical aspect of implant care—social participation and inclusion in different areas of the life of individuals with health impairments. One participant (post-lingually deafened) with a **cochlear** implant also related to experiencing tensions in social interactions due to their impairment and wrote in their diary:

"Either I counter, or I withdraw. Already at home I was not "welcome" with my hearing impairment and rather an outsider. Others only talk to my wife, even about me. Even when I'm standing next to her. According to the motto: He can't hear anything anyway." (DCI1)

Despite negative and discriminating experiences in social interactions, all study participants wearing cochlear implants reported that being able to hear by means of the implant strengthened their ability to stand up for themselves and live in a self-determined manner, reinforced their self-confidence, and increased their autonomy. One participant described their experiences as follows:

"Yes, you can stand up for yourself again [...] and that makes the whole thing fairer with the implant. That was always the problem beforehand, especially in my professional life. I was always a bit ignored or I couldn't stand up for myself because I just didn't understand that, or [...] then the situation was already over and this way you can [...] defend yourself better [...]." (GD1CIA1)

Likewise, the **cardiovascular** implant enabled individuals to participate and regain activities. One participant also described feeling like a part of the community again because of the improved health:

"After the rainstorm of the night, the traces of the flooded underground car park were removed together with the house owners. This took several hours and required some persistent physical effort. Without an implant, I would have not been any help to the community, I realised. I did not have air or endurance problems." (DC2)

Comparing the data among the three different implant groups shows that ethically relevant values may differ, depending on the specifics of the implant technology or on the disease. Nevertheless, it became clear that ethically relevant dimensions in implant care and in life with an implant play a major role in both individual's experiences in everyday life and the shaping of their lifeworld in all three implant groups.

3.4. Synthesis of the Study Results for Each Implant Type

We mainly gained insights into the individual perceptions on technology and health, sources and appraisal of information, the factors influencing dependence and responsibility, and individual values. These aspects influence decision-making processes, health behaviour, but also self-perception in the sense of one's own identity. In the following table (Table 5), some key findings for each implant field are summarised.

Table 5. Overview of the collective orientation patterns for each implant type.

	Selected Key Findings	Summary
Cochlear	Rapid development of technology Dependence on technological functioning (vicarious) Decision-making process Identity and participation	In the GDs, the decision-making process regarding the implant, keeping up with the ongoing technical development and communication and identity issues were particularly relevant. The parents' group differed slightly from the other two groups, although decision making was especially challenging here, due to its vicarious nature. The diaries revealed, primarily, challenges that all three cochlear groups encountered in their daily lives, which mainly concerned technology (damage prevention, responsibility), social environment and communication. Overall, the patients felt that they could live a more self-determined life because of hearing through the implant. In the context of care, it was striking that patients felt they had to be firm and demanding to make their claims successfully.
Glaucoma	Holistic view of the disease Marbled experiences in the healthcare setting Fear of disease progression Adherence to drug therapy	In the group without a stent, participants agreed above all that there are deficits in the doctor–patient relationship, due to low level of sensitivity and empathy on the part of the medical profession. This was overcome mainly by the exchange of experiences within the group and exertion of personal responsibility in the care context and in the procurement of information. The diaries accentuated the importance of successfully integrating drop therapy in everyday life. Uncertainty regarding the progression of the disease was perceived as burdensome and resulted in constant self-monitoring as a coping strategy. All participants pleaded for a more holistic approach to manage glaucoma.
Cardiovascular	Confrontation with mortality No alternative Fear vs. security Life planning	Patients with cardiovascular implants felt confronted with their own mortality, which was reflected in the pronounced need for exchange with others, in part to deal with concomitant psychological stress. Participants also stated that this promoted their own engagement within the care setting. Subjective quality of life (in interaction with physical and emotional symptom burden) depended on the balance between uncertainty, anxiety, acceptance, and gratitude. The disease and its treatment seemed to have a strong impact on the personal sense of security and confidence in one's own body, self-confidence and sense of normality of everyday life. The data showed that there was a difference regarding the perceived security and the acceptance of the implant between participants who were fitted with an implant out of an emergency situation and those who underwent a decision-making process regarding their implant.

4. Discussion

This study shows that individuals suffering chronic conditions where implants pose a therapeutic option see HL beyond the context of medical correctness concerning health or implant information and decision making. In addition, HL is related to the subjective appraisal of knowledge and information around the implant. These aspects are connected to the individual values regarding life with an implant and likewise affect them. Therefore, discussing HL in the context of implant care requires the illumination of the HL concept in its different facets regarding (1) dealing with information on the technology and the disease, (2) appraisal, dependence and responsibility and (3) ethically relevant values in the context of implant care. In the following, the main findings will be discussed along with the concepts presented in the introduction: functional and technology-oriented HL;

communicative and navigation HL; critical HL. These concepts are discussed both on individual and an organisational level. Furthermore, these findings will be contextualised and compared with existing research in this area, despite the paucity of data in the research landscape on this subject.

4.1. Technology and Health–Individual Perceptions, Attitudes and Information Needs

According to our findings, in implant care, functional HL [10,27] needs to be extended and replenished with technological understanding and the dealing with technical information. Here, we mainly relate to individual HL. Nevertheless, it is also the responsibility of the healthcare system to support individuals in their efforts to enhance their functional and technology-oriented health competences. With regard to the dynamics of technological progress as well as the opportunities and risks of innovative technologies, there is a need for a pronounced tolerance of ambiguity. Furthermore, strategies for dealing with rapidly changing or insufficient evidence or information must be developed. Tolerance of ambiguity, as described by Norton [28], is understood as the ability to handle "information marked by vague, incomplete, fragmented, multiple, probable, unstructured, uncertain, inconsistent, contrary, contradictory, or unclear meanings" and to not automatically perceive it as a source of psychological discomfort or threat. Hence, patients must also be able to recognise the dynamics of technological progress and technological developments and consider the associated uncertainties (e.g., low level of evidence due to innovation). Patients should be enabled to understand and apply implants' technological functionalities and corresponding background information to act in a self-determined and participatory manner.

Regarding **cochlear** implants, it is crucial that patients (or parents) comprehend the implant's technology, functionality and its impact on daily life prior to implantation, to be able to appropriately assess risks and benefits, further treatment options and make an informed decision. A study by Wheeler et al. (2007) showed that such deeper understanding of technology was lacking, even though individuals could successfully manage the CI in everyday life [29]. Our study shows that, in the everyday use of cochlear implants, basic understanding of technology and functional range (incl. accessories) and awareness of one's own responsibilities are essential for the successful use and protection of the implant in everyday live. Furthermore, patients *and* caregivers need to be aware of their own attitudes toward technology: especially in the light that one's own attitude towards integrating technological devices in the body can shape both the process of decision making and everyday experiences with the implant. The ambiguity of technical or risk information in the context of implant care may cause psychological stress among implant wearers and challenge their functional HL. There is some evidence, for example, that young individuals wearing **cochlear** implants with a low tolerance of ambiguity worry more about technological hazards [30]. Other studies have also addressed technology failure and damage prevention [29,31–34].

In the case of **glaucoma** treatment (e.g., drops and/or implant), patients are challenged to understand the consequences for everyday life associated with the respective treatment option (e.g., regular administration of eye drops and check-up appointments). This is not only relevant to decision making but also for implant care. E.g., understanding the consequences of not taking the drops can motivate and facilitate adhering to daily glaucoma medication [35]. In this respect, other studies revealed that eye drops were a factor that reinforced the decision for implantation [12]. Compared to cochlear implants, the needed information is less technology-dominated, but decision making still requires awareness of the individual attitude towards eye stents and understanding of their function and surgery-related specifics. Since technical information often requires the use of complex language and specific terms, insufficient individual HL may be a "by-product" of differences in the levels of knowledge and spoken language [18] between patients and their doctors. Therefore, such insufficiencies do not necessarily reflect information deficits of implant wearers. Stress may be caused by regional–urban differences in the quality of care, insufficient knowledge about the cause of the disease and thereby correspondingly uncertain prospects for treatment success. This was also reported by another study that stated that glaucoma as a disease brings some degree of uncertainty due to its "unknown nature and symptoms associated" [12]. This is additionally aggravated by missing transparency regarding clinics' implantation experience. Handling the ambiguity of such an information situation is part of individual HL and may support individuals in coping with stress.

In the context of the successful long-term disease management of **cardiovascular** diseases, it is essential for patients to develop strategies for dealing with stress (such as self-monitoring), i.e., to recognise their own needs and act accordingly. In addition, information about both the disease and the implant helps patients to manage their disease adequately. Furthermore, the skill of finding well-founded and sufficient information may increase individuals' confidence and sense of security. Other studies recommended considering quality-of-life aspects and patient-reported outcomes when evaluating a patient for a certain type of procedure (e.g., SAVR versus TAVI) [13,36]. On an organisational level, it is important that health professionals create realistic expectations for patients, since the patients' health and life might still be impacted by existing comorbidities [13,36]. In the case of heart valve surgery, studies show that there is not only the question regarding the type of procedure, but also the choice between biological and mechanical valve; too little knowledge and ability to assess information were seen as causes for difficulties in weighing up a decision [37,38]. Additionally, the peer-group exchange of information and individual experiences concerning, e.g., comorbidities or therapy side-effects, is perceived as helpful (which is in contrast to the findings of Schmied et al. (2015), that social support or peers were sources to which little recourse was made) [39]. Its promotion may indirectly contribute to the development of individual HL, especially in the context of existing comorbidities (since there is evidence that comorbidities among patients with implantable cardioverter defibrillators and pacemakers are associated with inadequate HL [40]).

Health prevention and promotion play a central role in patients' HL. Therefore, knowledge about and the willingness and ability to implement health-promoting measures in everyday life form a fruitful ground for individual HL, but also require a certain degree of autonomy and commitment. In order to be able to meet patients' pronounced need for exchange with peers, the healthcare system needs to inform about available possibilities, also outside the care setting. Decentralised platforms with curated information and possibilities of a direct exchange with professionals or self-help groups can promote needed skills for successfully handling and contextualising health and implant information.

4.2. Appraisal, Dependence and Responsibility–Building the Bridge to HL Competences

Our results show that patients can positively influence their implant care by assuming a demanding, informed and, above all, active patient role and exhibiting assertiveness skills. Such an active patient role may be associated with high individual HL, as a counterpart to the summary of evidence provided by Watson [3] on patients with low HL (asking few questions during medical consultations, lower adherence to medical advice, experiencing worse overall health outcomes). The study participants described that exactly those who act "more passively" and "less assertively" in the care delivery process have many more difficulties in obtaining adequate implant care. For example, appropriately assessing one's own level of medical knowledge allows patients to build trust in those treating them and to meaningfully combine the provided information with their subjective risk assessment. Especially in implant care, medical knowledge and information can be ambiguous. Additionally, successful implant care and disease management require patients to (autonomously) deal with the disease and adjust their care management accordingly. This is driven by a pronounced degree of proactive behaviour, including the willingness and ability to obtain information and to co-shape the diagnosis and treatment processes in implant care.

Our results reveal two main dimensions of HL, which are considered to be essential prerequisites for implant wearers' confidence in handling their health condition. On the one hand (1) communicative competences–as skills to participate in everyday life and to extract information and meaning making from different forms of communication and to apply this meaning to varying situations [9]. In addition, on the other hand, (2) navigation HL, described by Griese et al. (2020) as the ability to handle information in a way that enables navigating through the healthcare system on an individual level and in dependence of its complexity on an organisational level [10]. Both facets are related to the responsivity of the healthcare system to individuals' information and negotiation needs (i.e., the nature of the doctor–patient communication and the officially distributed information, e.g., leaflets or presentations). Moreover, they are related to implant wearers' needs regarding their efforts in navigating through the healthcare system and balancing among many different health services (i.e., coordination of the information flow between control examinations, additional therapies and hospital visits, as well as planning efforts and information needs). In the three different types of implants introduced here, the facets of communicative and navigation HL are emphasised differently on an organisational level.

From the perspective of **cochlear**-implant wearers, the ability of healthcare providers to enable participation and deliver responses to the needs of individuals related to their subjective experiences. This can incorporate, e.g., offering communication training or advice on how to deal with the new sense of hearing. In line with existing research [41–43], implant wearers had to adjust to the device and the "new" hearing experience with the implant, which required great effort. Furthermore, for successfully navigating through the healthcare system, implant wearers need to be able to understand and evaluate the importance of certain technical choices (e.g., the brand of the implant), make informed decisions on surgery or to decide among different health services and providers [32,44–47]. As outlined in the previous (Section 4.1) cochlear-implant wearers need information on technical and acoustics-related information. Such specific and often complex information require the system's responsivity, offering training and advice for the ways of successfully navigating between medicine and technology. A study by Sach and Whynes (2005) reported that prospective implant wearers felt that they were merely handed off to the implant centre by their physician, which was perceived as stressful because it triggered uncertainty about implantation [48]. This aspect also correlates with technology-related HL (see Section 4.1). Another important aspect of organisational HL from the perspective of cochlear-implant wearers is the provision of spaces for the exchange of experiences and information with others who are faced with similar challenges, problems and questions, both regarding decision making [33,49] and the period after surgery [33]. A health-literate action on an organisational level is characterised, e.g., by providing sufficient information [44,50] that patients need for acquiring medical knowledge. This enables an informed interaction with the healthcare system [33,51]—being able to articulate one's needs in a proper manner helps patients to make informed decisions on the variety of care options.

Since there is limited evidence on the success rate of the therapy with a **glaucoma** stent, the healthcare system needs to provide patients with specialists with high communicative HL who can assist patients in the process of risk assessment and decision making. Implant wearers emphasise their need to handle the glaucoma stent and the disease applying a holistic approach (glaucoma as a systemic disease) and wish to find this approach mirrored not only when searching for information themselves (see Section 4.1), but also by the healthcare system and the provided services. In line with these implications, studies indicated that the patient–doctor relationship plays a significant role where, especially, trust in one's own healthcare provider and the perception of a shared decision-making process are influential factors [12,52]. The systemic character of the disease challenges individuals' abilities to coordinate their diagnostic process and therapy and navigate through the healthcare system. Organisational HL should support individuals in their navigation efforts and offer paths for handling risk information based on scarce evidence.

With respect to passive **cardiovascular** implants, organisational HL is characterised by the transparent and comprehensible presentation of information, as well as low access barriers of care offers to enable patients to successfully coordinate their treatment. Since, in the case of heart diseases, patients are directly confronted with concerns regarding their own mortality and survival, organisational HL should be characterised by the responsivity of the health organisation to the individual and often vulnerable situation of the patient. For example, a study by Astin et al. (2017) found that, especially, the consultation between doctor and patient enforced the potential consequence of dying [13]. Moreover, concerns related to dependence on the functioning of the implant, psychological stress, risk assessments and mortality should be accounted for. Organisational HL should also include the provision of resources (information, time, offer of discussion) by professionals with high communicative HL to enable patients to deal successfully and make informed decisions in such an emotionally tensed field. This is highlighted by a case study of a patient, who reported that he felt overwhelmed and wanted to be "relieved of this decision". Furthermore, he depicted the decision as a method to free himself from an adverse mental state regardless of the actual medical urge [53].

Organisational HL needs to enable empowerment and support patients in the process of navigation through the healthcare system (e.g., by providing relevant information, offering opportunities for discussion and enabling access to courses). Health care providers need to be aware of the individual situation of the (prospective) implant wearer, taking into account the (prospective) implant wearer's dependence on the implant and the healthcare system, e.g., in counselling. This dependence is strongly related to the process of critically appraising information and individual responsibility. Therefore, the healthcare system needs to provide patients with sufficient space for negotiating individual responsibility and dependence regarding the provision of adequate patient care and thus promoting HL.

4.3. Implant-Related Values as Part of HL

The main findings of this study showed that knowledge about and the reflection on the implant may be a source of a subjective feeling of security (or insecurity) and self-confidence, strengthening the ability to act in a self-determined way in the care context. The lack thereof may have a negative effect on individuals' care management and, thus, on the successful handling of the implant. In the process of care-related decision making in the long term, it is essential for both implant wearers and caregivers to be aware of their own moral values and convictions (e.g., in terms of technology and health, identity, disability and ability, and participation, etc.). It can be challenging for patients to reconcile the decision for (or against) an implant with their own moral values, life planning and self-perception. Uncertainties arising in this setting can become a heavy burden for some individuals.

In connection with proxy decisions for or against an implant, as is the case for parents' deciding on a **cochlear** implant for their child, it is important to reflect on the ethical dimension of the long-term effects of the implants on the child's everyday life and identity. Furthermore, the wish to provide the child (or oneself) with the best possible treatment as a precondition for a successful life is often accompanied by various other decisions regarding social participation, education, acceptance and inclusion, which need to be constantly (re)appraised. These aspects are also shown in other articles where parental decision making was perceived as emotionally burdensome [31,47,54,55]. Ultimately, the decision for an implant was considered as beneficial for the child [31,32,47]. Hearing with the support of the implant reinforces a sense of autonomy and implant wearers feel empowered. Through this, patients are enabled to act in a more self-determined manner (e.g., proactively claiming on health services), which is significant from an ethical point of view. This is also reflected in a study in which implants were used frequently by a younger generation, which was attributed to the fact that they are perceived as valuable for them [29].

In the case of **glaucoma**, HL enables individuals to act autonomously in the field of healthcare in accordance with their individual values and lifeworlds, e.g., while coordinating health services according to their individual feeling of security or proactively claiming for an early treatment. The scarce evidence regarding the therapy of glaucoma and the knowledge gaps in relation to the origin and background of the disease manifest in an emotional burden but also restrict the patients in their subjective quality of life. This is intensified by the possibility of concomitant drug therapies as a temporary alternative to the implant, which can hamper the patient's decision-making process. This circumstance can present itself as a dilemma in the decision-making process. The handling of the disease requires a high degree of organisational HL (in terms of the responsibility in providing transparent und sufficient information) and individual critical HL (in terms of risk assessment and decision making) reflecting on ethical values. These findings are in line with Ontario Health (2019), which showed that individual values and experiences shaped the decision-making process, i.e., individuals' perceptions of living as a blind person [12].

In the field of **cardiovascular** implants, HL is related to subjective quality of life and involves an informed and evidence-guided risk–opportunity assessment in accordance with individual and societal values and life planning. The trade off between lifelong drug therapy, open-heart surgery or implant longevity requires value-oriented thinking. In this context, implant wearers benefit from a strengthened HL in terms of tolerance of ambiguity, adaptability and acceptance. In regard to this, it was recommended that patients must be informed to be able to weigh risk and benefits adequately and to understand all short-term and long-term consequences [37,56]. Hereby, especially, the emotional needs and circumstances of older people in particular should be considered [57]. Individual HL enables patients to adapt to their new life situation with the implant not only on a physical level, but can also help them to understand and embrace their new identity. Organisational HL interventions should therefore offer spaces for considering the individual situation of prospective implant wearers during consultancy and decision making. In contrast to this aspect, other findings suggested that participants did not want to be part of the direct decision but rather, in general, be emotionally supported by friends [37,58]. Then again, some studies showed that health professionals were valued in the decision-making process as "co-deciders" who take part in the decision or even take it from the patient [39,53,59]. Astin et al. (2017) recommend to explore patients' beliefs and preferences concerning quality and quantity of life in consultations [13]. This might enable patients to become aware of their values and create ideas of a good life, developing individual HL in this regard.

Against this background, given these diverse needs and preferences, value-oriented HL plays an essential role in informed decision-making, offering space for addressing the impact of the implant on an individual's identity and lifeworld, including the notion of mortality or issues of social participation. HL can empower implant wearers not only in terms of self-determination but also in their educational role—in sharing their experience with and knowledge about the disease and the implant with individuals who face similar challenges. Such felt responsibility of the individual contains an ethical dimension, which should be embraced and framed within the context of care and for which a framework must be set. Value-oriented HL should increase awareness, especially with regard to the major impacts of implants on identity, quality of life and life planning. From a moral perspective, health organisations' responsibilities lie in "examining and modifying their own activities, assumptions, and environments to remove HL–related barriers that hinder access to information, navigation of services, and decision making" [60], while constantly negotiating the system's underlying values on implants, health and disease against the values of their patients.

5. Practice Implications

The discussion of the findings of the current article provides some starting points for the development of individual and organisational health literacy in the context of implant care from both ethical and patient-oriented perspectives. In the following, the communicated needs of the study participants and the theoretical conclusions of their analysis are boiled down to a list of recommendations for future research and practice (see Table 6).

Table 6. Individual and organisational HL development at a glance.

Patients' Needs	Ethical Dimension	Future Research Topics	Practice
(1) Information and perceptions regarding the implant, technology and disease			
Improvement in health knowledge Comprehension of disease and risk factors Understanding actionability in terms of prevention	Empowerment in the field of decision making Responsibility of the system to provide understandable information and promote patients' skills in handling it	Development and assessment of such interventions and use of stronger designs [61].	Interventions on understanding, comprehension, actionability, and satisfaction [3] that are tailored to the needs of patients, addressing functional, interactive and critical skills without using difficult animated spoken text [61].
Improvement in technological knowledge on implants function on functional range on surgery specifics	Empowerment in the field of decision making Information responsibility of the system	Relevance of technology-oriented HL in implant care and ways of integrating it in the healthcare system.	Interventions on informing, training and discussing technology-related themes.
Increasing awareness towards one's own perceptions on technology and health	Empowerment—identity and decision making Value-oriented HL	Moral dimensions of HL and the impacts on individuals' attitudes to decision making.	Interventions on increasing awareness for moral and ethical questions among affected individuals, their doctors and technicians.
(2) Appraisal, dependence and responsibility			
Increasing individuals' tolerance of ambiguity	Empowerment in the field of decision making Information and communicative responsibility of the system	Factors that enable handling ambiguous technological and health information.	Interventions on an individual level—improving skills of handling ambiguous information—and on organisational level—offering paths and orientation frameworks.
Information needs on how to cope with psychological stress	Empowerment in the field of decision making Information responsibility of the system Value-oriented HL	Impact of psychological stress on decision making and the relation between technological risks and stress in the field of HL and health prevention.	Interventions for stress reduction in the context of implant care delivery and offering information and advice on coping strategies as well as possible supporting interventions (e.g., therapy, self-help groups, etc.).
Active involvement in health prevention and promotion	Empowerment Value-oriented HL	Effective ways of collecting and assessing fast-changing information on technical innovations and new therapies.	Interventions for increasing individual's responsibility in terms of health prevention and promotion, providing holistic information on disease, and health and technology.
Supporting objective and subjective risk assessment	Empowerment Value-oriented HL	Factors that impact subjective risk assessment in the context of health and technology (especially in the context of technical and medical innovations).	Interventions that include the provision of resources (information, time, offer of discussion) by specialists with high communicative HL who can assist patients in the process of risk assessment and decision making.

Table 6. Cont.

Patients' Needs	Ethical Dimension	Future Research Topics	Practice
Communicative skills both from providers and patients that enable individuals to interact with their doctors and extract and provide the necessary information through communication	Empowerment in the field of decision making Information responsibility of the system	Communicative action between doctors and patients.	Interventions for increasing individual HL through language (e.g., plain language), pedagogical techniques and clinical skills (e.g., shared decision making) [3].
(3) Implant-related values			
Skills of increasing the subjective quality of life	Empowerment Value-oriented HL Self-determination	Social, psychological and cultural aspects of implant development and implant care as well as the consequences for individuals after implantation.	Individual HL can be developed with interventions that, e.g., offer communication trainings or advice of how to deal with the new sense of hearing or a feeling of a foreign body in the eye, etc.
Ability to reconcile the individual values with the values of medicine and society	Empowerment Value-oriented HL Equity	Increasing the awareness of the moral dimension of individual and organisational HL in research may underline the importance of the co-construction of the concept using participatory approaches.	Interventions on HL development should raise awareness with regard to the major impact on identity, quality of life and life planning. From a moral perspective, organisations need to remove HL-related barriers that hinder "access to information, navigation of services, and decision making" [60].
Perceiving implant care as fair and affordable	Value-oriented HL Equity	Values of social justice and going beyond an individual and national cost benefit analysis [17].	Interventions on individual HL development should contain "meta-cognitive skills around critical thinking, self-awareness and citizenship rather than lists of practical skills" [17] and be open to revealing the power relations in their own framework (e.g., through intercultural comparisons, or case studies).

On a political level, the insights from this study, including the ethical aspects of implant care, suggest the promotion of research and interventions on HL development regarding implants, to strengthen integrated healthcare from physicians and implant centres and, not least, to include the education of the communications skills of healthcare professionals in several stages of their professional development. Furthermore, ethical aspects should inform the technical development of innovative implantable technology.

6. Strengths and Limitations

A methodological strength of the study is that research gaps were narrowed in two respects: on the one hand, the development of a qualitative method, here the GD, in the online setting and, on the other hand, the triangulation approach of grounded theory and the documentary method in the analytical evaluation of the study. A method that is traditionally conducted face to face (GD) was successfully adapted and could be additionally evaluated. The evaluations were mostly positive. Since there is still little empirical evidence in the literature concerning online GD, this study contributed not only on content but also on a methodological level to existing research on HL and qualitative approaches [14].

Furthermore, the methodological triangulation by GD and DS was a strength in itself and condensed the collected data and findings.

Due to the pandemic situation during the period of study planning and conduction, the recruiting of study participants was aggravated. In order to increase the number of participants and include those who had technical difficulties and could not attend the discussion via *GoToMeeting*, the GD with cardiovascular-implant wearers had to be supplemented by two interviews, which led to a certain level of inconsistency in the methodical evaluation (even though efforts were made to minimise the discrepancy as far as possible). Moreover, due to recruiting difficulties, two participants (one cochlear implant wearer and one having a cardiovascular implant) participated in both the GD and the DS; in addition, in one case, the inclusion criteria for glaucoma participants were not as strictly adhered to (one participant had a normal-pressure glaucoma instead of open-angle glaucoma).

Concerning the study sample, few limitations need to be outlined. The sample size of the GD study was smaller than intended by the researchers due to the following two reasons: (1) wearers of glaucoma and cardiovascular implants were very hard to reach and in spite of the various intensive attempts of the researchers to reach potential participants, there were few individuals interested in taking part in the study and (2) the pandemic situation may have influenced individual's willingness to take part in studies in general. One participant from the already very limited pool of participants with a cardiovascular implant appeared psychologically highly stressed, which may be an individual case and not necessarily representative of this patient group. Due to the significantly smaller pool of interested participants in the field of glaucoma and cardiovascular implants, the sample was not as diverse as in the case of cochlear-implant wearers (or parents of children with cochlear implants). For example, most participants with cardiovascular implants were male, which could be also due to the fact that cardiovascular diseases are still widely seen as male-typical diseases. As a result, such diseases are misrecognised in women or are discovered only at a late stage; the relative proportion of women who die from cardiovascular diseases is higher than of men [62,63]. It was also noticeable that all parents of children wearing cochlear implants who participated in the study were female, which can be seen as bias due to a gender imbalance in this sub-group. Furthermore, as the approach was based on open recruitment calls by project partners, and other institutions such as self-help groups, a bias could have risen from the fact that, mainly, people participated in the studies who are interested in their disease and concerned with their body and health.

A strength of the study is that there was no drop-out in either the GD or the DS. We attribute this to careful methodological preparation and close contact with the participants during the study period. The manageable number of participants in both parts of the study enabled the research team to continuously provide personal assistance to a high degree.

7. Conclusions

Given the innovation character of implant care in the context of chronic conditions, this study shows the role of implantable technology as a challenging factor for both individual and organisational HL. Individuals need to handle health- and technology-related information, staying up to date with the high speed of implant developments. Affected individuals need to find their way around the healthcare system, assess risks and act in a self-determined manner in the context of implant care. Furthermore, patients search for ways of integrating the implant in their everyday life, building on an emerging implant or disease-related identity and need to be supported in their efforts to reconcile their feeling of dependence with individual responsibility through critical and value-oriented appraisal of medical and technical information.

Such a complex interplay of competences, experiences and needs related to life with an implant requires from health providers to create efficient frameworks for orientation in a field dominated by ambiguous information and fast-changing evidence. From an ethical point of view, it is not enough to make implant care comprehensible, consulting implant wearers in a purely medical way. It must be acknowledged that an implantation may infiltrate various spheres of an individual's body and lifeworld. Such *infiltration* touches on ethically relevant dimensions and values that need to be considered in the care context, increasing ethical awareness in the fields of HL development and in health-care practice. Finding place for reflection on the individual values of (prospective) implant wearers and the underlying convictions in implant care constitutes an essential task for organisational HL development.

Our study results demonstrated the interconnectedness between the acquisition and appraisal of technology-related information and knowledge about one's own disease, the interactions within implant care between system and individual, the acceptance and adaptation of the implant in relation to one's own body perception, on one hand, and ethically relevant dimensions such as dependency, responsibility and self-determination that accompany these aspects, on the other hand. Moreover, they emphasise the importance of individual and organisational HL, which must be, as a concept, sensibilised to ethically relevant dimensions in implant care.

For the development in individual and organisational HL, this demands a participative approach, and more attention to the technological layer of information and its role in supporting empowerment. Furthermore, if perceived as a hazard, the technology of the implant may impact HL and decision making. Interventions on HL should therefore provide advice and training on how to handle stress caused by too much, too complex or too ambiguous information. The continuous trade off between dependence (on the implant in everyday life and the health system) and responsibility (in terms of empowerment, decision making and critical appraisal) seems to be a core element of individual and organisational HL among implant wearers. Since values on health and disease play a central role in implant care, it is essential to pay closer attention to the ethical aspects of implant care and contribute to the promotion of a value-oriented HL. Since promoting HL may enable individuals to realise fundamental ethical values, HL development is an ethic responsibility itself.

Author Contributions: Conceptualisation, C.H. and M.L.; Methodology, C.H., M.L., L.H., S.S., S.J., A.B. and S.F.; Validation, C.H., M.L. and S.S.; Formal analysis, C.H., M.L. and S.S.; Investigation, C.H., M.L., L.H., S.S., S.J., A.B. and S.F.; Writing—original draft preparation, C.H. and M.L.; Writing—review and editing, L.H., S.S., S.J., C.W., A.B. and S.F.; Visualisation, C.H., M.L. and S.S.; Supervision, C.W.; Conceptualisation of the study and project administration, S.J. and C.W.; Funding acquisition, C.W. All authors have read and agreed to the published version of the manuscript.

Funding: This research was funded by the Federal Ministry of Education and Research, Germany (Bundesministerium für Bildung und Forschung, BMBF), grant number 03ZZ0923D. The sponsor did not influence the conception or course of the study nor the reporting of results.

Institutional Review Board Statement: The study was conducted in accordance with the Declaration of Helsinki, and approved by the Ethics Committee of the Medical Faculty of the University of Cologne (protocol code: 20-1176 and date of approval: 1 November 2020).

Informed Consent Statement: Informed consent was obtained from all subjects involved in the study.

Data Availability Statement: Not applicable.

Acknowledgments: We are obliged to our participants for their time, interest and strong engagement in the research process and thank them for their openness. This project was conducted at the Cologne Center for Ethics, Rights, Economics and Social Sciences of Health (CERES) under the leadership of Christiane Woopen in cooperation with the Hannover Medical School and Rostock University Medical Center. We are very grateful for the support of Thomas Lenartz, Tobias Schilling and Rudolf F. Guthoff in the definition of the inclusion and exclusion criteria, in the recruitment process and for the valuable input and medical advice. We also thank Meike Hartmann for her valuable contribution as part of our team, and our RESPONSE Partners for the project synergy and exchange.

Conflicts of Interest: The authors declare no conflict of interest.

Appendix A

Table A1. Group discussion: adapted to each implant type.

What Comes to Your Mind in Connection with the Implant and Medical Care When You Hear the Following Term?
Justice
Quality of Life
Safety
Technology
Self-determination
Acceptance
Damage prevention
Patient well-being
Health
Powerlessness
Question Block 1: Previous history: decision for an implant, information, expectations, personal feelings
When and how did you first become aware of the possibility of receiving an implant?
Question Block 2: Present: How do you experience everyday life/your life with the implant?
How did you experience the counselling and care regarding your implant?
Question Block 3: Future: prospects, expectations, wishes, fears
Do you feel that your needs are adequately addressed in the health system? How do you see the future with regard to your life with an implant?

Appendix B

Table A2. "Inspiration sheet" for the diaries: adapted to each implant type.

Diary Study "(Everyday) Life with an Implant" Inspirations for Your Diary	
What situations were relevant for you today in relation to your implant? Describe these situations! What did they trigger in you? When you think back to today, what thoughts about your implant were on your mind?	The implant
What feelings did you have about your implant today? How did you perceive yourself with your implant? Can you relate these feelings to a specific situation or trigger? How did you deal with these feelings and situations? What were you satisfied with and what would you perhaps like to do differently next time?	Emotions
In a certain situation, did your implant have an influence on how you planned or organised something in everyday life? What has changed for you in relation to it, i.e., improved or worsened? Has your quality of life today been influenced by the implant? How? Did you feel limited or restricted by the implant today, or did you feel supported in a particular way? In which situations?	Quality of Life
Did you have any questions, problems or concerns about the implant technique today? How did you address them?	Technology
Have you communicated with anyone today about the implant? With whom and why? Was there anything you would like to report in relation to it?	Care

Appendix C

Table A3. Structure of the collective orientation patterns of GD and DS.

Cochlea	
Group Discussion	**Diary Study**
Information and perceptions regarding the implant, technology and disease	
Perceptions on the implant as a physical object	
Sensory perception; everyday life; implant as part of the person	Everyday life
Perceptions on the implant's functioning and damage prevention	
Features and functions	Equipment and features; mobility and safety; planning and preparation; damage prevention
Information and knowledge related to the implant and the disease	
Differences between implant brands; fast development of technology; exchange of experiences; initiation to technology	Exchange of experiences; individual hearing story
Appraisal, dependence and responsibility	
Appraisal of information and disease	
Decision-making; attitudes towards technology	Decision-making; individual attitudes towards technology; physical and psychological effects; sense of hearing
The role of the active patient	
Proactive behaviour in care management	Navigation coping strategies
Dependence on the healthcare system and the implants	
Implant vs. other/future therapy options; (dependence on) technology; counselling and education; aggravated diagnosis of other diseases; quality of care	(dependence on) Technology; care; needs and wishes
Attitudes, coping and responsibility	
Implant education; implant handling	Coping strategies; implant handling; parental handling regarding children's CI
Implant related values	
Self-determination in the context of treatment irreversibility and perceptions of good life	
Proxy decision-making for a child; autonomy in use of technology	Independence; limitations and challenges of the implant
Identity and participation	
(collective) Identity; participating in life (again); standing up for oneself; social dynamics and adaptation; competences	Activities and inclusion; support; non-hearing and the environment; reactions from the environment; sign language; CI wearer about CI in contact with others; restrictions and aids in communication
Glaucoma	
Group Discussion	**Diary Study**
COP: Information and perceptions regarding the implant, technology and disease	
Perceptions on the implant as a physical object	
Implant and prevention	Implant perception
Perceptions on the implant's functioning and damage prevention	

Table A3. Cont.

Implant and prevention	Functionality; influencing factors; vision/visual acuity
Information and knowledge related to the implant and the disease	
Information; little knowledge about the disease in the (medical) environment; early detection and diagnosis; inner ocular pressure (IOP)	Information and education; comorbidities; exchange and communication; family history
COP: Appraisal, dependence and responsibility	
Appraisal of information and disease	
Quality of life and symptoms; decision-making; research and treatment options; holistic treatment approach	Experiencing glaucoma; accompanying symptoms
The role of the active patient	
Coordination of treatment and follow-up; assertiveness and HL; individual initiative (treatment and information)	Exchange and communication
Dependence on the healthcare system and the implants	
Doctor-patient relationship; education and instructions; drop therapy and measuring IOP; healthcare system and financing; quality of care	Operation, pre- and aftercare
Attitudes, coping and responsibility	
Drop therapy; stress; self-help groups; educating the surroundings	Handling symptoms; drop therapy and pressure control; aids; coping strategies
COP: Implant related values	
Self-determination in the context of treatment irreversibility and perceptions of good life	
Self-determination	Independence; quality of life
Identity and participation	
Self-determination	Personal environment

Cardiovascular

Group Discussion	Diary Study
COP: Information and perceptions regarding the implant, technology and disease	
Perceptions on the implant as a physical object	
Perceptions on the implant	Effects on everyday life (post-op)
Perceptions on the implant's functioning and damage prevention	
Safety; functioning of the implant	Preventative action; heart problems and implant
Information and knowledge related to the implant and the disease	
Age and gender; education; implant type and innovation	Information gathering
COP: Appraisal, dependence and responsibility	
Appraisal of information and disease	
Emergency situation or already known heart problems; decision-making	Medication; comorbidities
The role of the active patient	
Doctor-patient relationship; patient role	Patient role
Dependence on the healthcare system and the implants	

Table A3. *Cont.*

Quality of care; treatment/implantation; coordination of treatment and follow-up	Quality of care; additional treatments
Attitudes, coping and responsibility	
Psychological coping; educating; respect for own health	Coping strategies; anxiety and concerns
COP: Implant related values	
Self-determination in the context of treatment irreversibility and perceptions of good life	
Quality of life; gratitude	Attitudes towards the implant
Identity and participation	
Role of family; role of self-help groups; (collective) identity	Family and friends; burden vs. support for others; volunteering and engagement; effects on personality and self-image

References

1. Apter, A.J.; Paasche-Orlow, M.K.; Remillard, J.T.; Bennett, I.M.; Ben-Joseph, E.P.; Batista, R.M.; Hyde, J.; Rudd, R.E. Numeracy and Communication with Patients: They Are Counting on Us. *J. Gen. Intern. Med.* **2008**, *23*, 2117–2124. [CrossRef]
2. Hoffmann, T.; Del Mar, C. Patients' Expectations of the Benefits and Harms of Treatments, Screening, and Tests. *JAMA Intern. Med.* **2015**, *175*, 274–286. [CrossRef] [PubMed]
3. Watson, J.C. Talking the Talk: Enhancing Clinical Ethics with Health Literacy Best Practices. *HEC Forum* **2019**, *31*, 177–199. [CrossRef]
4. Sørensen, K.; Van den Broucke, S.; Fullam, J.; Doyle, G.; Pelikan, J.; Slonska, Z.; Brand, H.; (HLS-EU) Consortium Health Literacy Project European. Health literacy and public health: A systematic review and integration of definitions and models. *BMC Public Health* **2012**, *12*, 80. [CrossRef]
5. Frosch, D.L.; Elwyn, G. Don't Blame Patients, Engage Them: Transforming Health Systems to Address Health Literacy. *J. Health Commun.* **2014**, *19*, 10–14. [CrossRef] [PubMed]
6. Nutbeam, D. The evolving concept of health literacy. *Soc. Sci. Med.* **2008**, *67*, 2072–2078. [CrossRef] [PubMed]
7. Chinn, D.; McCarthy, C. All Aspects of Health Literacy Scale (AAHLS): Developing a tool to measure functional, communicative and critical health literacy in primary healthcare settings. *Patient Educ. Couns.* **2013**, *90*, 247–253. [CrossRef]
8. Chinn, D. Critical health literacy: A review and critical analysis. *Soc. Sci. Med.* **2011**, *73*, 60–67. [CrossRef] [PubMed]
9. Nutbeam, D. Health literacy as a public health goal: A challenge for contemporary health education and communication strategies into the 21st century. *Health Promot. Int.* **2000**, *15*, 259–267. [CrossRef]
10. Griese, L.; Berens, E.-M.; Nowak, P.; Pelikan, J.M.; Schaeffer, D. Challenges in Navigating the Health Care System: Development of an Instrument Measuring Navigation Health Literacy. *Int. J. Environ. Res. Public Health* **2020**, *17*, 5731. [CrossRef]
11. WHO. Constitution of the World Health Organization. Available online: https://www.who.int/about/governance/constitution (accessed on 15 February 2022).
12. Ontario Health (Quality). *Minimally Invasive Glaucoma Surgery: A Budget Impact Analysis and Evaluation of Patients' Experiences, Preferences, and Values*; Ontario Health (Quality): Toronto, ON, Canada, 2019; Volume 19, pp. 1–57. Available online: https://www.hqontario.ca/Evidence-to-Improve-Care/Health-Technology-Assessment/Journal-Ontario-Health-Technology-Assessment-Series (accessed on 15 February 2022).
13. Astin, F.; Horrocks, J.; McLenachan, J.; Blackman, D.J.; Stephenson, J.; Closs, S.J. The impact of transcatheter aortic valve implantation on quality of life: A mixed methods study. *Heart Lung* **2017**, *46*, 432–438. [CrossRef]
14. Hübner, C.; Hartmann, M.; Harzheim, L.; Junger, S.; Lorke, M.; Schulz, S.; Woopen, C. Konzeption und Durchführung qualitativer Erhebungen im Online-Setting am Beispiel von Gruppendiskussionen. In Proceedings of the Deutscher Kongress für Versorgungsforschung (DKVF), Online, 6–8 October 2021. [CrossRef]
15. Levin-Zamir, D. IUHPE Positionspapier zur Gesundheitskompetenz: Eine praktische Vision für eine gesundheitskompetente Welt. In *Health Literacy im Kindes-Und Jugendalter: Ein-Und Ausblicke*; Bollweg, T.M., Bröder, J., Pinheiro, P., Eds.; Springer Fachmedien Wiesbaden: Wiesbaden, Germany, 2020; pp. 599–619.
16. Ernstmann, N.; Bauer, U.; Berens, E.-M.; Bitzer, E.M.; Bollweg, T.M.; Danner, M.; Dehn-Hindenberg, A.; Dierks, M.L.; Farin, E.; Grobosch, S.; et al. DNVF Memorandum Gesundheitskompetenz (Teil 1)—Hintergrund, Relevanz, Gegenstand und Fragestellungen in der Versorgungsforschung. *Das Gesundh.* **2020**, *82*, e77–e93. [CrossRef]
17. Paakkari, L.; George, S. Ethical underpinnings for the development of health literacy in schools: Ethical premises ('why'), orientations ('what') and tone ('how'). *BMC Public Health* **2018**, *18*, 326. [CrossRef] [PubMed]
18. Tauqeer, Z. To Understand and Be Understood: The Ethics of Language, Literacy, and Hierarchy in Medicine. *AMA J. Ethic* **2017**, *19*, 234–237. [CrossRef]

19. Covan, E.K. Decisions in the context of maternal health: Musing politics, health literacy, emotions, ethics, and technology. *Health Care Women Int.* **2018**, *39*, 1161–1162. [CrossRef] [PubMed]
20. Gazmararian, J.A.; Curran, J.W.; Parker, R.; Bernhardt, J.M.; DeBuono, B.A. Public health literacy in America: An ethical imperative. *Am. J. Prev. Med.* **2005**, *28*, 317–322. [CrossRef] [PubMed]
21. Janssens, K.A.M.; Bos, E.H.; Rosmalen, J.G.M.; Wichers, M.C.; Riese, H. A qualitative approach to guide choices for designing a diary study. *BMC Med. Res. Methodol.* **2018**, *18*, 140. [CrossRef]
22. Kühn, T.; Koschel, K.-V. *Gruppendiskussionen: Ein Praxis-Handbuch*, 1st ed.; VS Verlag für Sozialwissenschaften: Wiesbaden, Germany, 2011. Available online: https://link.springer.com/content/pdf/10.1007%2F978-3-531-93243-9.pdf (accessed on 16 November 2021).
23. Bohnsack, R.; Nentwig-Gesemann, I.; Nohl, A.-M. *Die Dokumentarische Methode und Ihre Forschungspraxis*; VS Verlag für Sozialwissenschaften: Wiesbaden, Germany, 2013. Available online: https://link.springer.com/content/pdf/10.1007%2F978-3-531-19895-8.pdf (accessed on 20 October 2021).
24. Strauss, A.; Corbin, J.M. *Grounded Theory in Practice*; San Jose State University; SAGE Publications, Inc.: Thousand Oaks, CA, USA, 1997. Available online: https://us.sagepub.com/en-us/nam/grounded-theory-in-practice/book6165 (accessed on 20 October 2021).
25. Schmitt-Howe, B. Triangulation durch Dokumentarische Methode und Grounded Theory Methodology (GTM) auf der Basis von problemzentrierten (Gruppen-)Interviews. In *Dokumentarische Methode: Triangulation und Blinde Flecken*; Dörner, O., Loos, P., Schäffer, B., Schondelmayer, A., Eds.; Verlag Barbara Budrich: Leverkusen, Germany, 2019; pp. 33–50. Available online: https://library.oapen.org/bitstream/handle/20.500.12657/23741/1006403.pdf?sequence=1&isAllowed=y (accessed on 15 February 2022).
26. Aguado, K. Grounded Theory und Dokumentarische Me-thode. In *Forschungsmethoden in der Fremdsprachendidaktik*; Handbuch, E., Caspari, D., Klippel, F., Legutke, M., Schramm, K., Eds.; Narr Francke Attempto: Tübingen, Germany, 2016; pp. 243–256.
27. Institute of Medicine. *Health Literacy: A Prescription to End Confusion*; National Academies Press: Washington, DC, USA, 2004. Available online: https://www.nap.edu/catalog/10883/health-literacy-a-prescription-to-end-confusion (accessed on 15 February 2022).
28. Norton, R.W. Measurement of Ambiguity Tolerance. *J. Pers. Assess.* **1975**, *39*, 607–619. [CrossRef]
29. Wheeler, A.; Archbold, S.; Gregory, S.; Skipp, A. Cochlear Implants: The Young People's Perspective. *J. Deaf Stud. Deaf Educ.* **2007**, *12*, 303–316. [CrossRef] [PubMed]
30. Myers, J.R.; Henderson-King, D.H.; Henderson-King, E.I. Facing Technological Risks: The Importance of Individual Differences. *J. Res. Pers.* **1997**, *31*, 1–20. [CrossRef]
31. Hallberg, L.R.-M.; Ringdahl, A. Living with cochlear implants: Experiences of 17 adult patients in Sweden. *Int. J. Audiol.* **2004**, *43*, 115–121. [CrossRef] [PubMed]
32. Fitzpatrick, E.M.; Jacques, J.; Neuss, D. Parental perspectives on decision-making and outcomes in pediatric bilateral cochlear implantation. *Int. J. Audiol.* **2011**, *50*, 679–687. [CrossRef]
33. Watson, V.; Verschuur, C.; Lathlean, J. Exploring the experiences of teenagers with cochlear implants. *Cochlea- Implant. Int.* **2016**, *17*, 293–301. [CrossRef] [PubMed]
34. Vieira, S.D.S.; Dupas, G.; Chiari, B.M. Cochlear implant: The family's perspective. *Cochlea- Implant. Int.* **2018**, *19*, 216–224. [CrossRef] [PubMed]
35. Frech, S.; Guthoff, R.; Gamael, A.; Helbig, C.; Diener, A.; Ritzke, M.; Wollny, A.; Altiner, A. Patterns and Facilitators for the Promotion of Glaucoma Medication Adherence—A Qualitative Study. *Healthcare* **2021**, *9*, 426. [CrossRef] [PubMed]
36. Ontario Health (Quality). Transcatheter Aortic Valve Implantation in Patients with Severe Aortic Valve Stenosis at Low Surgical Risk: A Health Technology Assessment. In *Ont. Health Technol. Assess. Ser.*; 2016; 16, pp. 1–94. Available online: https://www.ncbi.nlm.nih.gov/pmc/articles/PMC7670297/ (accessed on 15 February 2022).
37. Korteland, N.M.; Bras, F.J.; A van Hout, F.M.; Kluin, J.; Klautz, R.J.M.; Bogers, A.J.J.C.; Takkenberg, J.J.M. Prosthetic aortic valve selection: Current patient experience, preferences and knowledge. *Open Heart* **2015**, *2*, e000237. [CrossRef]
38. Frankel, N.Z. Surgical Aortic Valve Replacement vs Transcatheter Aortic Valve Replacement. *JAMA Intern. Med.* **2014**, *174*, 495–496. [CrossRef]
39. Schmied, W.; Schäfers, H.J.; Köllner, V. Lebensqualität oder Lebenserwartung? Kriterien und Informationsquellen für die Entscheidungsfindung bei Patienten im Vorfeld von Aortenklappenoperationen/ Quality of life or life expectancy? Criteria and sources of information in the decision-making of patients undergoing aortic valve surgery. *Z. Für Psychosom. Med. Psychother.* **2015**, *61*, 224–237.
40. Hickey, K.T.; Sciacca, R.R.; Gonzalez, P.; Castillo, C.; Frulla, A. Assessing Health Literacy in Urban Patients With Implantable Cardioverter Defibrillators and Pacemakers. *J. Cardiovasc. Nurs.* **2015**, *30*, 428–434. [CrossRef]
41. Dornhoffer, J. An Otologist's Experience as a Cochlear Implant Patient-The Power of Neuroplasticity. *JAMA Otolaryngol. Neck Surg.* **2019**, *145*, 401–402. [CrossRef] [PubMed]
42. Finlay, L.; Molano-Fisher, P. 'Transforming' self and world: A phenomenological study of a changing lifeworld following a cochlear implant. *Med. Health Care Philos.* **2007**, *11*, 255–267. [CrossRef] [PubMed]
43. Hilton, K.; Jones, F.; Harmon, S.; Cropper, J. Adolescents' Experiences of Receiving and Living with Sequential Cochlear Implants: An Interpretative Phenomenological Analysis. *J. Deaf Stud. Deaf Educ.* **2013**, *18*, 513–531. [CrossRef]

44. Athalye, S.; Mulla, I.; Archbold, S. The experiences of adults assessed for cochlear implantation who did not proceed. *Cochlea-Implant. Int.* **2014**, *15*, 301–311. [CrossRef]
45. Aloqaili, Y.; Arafat, A.S.; Almarzoug, A.; Alalula, L.S.; Hakami, A.; Almalki, M.; Alhuwaimel, L. Knowledge about cochlear implantation: A parental perspective. *Cochlea-Implant. Int.* **2018**, *20*, 74–79. [CrossRef]
46. Dillon, B.; Pryce, H. What makes someone choose cochlear implantation? An exploration of factors that inform patient decision making. *Int. J. Audiol.* **2019**, *59*, 24–32. [CrossRef]
47. Incesulu, A.; Vural, M.; Erkam, U. Children with Cochlear Implants: Parental Perspective: Otology & Neurotology. *Otol. Neurotol.* **2003**, *24*, 605. Available online: https://journals.lww.com/otology-neurotology/fulltext/2003/07000/children_with_cochlear_implants__parental.13.aspx (accessed on 15 February 2022). [PubMed]
48. Sach, T.H.; Whynes, D.K. Paediatric cochlear implantation: The views of parents. *Int. J. Audiol.* **2005**, *44*, 400–407. [CrossRef]
49. Jeffs, E.; Redfern, K.; Stanfield, C.; Starczewski, H.; Stone, S.; Twomey, T.; Fortnum, H. A pilot study to explore the experiences of congenitally or early profoundly deafened candidates who receive cochlear implants as adults. *Cochlea-Implant. Int.* **2015**, *16*, 312–320. [CrossRef] [PubMed]
50. Mäki-Torkko, E.M.; Vestergren, S.; Harder, H.; Lyxell, B. From isolation and dependence to autonomy—Expectations before and experiences after cochlear implantation in adult cochlear implant users and their significant others. *Disabil. Rehabil.* **2014**, *37*, 541–547. [CrossRef] [PubMed]
51. Ng, Z.Y.; Lamb, B.; Harrigan, S.; Archbold, S.; Athalye, S.; Allen, S. Perspectives of adults with cochlear implants on current CI services and daily life. *Cochlea-Implant. Int.* **2016**, *17*, 89–93. [CrossRef]
52. Cross, V.; Shah, P.; Glynn, M.; Chidrawar, S. ReGAE 5: Can we improve the surgical journey for African-Caribbean patients undergoing glaucoma filtration surgery? Some preliminary findings. *Clin. Ophthalmol.* **2008**, *3*, 1–12. [CrossRef]
53. A Rauen, J.; A Rauen, C. A patient's bold voice: A journey through cardiac surgery. *AACN Adv. Crit. Care* **2006**, *17*, 133–144. [CrossRef]
54. Beattie, R.; Ritter-Brinton, K.; Snart, F. A Mother and Son Cochlear Implant Case Study: Making the Decision Twice. *Adv. Oto-Rhino-Laryngol.* **2000**, *57*, 141–144. [CrossRef]
55. Bruin, M.; Nevøy, A. Exploring the Discourse on Communication Modality after Cochlear Implantation: A Foucauldian Analysis of Parents' Narratives. *J. Deaf Stud. Deaf Educ.* **2014**, *19*, 385–399. [CrossRef]
56. Boothroyd, L.J.; Spaziano, M.; Guertin, J.R.; Lambert, L.J.; Rodés-Cabau, J.; Noiseux, N.; Nguyen, M.; Dumont, E.; Carrier, M.; de Varennes, B.; et al. Transcatheter Aortic Valve Implantation: Recommendations for Practice Based on a Multidisciplinary Review Including Cost-Effectiveness and Ethical and Organizational Issues. *Can. J. Cardiol.* **2013**, *29*, 718–726. [CrossRef]
57. Skaar, E.; Ranhoff, A.H.; Nordrehaug, J.E.; E Forman, D.; Schaufel, M.A. Conditions for autonomous choice: A qualitative study of older adults' experience of decision-making in TAVR. *J. Geriatr. Cardiol.* **2017**, *14*, 42–48. [CrossRef] [PubMed]
58. Olsson, K.; Näslund, U.; Nilsson, J.; Hörnsten, A. Patients' experiences of the transcatheter aortic valve implantation trajectory: A grounded theory study. *Nurs. Open* **2018**, *5*, 149–157. [CrossRef] [PubMed]
59. Lauck, S.B.; Baumbusch, J.; Achtem, L.; Forman, J.M.; Carroll, S.; Cheung, A.; Ye, J.; A Wood, D.; Webb, J.G. Factors influencing the decision of older adults to be assessed for transcatheter aortic valve implantation: An exploratory study. *Eur. J. Cardiovasc. Nurs.* **2016**, *15*, 486–494. [CrossRef]
60. Goeddel, L.A.; Porterfield, J.R.; Hall, J.D.; Vetter, T.R. Ethical Opportunities with the Perioperative Surgical Home. *Anesthesia Analg.* **2015**, *120*, 1158–1162. [CrossRef]
61. Visscher, B.B.; Steunenberg, B.; Heijmans, M.; Hofstede, J.M.; Devillé, W.; Van Der Heide, I.; Rademakers, J.; Visscher, B.B.; Steunenberg, B.; Heijmans, M.; et al. Evidence on the effectiveness of health literacy interventions in the EU: A systematic review. *BMC Public Health* **2018**, *18*, 1414. [CrossRef]
62. Townsend, N.; Nichols, M.; Scarborough, P.; Rayner, M. Cardiovascular disease in Europe—Epidemiological update. *Eur. Heart J.* **2015**, *36*, 2696–2705. [CrossRef] [PubMed]
63. Maas, A.H.; van der Schouw, Y.T.; Regitz-Zagrosek, V.; Swahn, E.; Appelman, Y.E.; Pasterkamp, G.; Cate, H.T.; Nilsson, P.M.; Huisman, M.V.; Stam, H.C.; et al. Red alert for women's heart: The urgent need for more research and knowledge on cardiovascular disease in women: Proceedings of the Workshop held in Brussels on Gender Differences in Cardiovascular disease, 29 September 2010. *Eur. Heart J.* **2011**, *32*, 1362–1368. [CrossRef]

MDPI
St. Alban-Anlage 66
4052 Basel
Switzerland
Tel. +41 61 683 77 34
Fax +41 61 302 89 18
www.mdpi.com

International Journal of Environmental Research and Public Health Editorial Office
E-mail: ijerph@mdpi.com
www.mdpi.com/journal/ijerph

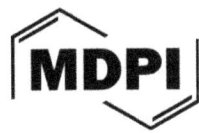

www.ingramcontent.com/pod-product-compliance
Lightning Source LLC
LaVergne TN
LVHW070643100526
838202LV00013B/867

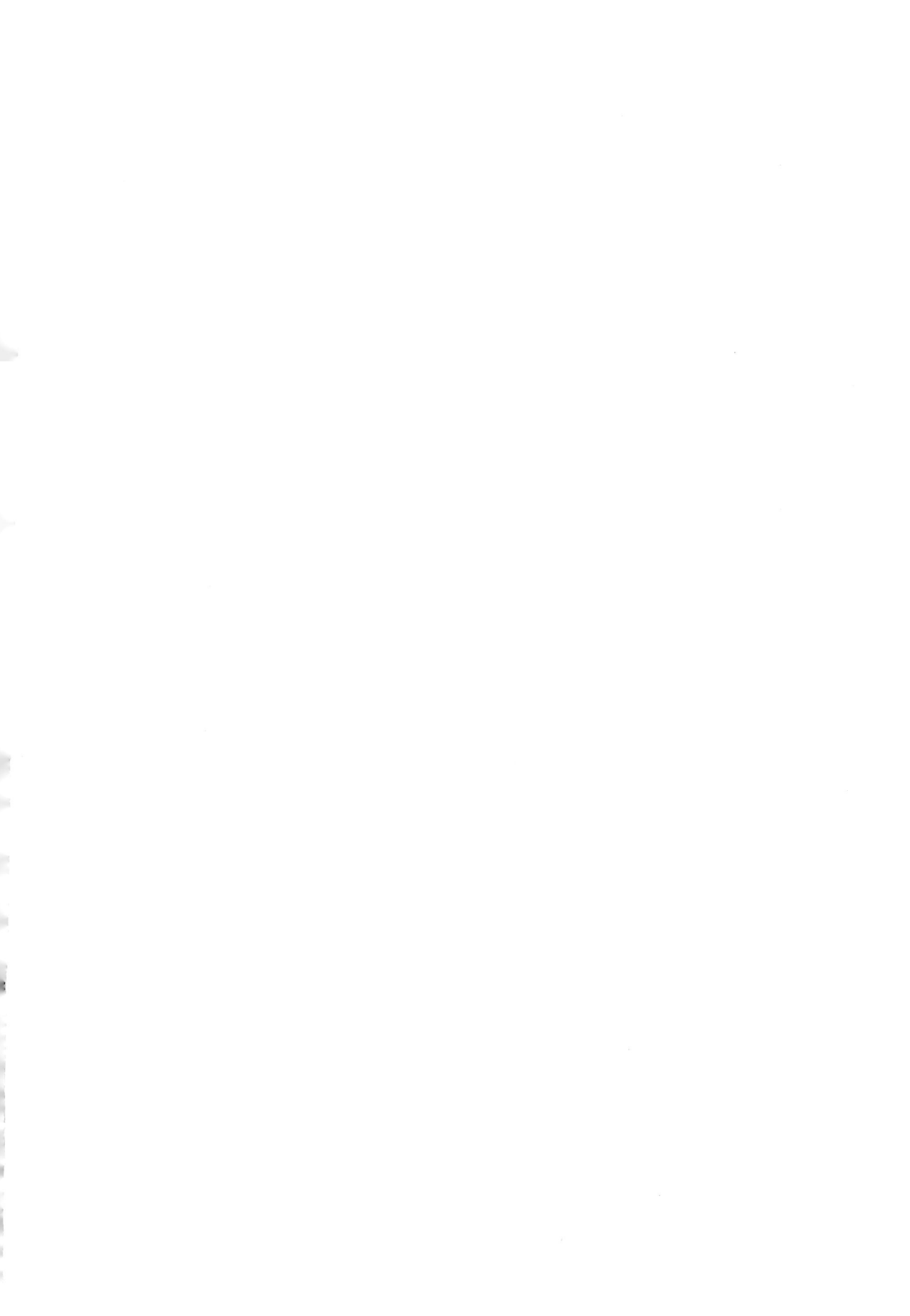